T0192361

Pharmaceutical Extrusion Technology

Second Edition

DRUGS AND THE PHARMACEUTICAL SCIENCES
A Series of Textbooks and Monographs

Series Executive Editor

James Swarbrick

PharmaceuTech, Inc.
Pinehurst, North Carolina

Recent Titles in Series

Pharmaceutical Extrusion Technology, Second Edition, *Isaac Ghebre-Sellassie, Charles E. Martin, Feng Zhang, and James Dinunzio*

Biosimilar Drug Product Development, *Laszlo Endrenyi, Paul Declerck, and Shein-Chung Chow*

High Throughput Screening in Drug Discovery, *Amancio Carnero*

Generic Drug Product Development: International Regulatory Requirements for Bioequivalence, Second Edition, *Isadore Kanfer and Leon Shargel*

Aqueous Polymeric Coatings for Pharmaceutical Dosage Forms, Fourth Edition, *Linda A. Felton*

Good Design Practices for GMP Pharmaceutical Facilities, Second Edition, *Terry Jacobs and Andrew A. Signore*

Handbook of Bioequivalence Testing, Second Edition, *Sarfaraz K. Niazi*

Generic Drug Product Development: Solid Oral Dosage Forms, Second Edition, *edited by Leon Shargel and Isadore Kanfer*

Drug Stereochemistry: Analytical Methods and Pharmacology, Third Edition, *edited by Krzysztof Jozwiak, W. J. Lough, and Irving W. Wainer*

Pharmaceutical Powder Compaction Technology, Second Edition, *edited by Metin Çelik*

Pharmaceutical Stress Testing: Predicting Drug Degradation, Second Edition, *edited by Steven W. Baertschi, Karen M. Alsante, and Robert A. Reed*

Pharmaceutical Process Scale-Up, Third Edition, *edited by Michael Levin*

Sterile Drug Products: Formulation, Packaging, Manufacturing and Quality, *Michael J. Akers*

Freeze-Drying/Lyophilization of Pharmaceutical and Biological Products, Third Edition, *edited by Louis Rey and Joan C. May*

Oral Drug Absorption: Prediction and Assessment, *edited by Jennifer B. Dressman and Christos Reppas*

Generic Drug Product Development: Specialty Dosage Forms, *edited by Leon Shargel and Isadore Kanfer*

*A complete listing of all volumes in this series can be found at **www.crcpress.com***

Pharmaceutical Extrusion Technology

Second Edition

Edited by
Isaac Ghebre-Sellassie
Charles Martin
Feng Zhang
James DiNunzio

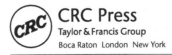

CRC Press
Taylor & Francis Group
Boca Raton London New York

CRC Press is an imprint of the
Taylor & Francis Group, an **informa** business

CRC Press
Taylor & Francis Group
6000 Broken Sound Parkway NW, Suite 300
Boca Raton, FL 33487-2742

First issued in paperback 2020

ISBN-13: 978-1-4987-0491-5 (hbk)
ISBN-13: 978-0-367-73508-1 (pbk)

Library of Congress Cataloging-in-Publication Data

Names: Ghebre-Sellassie, Isaac, 1947- editor. | Martin, Charles, M.B.A., editor.
Title: Pharmaceutical extrusion technology / [edited by] Isaac Ghebre-Sellassie, Charles E. Martin, Feng Zhang and James Dinunzio.
Description: Second edition. | Boca Raton : CRC Press, [2018] | Series: Drugs and the pharmaceutical sciences | Revised edition of: Pharmaceutical extrusion technology / edited by Isaac Ghebre-Sellassie, Charles Martin. New York : M. Dekker, 2003. | Includes bibliographical references and index.
Identifiers: LCCN 2017049196| ISBN 9781498704915 (hardback : alk. paper) | ISBN 9781351129015 (ebook)
Subjects: LCSH: Pharmaceutical technology. | Extrusion process.
Classification: LCC RS192 .P4618 2018 | DDC 615.1/9--dc23
LC record available at https://lccn.loc.gov/2017049196

Visit the Taylor & Francis Web site at
http://www.taylorandfrancis.com

and the CRC Press Web site at
http://www.crcpress.com

To my kiddos, Adam & Isabella, this one is for you!

James DiNunzio

*This is for you, my wife Amleset and my children
Mesfin, Sarona and Joseph*

Isaac Ghebre-Sellassie

*To James W. McGinity, you are a fantastic mentor. I would not
be where I am today without your guidance and support!*

Feng Zhang

In memory of my father and mother, Red and Mary Ann

Charles Martin

Contents

Preface to the Second Edition

Extrusion is a process in which materials are intimately mixed and pumped under controlled conditions of temperature, shear, and pressure to generate a variety of in-process and finished products using pieces of equipment collectively known as extruders. Most of the early applications of this technology were limited to industrial processes that ranged from compaction of clay and straw to the mastication of rubber and plastics. Since the 1960s, extrusion has dominated the plastics industry as compared to other available batch type devices. Prominent in its absence throughout this period was the application of extrusion in the development and manufacture of pharmaceutical products. Over the last several decades, the technology has emerged as a leading production platform for a range of pharmaceutical products covering a number of delivery modalities. The range of pharmaceutical products produced using hot-melt extrusion highlights the versatility of the platform and the potential to develop systems beyond the standard tablets and capsules for oral administration. As the field has evolved in terms of practical application, the science of pharmaceutical extrusion has also grown. The intent of this book is to provide pharmaceutical scientists and engineers with basic principles and fundamentals of extrusion technology and a detailed description of the practical applications of extrusion processes using state-of-the-art examples and scientific understanding.

The book is sectioned into several major themes covering: introductory material, process-specific considerations, and drug delivery applications. In the introductory section, elements of history, equipment design, and general process considerations are described. Opening with a historical overview of extruders and extrusion technology, a detailed overview of the evolutionary development of the technology is provided. Early patents that formed the basis for the widespread use of the technology are highlighted. Extrusion design features that are common to general industrial applications, but also uniquely applicable to the pharmaceutical industry, including cleanability of the product contact parts, are discussed. Designing robust control strategies to include collection, rejection, quality, and traceability for continuous twin screw extrusion processes will ensure that a consistent product is formed over the total operation time. These techniques are extensively discussed along with examples for distilling these principles into practice.

As the text develops, a more detailed discussion of equipment design is provided. Co-rotating and counterrotating twin-screw compounding extruders are mass transfer devices that are used to mix together two or more materials into a homogeneous mass in a continuous process. This is accomplished through distributive and dispersive mixing of the various components in a formulation. These aspects as well as screw designs specific to twin screw extruders are discussed in depth. Extrusion dies, located at the exit end of the barrel assembly, are critical parts of the extrusion system that can help to form a successful process, particularly during the manufacture of controlled-release dosage forms and shaped drug products. The success of a given process depends on, among other factors, die design. While some dies may be simple, others can be extremely complex with features that are critical to enable uniform production. Recognizing that most extruders are operated in a starve-fed mode, the use of feeders to accurately meter material to the extruder also represents a critical component of the process that can directly impact product uniformity and residence time. Both upstream and downstream considerations of the process are reviewed to highlight the importance of these elements in the design of a successful extrusion process.

During extrusion, liquids and powders must be fed accurately in a continuous manner throughout the run time, including the refill period, to ensure formulation consistency, constant throughput, proper order of mixing of ingredients, and regulated mass transfer. Beyond the engineering considerations, it is necessary to account for formulation properties which can be evaluated through rheological and physical property characterization. A detailed description of torque rheometers, instruments that are essential for the characterization of formulations and processing parameters, and techniques that help elucidate the rheological properties of melts are presented. New sections covering emerging applications of foam extrusion are also provided. Cell nucleation, materials, and applications are all discussed. Downstream processing is also covered, with particular focus on multiparticulate manufacture via pelletization.

As the text continues to evolve, a discussion on drug release from extruded controlled release dispersions is presented, focusing on the drug release mechanism of extended-release dosage forms, and the application of the twin screw extrusion process to prepare various extended-release dosage forms. One advantage of extended-release drug delivery systems is higher patient compliance due to less frequent dosing. Shape extrusion involving solid or hollow structures which support a range of advanced controlled release products is also discussed. Other shaped systems, including sheets and laminates, which have applications in transdermal drug delivery and fast-dissolving films intended for oral drug delivery are described. Beyond these emerging areas of extrusion application, there is a detailed discussion of the application of extrusion for the production of amorphous solid dispersions for solubility enhancement. New sections covering the application of simulation technology to aid in the design of these products have been added, which specifically discuss the application for the assessment of residence time and mixing efficiency. Additional discussion around non-traditional applications such as devolatilization helps to provide insight into emerging areas of extrusion while highlighting the versatility of the platform. Closing out the text are sections on installation, commissioning, and qualification requirements for extruders employed in the pharmaceutical industry. Control systems and instrumentation, which provide efficient mechanisms to control and monitor key process variables and data-acquisition systems, are also discussed.

Given the well-documented advantages that extrusion technology offers, continued expansion is expected, thereby challenging equipment manufacturers and process engineers to further refine and expand the application of the technology in the development and manufacturing of pharmaceutical dosage forms, with particular emphasis on equipment design and configurations. Additionally, new areas of equipment scale down and realization of process simulation are expected to grow and facilitate a new generation of products using extrusion. This will help to enable new products that utilize extrusion for a range of applications including:

- Melt extruded amorphous dispersions and controlled release systems for oral delivery
- Development of multi-functional devices that combine functional and therapeutic benefits
- Increased usage of supercritical fluid injection for a variety of benefits: plasticizing, foaming, devolatilization, and microstructural control for novel drug delivery applications
- Continued application of wet and melt granulation for more efficient drug development and manufacturing

The first edition of this book was the first of its kind that extensively explored the well-developed science of extrusion technology as applied to pharmaceutical drug product development and manufacturing. By covering a wide range of relevant topics, the current text brings together all technical information necessary to develop and market pharmaceutical dosage forms that meet current quality and regulatory requirements. As extrusion technology continues to be refined, the usage of extruder systems and the array of applications will continue to expand, but the core technologies as represented in Pharmaceutical Extrusion Technology will remain the same.

Isaac Ghebre-Sellassie
Charles Martin
Feng Zhang
James DiNunzio

Preface to the First Edition

Extrusion is a process in which materials are mixed intimately under controlled conditions of temperature, shear, and pressure to generate a variety of in-process and finished products using pieces of equipment collectively known as extruders. Most of the early applications of this technology were limited to industrial processes that ranged from compaction of clay and straw to the mastication of rubber and plastics. Prominent in its absence throughout this period was the application of extrusion in the development and manufacture of pharmaceutical products. As a result, until recently, the pharmaceutical industry contributed very little to the technological advances made either in the improvement of existing extrusion equipment or in the design of specialized extruders that satisfy its highly regulated sphere of operation. However, as soon as work started on the applicability of the technology in pharmaceutical dosage from development, it became apparent that extrusion processes not only improve the efficiency of pharmaceutical manufacturing processes, but also can significantly enhance the quality of manufactured products owing to the mixing efficiency of extruders. The intent of this book is, therefore, to provide pharmaceutical scientists and technologies with basic principles and fundamentals of extrusion technology and a detailed description of the practical applications of extrusion processes.

Chapter 1 provides a historical overview of extruders and extrusion technology, and describes the evolutionary development of the technology in an attempt to address the processing needs of the time. Early patents that formed the basis for the widespread use of the technology are highlighted. Extrusion design features that are common to general industrial applications, but also uniquely applicable to the pharmaceutical industry, including cleanability of the product contact parts, are discussed in Chapter 2. Single-crew extruders, the first family of extruders to be widely introduced into the market, are continuous, high-pressure generating pumps that also perform limited mixing and devolatilization functions. These extruders, as well as the impact of different system configurations on the processability of various formulations, are extensively discussed in Chapter 3. Chapter 4 addresses twin-screw extruders. Corotating and counterrotating twin-screw compounding extruders are mass transfer devices that are used to mix together two or more materials into a homogeneous mass in a continuous process. This is accomplished through distributive and dispersive mixing of the various components in a formulation. These aspects as well as screw designs specific to twin-screw extruders are discussed in depth.

Extrusion dies, located at the exit end of the barrel assembly, are critical parts of the extrusion system that can literally make or break a process, particularly during the manufacture of controlled-release dosage forms. Success of a given process depends on, among other factors, die design. While some dies may be simple, others can be extremely complex. These and some of the techniques employed in die design are reviewed in Chapter 5. Chapter 6 covers material handling and feeder technology. During extrusion, liquids and powders must be fed accurately in a continuous manner throughout the run time, including the refill period, to ensure formulation consistency, constant throughput, proper order of mixing of ingredients, and regulated mass transfer. Feeders are hence critical components of the extrusion line that need to be evaluated carefully. A detailed description of torque rheometers, instruments that are essential for the characterization of formulations and processing parameters, and techniques that help elucidate the rheological properties of melts, are presented in Chapter 7.

Chapter 8 describes general extrusion processes and troubleshooting, and delineates the impact each process parameter has on the characteristics of the overall manufacturing process. Chapter 9 covers melt pelletization processes, and provides a review of the various pelletizers that have been in use since the 1950s. Chapter 10 focuses specifically on critical formulation parameters that affect the development of melt-extruded controlled release pellets, with particular emphasis on the effect of various formulation components on the release profiles of oral solid dosage forms. Shape extrusion involving solid or hollow structures is discussed in Chapter 11. Chapter 12 describes in detail technologies relevant to the manufacturing of sheets and laminates, materials that could have extensive application in transdermal drug delivery and fast-dissolving films intended for oral drug delivery. The enhancement of dissolution rates, and hence bioavailabilities, of poorly water-soluble drug substances formulated as melt-extruded molecular and particulate dispersions is discussed in Chapters 13 and 14.

Chapter 15 covers recent advances made in the area of extrusion/spheronization, a popular solvent-based pelletization process that is employed, in the majority of cases, to manufacture high-potency pellets. Key process variables and formulation factors that determine the quality of pellets are highlighted. Wet granulation processes, which traditionally have employed planetary and high-shear mixers, can also be carried out using modified twin-screw extruders. Extruders, being high-intensity, small-volume mixers, produce very uniform granulations that allow the manufacture of precisely designed oral dosage forms and are discussed in Chapter 16. Control systems and instrumentation, which provide efficient mechanisms to control and monitor key process variables and data-acquisition systems, are discussed in Chapter 17. Chapter 18 provides an overview of the installation, commissioning, and qualification requirements for extruders employed in the pharmaceutical industry. Given the advantages that extrusion technology offers, interest in the technology is expected to grow, thereby challenging equipment manufacturers and process engineers to further refine and expand the application of the technology in the development and manufacturing of pharmaceutical dosage forms, with particular emphasis on equipment design and configurations. Some of these potential future developments and benefits are summarized in Chapter 19.

This book is the first of its kind that discusses extensively the well-developed science of extrusion technology as applied to pharmaceutical drug product development and manufacturing. By covering a wide range of relevant topics, the text brings together all technical information necessary to develop and market pharmaceutical dosage forms that meet current quality and regulatory requirements. As extrusion technology continues to be refined further, usage of extruder systems and the array of applications will continue to expand, but the core technologies as represented in *Pharmaceutical Extrusion Technology* will remain the same.

Isaac Ghebre-Sellassie
Charles Martin

About the Editors

James DiNunzio is a Principal Scientist in the Formulation Sciences Group at Merck & Co., Inc. and currently leads the Hot-Melt Extrusion Subject Matter Expert team. He received his Ph.D. from the University of Texas at Austin in Pharmaceutics. He has published numerous research articles, book chapters, and is a co-inventor on multiple patents and patent applications. His current research interests include formulation design for melt extruded systems and the development of continuous manufacturing processes.

Charles Martin is President/General Manager of Leistritz Extrusion. He is responsible for the management of a company that provides manufacturing equipment and engineering services to the plastics, medical and pharmaceutical industries in the USA and around the world. Extensively published in trade publications, textbooks and journals, Charlie has delivered 100+ technical presentations at wide-ranging international events, and was the co-editor of the 1st edition of the textbook Pharmaceutical Extrusion Technology. He has been awarded 2 extrusion-related patents. Charlie earned his undergraduate degree from Gettysburg College, Gettysburg, Pennsylvania and MBA from Rutgers University, New Brunswick, New Jersey.

Feng Zhang is an assistant professor at the University of Texas at Austin. Dr. Zhang is the author and coauthor of more than 40 publications and more than 10 patents. A member of American Association of Pharmaceutical Scientist, he received his Ph.D. degree (1999) in Pharmaceutical Science from the University of Texas at Austin, Austin, Texas.

Isaac Ghebre-Sellassie is President, Pharmaceutical Technology Solutions, Morris Plains, New Jersey, and Executive Director and Chief Scientific Officer, MEGA Pharmaceuticals, Asmara, Eritrea. Dr. Ghebre-Sellassie is the author or coauthor of more than 50 professional publications, including Multiparticulate Oral Drug Delivery and Pharmaceutical Pelletization Technology (both titles, Marcel Dekker Inc.), and the holder of 17 patents. A member of the American Association of Pharmaceutical Scientists and the International Society for Pharmaceutical Engineering, he received his M.S. (1978) and Ph.D. (1981) degrees from Purdue University, West Lafayette, Indiana.

Contributors

Bob Bessemer
Conair Group
Cranberry Township, Pennsylvania

Christopher C. Case
Reduction Engineering
Pittsburgh, Pennsylvania

Sharmista Chatterjee
Food and Drug Administration
Center for Drug Evaluation and Research
Silver Spring, Maryland

Celia N. Cruz
Food and Drug Administration
Center for Drug Evaluation and Research
Silver Spring, Maryland

Dipen Desai
Kashiv Pharmaceuticals
Bridgewater, New Jersey

James DiNunzio
Merck & Co., Inc.
Kenilworth, New Jersey

Tom Dobbie
Porpoise Viscometers Ltd.
Lancashire, England

Adam Dreiblatt
Extrusioneering International, Inc.
Randolph, New Jersey

Thomas Durig
Ashland Inc.
Wilmington, Delaware

Bert Elliott
Leistritz Extrusion
Somerville, New Jersey

Niloufar Faridi
Polymer Processing Institute
Newark, New Jersey

Xin Feng
Department of Pharmaceutics and Drug
  Delivery
The University of Mississippi
Oxford, Mississippi

Brian Haight
Leistritz Extrusion
Somerville, New Jersey

Albrecht Huber
Leistritz Extrusionstechnik GmbH
Nuremberg, Germany

David Johnson
Merck & Co., Inc.
Kenilworth, New Jersey

Stuart J. Kapp
Leistritz Extrusion
Somerville, New Jersey

Pinak Khatri
G&W PA Laboratories
Sellersville, Pennsylvania

Bo Lang
Drug Product Science & Technology,
  Pharmaceutical Development
Bristol-Myers Squibb
New Brunswick, New Jersey

Tony Listro
Foster Delivery Science, Inc.
Putnam, Connecticut

Mayur Lodaya
GlaxoSmithKline
Research Triangle Park, North Carolina

Rapti Madurawe
Food and Drug Administration
Center for Drug Evaluation and Research
Silver Spring, Maryland

Charles Martin
Leistritz Extrusion
Somerville, New Jersey

Scott T. Martin
Thermo Fisher Scientific
Tewksbury, Massachusetts

Kathrin Nickel
Leistritz Extrusionstechnik GmbH
Nuremberg, Germany

Sharon Nowak
Coperion K-Tron
Pitman, New Jersey

Pete A. Palmer
Wolock & Lott
Branchburg, New Jersey

Gaurang Patel
Kashiv Pharmaceuticals
Bridgewater, New Jersey

Naresh Pavurala
Food and Drug Administration
Center for Drug Evaluation and Research
Silver Spring, Maryland

Rick Peng
Merck & Co., Inc.
Kenilworth, New Jersey

John Perdikoulias
Compuplast International Inc.
Williamsville, New York

Wantanee Phuapradit
Kashiv Pharmaceuticals
Bridgewater, New Jersey

Harpreet Sandhu
Kashiv Pharmaceuticals
Bridgewater, New Jersey

Navnit Shah
Kashiv Pharmaceuticals
Bridgewater, New Jersey

Richard Steiner
Düsseldorf, Germany

Graciela Terife
Merck & Co., Inc.
Rahway, New Jersey

William Thiele
Leistritz Extrusion
Somerville, New Jersey

Michael Thompson
Department of Chemical
  Engineering
McMaster University
Hamilton, Ontario, Canada

Atsawin Thongsukmak
Kashiv Pharmaceuticals
Bridgewater, New Jersey

Jaydeep Vaghashiya
Kashiv Pharmaceuticals
Bridgewater, New Jersey

Fengyuan Yang
Ashland Inc.
Wilmington, Delaware

Feng Zhang
College of Pharmacy
The University of Texas at
  Austin
Austin, Texas

1 Twin-Screw Extruders for Pharmaceutical Products from a Technical and Historical Perspective

Charles Martin

CONTENTS

1.1 INTRODUCTION

If the old saying "the best indication of future performance is past performance"
holds true, then the future for twin-screw extrusion to develop and manufacture

dosage forms will eventually dominate the pharmaceutical manufacturing landscape for new drug entities. Developed almost 100 years ago for food and natural rubber/plastics applications, twin-screw extrusion now generates some of the most cutting-edge drug delivery systems available.

Polymers are specified to function as thermal binders and act as drug depots and/or drug release retardants upon cooling and solidification. This means active pharmaceutical ingredients (APIs) need to be intimately mixed with a wide range of excipients. There are many mixing devices, but it will become evident that twin-screw extrusion processing offers significant advantages as compared to batch manufacturing techniques. An advantage is that solvents and water are generally not necessary for processing, which reduces the number of processing steps because expensive drying equipment and time-consuming drying steps can be eliminated.

After 100 or so years of usage, the well-characterized nature of the twin-screw extrusion process lends itself to ease of scale-up and process optimization, while also affording benefits of continuous manufacturing and adaptability to process analytical technology in an ever-changing regulatory and fiscal environment. What's occurring today for pharmaceuticals with regard to the implementation of extrusion technology to increase efficiencies and save costs is analog to what occurred 80 or so years ago in the plastics and food sectors of industry as batch processes were replaced by continuous manufacturing alternatives for reasons that are now obvious.

Almost every plastic has been processed at some stage in the manufacturing train on a twin-screw extruder (TSE) to mix materials to impart desired properties into a final part. Plastics is a major worldwide industry that plays a role in all facets of modern life, from health and well-being, nutrition, shelter, and transportation to safety and security, communication, sports, and leisure activities. Twin-screw extrusion is used for the production of every day products such as packaging films, fibers for carpets, car interiors and windshields, along with products like structural decking, space-shuttle parts, conductive parts, and even synthetic wine corks. These are all high-tech products!

This ability to mix materials to customize product performance caused visionary pharmaceutical scientists to consider extrusion to enable therapies of poorly soluble compounds through the generation of amorphous solid dispersions. The embrace of melt extrusion by the scientific community has led to further research efforts and understanding of how the technology can be applied. As a result, traditional plastics process techniques have been transferred to manufacturing novel dosage forms and unique multifunctional medical devices. It is now a fact that twin-screw extrusion can produce reliable and robust drug product manufacturing alternatives and shows unlimited potential for new, novel dosage forms.

1.2 EVOLUTION OF BATCH TO CONTINUOUS AND SINGLE- TO TWIN-SCREW EXTRUDERS IN THE PLASTICS INDUSTRY

The earliest commercial machines for mixing food and polymer melts (natural rubbers) were batch mixers. The first major mixer, a two-roll mill, was described in an 1836 patent. A side view of a two-roll mill is presented in Figure 1.1. It was not until the early 20th century that batch mixer designs stabilized with a ram containing

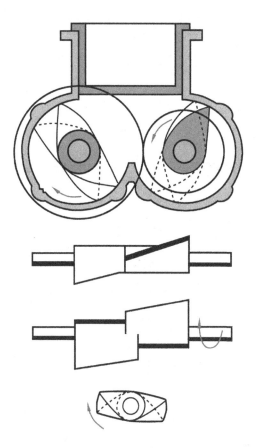

FIGURE 1.1 Side view of two-roll mill.

internal mixers. These were the same batch-mixing devices that dominated polymer and food industries into the 1960s. A side view of a conventional batch mixer is presented in Figure 1.2. Batch mixers are vessels in which polymers, oils, fillers, and additives are measured, introduced, and operated in an unfilled and largely unpressurized manner. In a starved unpressurized mixing chamber, the compounds may avoid the locally pressurized region of high shear between the rotor blades and chamber wall, which can result in a compound that has a wide distribution in states of agglomerate breakup and distribution. By definition, batch mixers are "large mass" discontinuous mixers.

Processing technologies that used single-screw pumping devices began to commonly appear in the mid- to late 1800s for products such as pasta, soap, and ceramic materials. These devices reflected the transition that was underway from batch to continuous processing. A schematic diagram of a single-screw extruder is presented in Figure 1.3. Why did this transition take place? Early issues were primarily related to "product quality," as evidenced by a patent on screw extrusion by Gray (1879) that involved extruding thermoplastic products for wire coating. Gray argued that the quality of the insulation properties was better than that produced by a ram (batch)

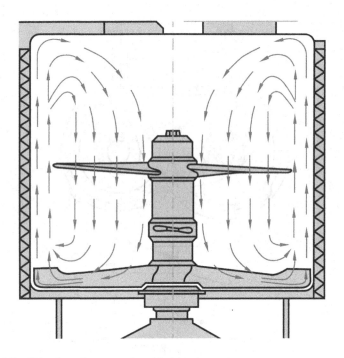

FIGURE 1.2   Side view of a conventional batch mixer.

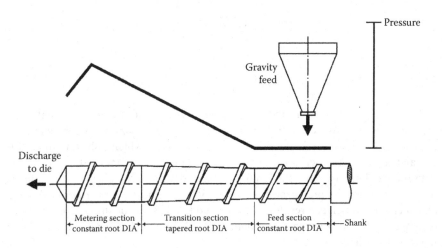

FIGURE 1.3   Single-screw extruder screw design with flood-fed feed throat and the associated pressure/pumping profile.

extruder. Interestingly, the issue of higher production rates was not raised, suggesting that improved pumping consistencies and quality drove the invention.

In the mid-1800s, continuous-mixing machines began to be used, but seemingly were not widely commercialized. Continuous mixers began appearing in patent literature from the 1920s to 1960s; however, it was only during the second half of

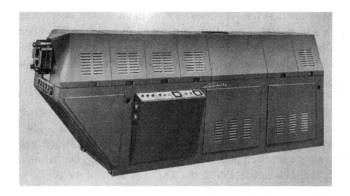

FIGURE 1.4 Photo of a 1960s-era TSE.

the 20th century that TSEs were accepted as the continuous mixer that most often produced a higher-quality, more uniform mix at reduced mixing/residence times and localized temperatures. The comparatively first-in, first-out nature of the TSE also meant the materials experienced a more uniform heat/shear history as compared to available batch-type devices.

In the 1950s and 1960s a lot of work was performed using single-screw extruders, with some success. A single-screw extruder, as the name implies, uses a one-piece screw inside a one-piece barrel driven by a motor/gearbox—a much simpler design as compared to a TSE. In the 1970s, a tipping point occurred and much of the food/plastic industries transitioned from batch to continuous processing, primarily via twin-screw extrusion. A photograph of a 1960s-era TSE is presented in Figure 1.4. Screw design of an early-stage counter-rotating intermeshing twin screw is shown in Figure 1.5. Interestingly, the processing section shrouding is similar to what is used in today's TSE for pharmaceutical applications.

In the early 1980s, the TSE became the most preferred continuous mixer used in compound plastics, primarily because TSEs are better mixers than single-screw

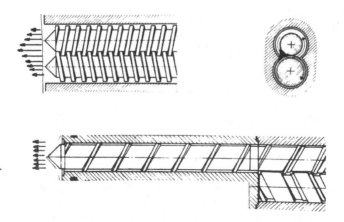

FIGURE 1.5 Screw design of early-stage counterrotating intermeshing TSEs.

extruders (SSEs) due to several features relating to interscrew interactions that make it significantly easier to successfully compound a formulation. That being said, the SSE maintains its place for low-intensity mixing applications and high-pressure pumping, which is why this device makes the most of the extruded items we see and use every day, e.g., drinking straws and packaging film.

During this time frame (1980s and 1990s), research activities on polymer mixing intensified at universities and research institutions such as the University of Akron, Polymer Processing Institute, and Ecole Polytechnique, to name a few. Exhaustive mixing studies were performed, thousands of papers were published, and many millions of dollars were invested in developing (and marketing) the "ultimate" continuous mixer. By the mid- to late 1990s, the TSE was deemed the device of choice for most mixing and many devolatilization processes.

Today, the TSE continues to dominate the market for continuous mixing and devolatilization, and SSE high-pressure pumping for the extrusion of parts such as film, sheet, profiles, tubes, fibers, coatings, etc. Interestingly, in terms of the number of units currently installed each year, there are approximately ten times as many SSEs compared to TSEs, implying there are still opportunities for usage of SSEs for therapeutic drug delivery systems, particularly for multifunctional medical devices.

1.3   HISTORY OF TWIN-SCREW EXTRUSION FOR PHARMACEUTICALS

Interest in extrusion by the pharmaceutical industry began in the 1980s. Some early work was performed by Goedecke GmbH in Germany that led to the installation of a 50-mm-class corotating TSE for a melt granulation process. The machine supplier, Leistritz, struggled with the paperwork and wondered why Goedecke chose such a funny color for the equipment, but not much more, and was unaware that a new market was beginning to unfold. The extrusion equipment remains in production today.

The case study of Rezulin™, the first drug manufactured via melt extrusion, provides enlightening history. In 1989, Isaac Ghebre-Sellassie of Parke-Davis/Warner-Lambert (PD/WL) was asked by management to convert a spray dried process for the solubilization of a poorly soluble drug substance, troglitazone, to an alternative organic solvent-free manufacturing. The spray drying process had been initially selected after all commonly used methods (fusing method, hot melt/solvent evaporation, and solvent evaporation process) were evaluated in order to improve the bioavailability of troglitazone. However, the drug substance and processes that included melting had to be abandoned, prompting atypical methodologies to be considered, which resulted in a laboratory-scale TSE being installed in the PD/WL labs.

As a result, the PD/WL staff began to explore melt extrusion as an alternative process that generated an amorphous dispersion of the drug in a polymeric matrix and simultaneously ensured the stability of the drug substance during processing. Since the TSE was available and recognized to offer superior mixing capabilities with a short residence time, a decision was made to assess the melt-extrusion (ME) process. The formulation and process were optimized using a Leistritz 34-mm TSE without degradation of the drug substance even when the formulation was processed above the melting temperature of the drug substance, due to the short residence time in the TSE of less than one minute.

The Rezulin™ process, as it became known, was then transferred to a Leistritz 50-mm production-scale TSE. The product was approved by the Federal Drug Administration (FDA) and introduced in 1997, becoming the first commercial product that utilized ME as a solubility enhancement manufacturing process. Interestingly, the initial batch size was 250 kg. Due to the consistency and reproducibility of the product, the batch size was eventually increased to 5000 kg over 500 hours. During the time the product was in the market, there were no batch failures. A U.S. patent for the formulation and process was issued in 2004 (USA Patent 6,677,362) (Ghebre-Sellassie I., 2015, Adoption of twin screw extrusion by pharmaceutical industry, personal communications). Somewhat similar work was performed in Europe by companies such as Knoll (later Abbott and Soliqs), Mundiepharma and Napp (Steiner R., 2015, Adoption of twin screw extrusion by pharmaceutical industry, personal communications).

Simultaneously in the early 1990s, under the auspices of Jim McGinity and the University of Texas (UT), vigorous and varied research efforts were exerted to develop alternative processes to solvent evaporation for the preparation of transdermal and transmucosal film delivery systems, which spawned UT's first poster at the annual meeting of American Association of Pharamceutical Scientists (AAPS) in 1994. Early success with the acrylic polymers was followed by work to prepare granules, pellets, and tablets with a wide variety of polymers and lipids (McGinity J., 2015, Investigation of twin screw extrusion by pharmaceutical scientists in academia, personal communications).

During this timeframe, UT graduates (John Koleng, Feng Zhang, Michael Crowley, and others) became the nucleus of the management team at PharmaForm, a UT incubator company that led pioneering efforts using melt extrusion as a manufacturing platform. At this time, melt-extrusion technology became recognized as a viable manufacturing platform.

In 2003 the first book on the subject matter, *Pharmaceutical Extrusion Technology*, edited by Isaac Ghebre Selassie and Charles Martin, was published by Informa Healthcare. In addition to some of the early pioneers from the pharmaceutical world, many of the chapters were provided by extrusion experts from the plastics industry, focusing on extrusion engineering principles.

Then a spark! The FDA's 2004 Process Analytical Technology (PAT) initiative provided drug makers a framework for pharmaceutical development, manufacturing, and quality assurance through in-line monitoring. In a nutshell, the PAT initiative encouraged considering extrusion for the manufacture of new dosage forms—the PAT initiative could have literally been written by a TSE equipment supplier, since it denotes attributes inherent with that device and continuous processing.

Another solubility-enhanced product that was approved by the FDA was Kaletra™, which was a reformulation of a drug to treat HIV (Breitenbach 2006) that provided a robust dosage form that did not require refrigeration to maintain stability. Kalletra™ applied melt-extrusion technology to improve the overall therapeutic efficacy of a drug and currently represents the most commercially successful melt-extruded dosage form to enhance oral bioavailability of poor water-soluble drugs.

Now the activities relating to melt-extrusion activity really began to accelerate. The seeds had been planted from the early development work at Parke-Davis, the ground had been fertilized at research institutions like the University of Texas to develop an understanding of melt extrusion, and the FDA's 2004 PAT initiative had provided the germination effect that allowed melt-extrusion usage to expand. In the early 1990s, there were only a handful of TSE pharmaceutical class installations worldwide. In the next 10 years, this number would dramatically increase into all niches of the pharmaceutical landscape, ranging from universities to large pharmaceutical companies, with Contract Research Organizations (CROs), Contract Manufacturing Organizations (CMOs), and generic drug companies all becoming users of melt extrusion.

By 2010 almost every major pharmaceutical company had installed TSEs into their R&D equipment portfolios. The use of SSEs had faded, as the comparative utility of TSEs for mixing and devolatilization became apparent. Research efforts across the board were intensified and several amorphous compositions were commercialized, leading to the general acceptance of melt extrusion as a viable technology.

In the last dozen years, Merck has become a leading proponent and has evolved into a cutting-edge innovator introducing, developing, and promoting various extrusion-related technologies in the areas of foaming, devolatilization, shape extrusion, and computer modeling. Novartis, GSK, BASF, Evonik, Dow Chemical, Grunenthal, and Ashland have all been active in developing and marketing extrusion processes. Bend Research, PharmaForm (now Formex), ExxPharma Therapeutics, Rottendorf, and Foster Delivery Science are examples of companies that offered contract services early on, with the list growing to 40-plus worldwide. In addition to UT, early research efforts began at the University of Mississippi and Massachusetts Institute of Technology, followed by St. John's, the New Jersey Institute of Technology, University of Pittsburgh, Instituto de Capacitación del Plástico y del Caucho (ICIPC), NOLL GmbH, Halle Plastic GmbH, and others.

While the majority of melt-extrusion applications have focused on oral delivery, commercially marketed melt-extruded products are already available that have changed the drug delivery paradigm. The most well-known is NuvaRing (Merck-Schering Plough), which uses a coextrusion process to imbed the API into an ethylene vinyl acetate (EVA) core matrix. Another melt-extrusion-shaped system is Lacrisert™, a rod inserted into the pocket of the patient's lower eyelid to minimize symptoms associated with dry eyes. Development efforts are currently being expended for transdermal patches, dissolvable films, and foamed and coextruded products that are made by the extrusion process. These products represent the most novel of melt-extrusion developments. A list of commercial products manufactured using the twin-screw melt-extrusion process is presented in Table 1.1.

1.4   BASICS FOR TSE

1.4.1   SCREW ELEMENTS

The same process tasks are performed in any TSE. Initially, materials are metered into the extruder feed throat and solids conveying occurs. The materials being

TABLE 1.1

Commercial Drug Products Manufactured Using TSE

Product	Indication	HME Purpose	Company
Rezulin (Troglitazone)	Diabetes	Amorphous dispersion	Wyeth
Onmel (Itraconazole)	Antifungal	Amorphous dispersion	Merz North America, Inc.
Zoladex (Goserelin Acetate)	Prostate cancer	Shaped system	AstraZeneca
Implanon (Etonogestrel)	Contraceptive	Shaped system	Merck
Lacrisert (HPC Rod)	Dry eye syndrome	Shaped system	Merck
Gris-PEG (Griseofulvin)	Antifungal	Crystalline dispersion	Pedinol Pharmacal
Palladone (Hydromorphone HCl)	Pain	Controlled release	Purdue Pharma
Nucynta (Tapentadol)	Pain	Controlled release	Depomed Inc.
Opana ER (Oxymorphone HCl)	Pain	Controlled release	Endo Pharmaceuticals
NevaRing (Etonogestrel, Ethinyl Estradiot)	Contraceptive	Shaped system	Merck
Norvir (Ritonavir)	Antiviral (HIV)	Amorphous dispersion	Abbvie
Kaleatra (Ritonavir/ Lopinavir)	Antiviral (HIV)	Amorphous dispersion	Abbvie
Eucreas (Vildagliptin/ Metformin HCl)	Diabetes	Melt granulation	Novartis
Zithromax (azithromycin)	Antibiotic	Melt granulation	Pfizer
Orzurdex (dexamethanone)	Macular edema	Shaped system	Allergan
Noxafil (posaconazole)	Antifungal	Amorphous dispersion	Merck
Belsomra (suvorexant)	Medication for insomnia	Amorphous dispersion	Merck

processed must pass through a series of pressurized, fully filled mixing regions. The materials are then melted via mixing elements and conveyed via flighted elements. Flighted elements discharge the melt through a die or other pressure-generating device into various shapes for downstream processing.

At the heart of any TSE process sections are the rotating screws contained within barrels. Screws are typically segmented and assembled on shafts, in which case the torque transmitted to the shaft is the limiting factor for the amount of power/torque that is available to process materials. Screws for TSEs can also be a one-piece design with significantly higher torque transmittal possibilities. Because of the complexity that occurs due to the many engineering variables in screw design, as well as the non-Newtonian nature of most polymeric materials that are processed, mathematical predictive modeling of material behavior in the TSE is quite difficult.

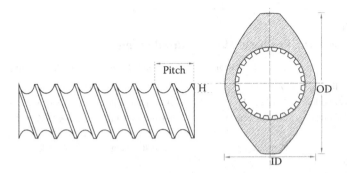

FIGURE 1.6   Illustration of pitch, outer diameter (OD), and inner diameter (ID).

The OD/ID ratio (outside screw diameter/inside screw diameter) and channel depth are important TSE design parameters, as these parameters dictate the available free volume and torque. A graphic illustration of the outer diameter, inner diameter, and flight depth of screw elements is presented in Figure 1.6. As the channel depth increases, the ID decreases and results in less attainable shaft torque. An optimum balance between free volume and torque is important as both represent boundary conditions that may limit attainable material throughput rates.

A TSE is generally referred to by the diameter of its screws. For instance, a "ZSE-18" model would reflect a TSE with an 18-mm screw outside diameter (OD) for each screw. In the plastics and food industries, ODs range from 12 to 400+ mm with outputs from 50 g to greater than 50,000 kg/hr. Pharmaceutical TSEs are generally in the 60–70-mm class and below, with research and development efforts performed on TSEs with screw ODs in the 10–30-mm range. Flight depths range from as little as 1–3 mm on a small lab extruder to approximately 15 mm on a 70-mm-class machine. Even a 140-mm-class TSE will only have a flight depth in the 25-mm range—hence the term small mass continuous mixer with short mass transfer distances.

There are seemingly an infinite number of possible screw variations. There are, however, only three basic types of screw elements: flighted elements, mixing elements, and zoning elements. Flighted elements forward material past barrel ports, through mixers, and out of the extruder through a die. Mixing elements facilitate the mixing of the various components being processed. Zoning elements isolate two operations. Some elements can be multifunctional.

Flighted elements are available with various angles for different conveyance attributes, depending upon location placement (Figure 1.7). The higher the pitch of the flight angle, the faster it pumps. Higher-volume feed elements and slotted elements that both pump and mix are available and matched to the unit operations as dictated by the process.

Kneading elements, the most common mixing element, are strategically placed along the length of the screws (Figure 1.8). Wider kneaders cause extension mixing and planar shear to be imparted into the materials being processed and are more dispersive in nature as compared to narrow kneaders that result in divisions and recombination of melt streams, and therefore facilitate distributive mixing. Other parameters regulating mixing intensity include the offset angle of the kneaders

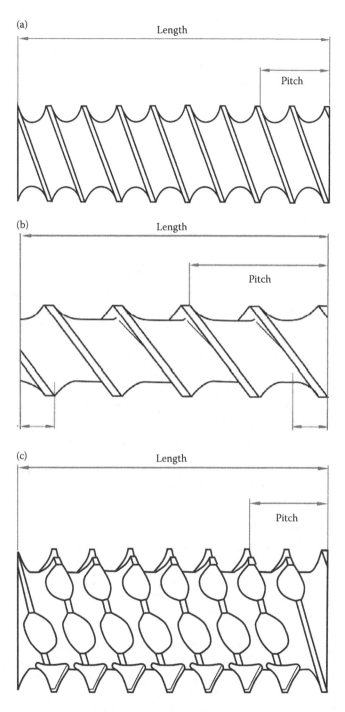

FIGURE 1.7 Examples of flighted elements: (a) small pitch conveying element; (b) large pitch conveying element; (c) slotted mixing/conveying element.

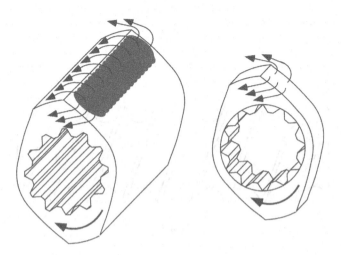

FIGURE 1.8   Examples of mixing (kneading) elements.

(30° or 60° forward or reverse) or neutral (90°). It should be noted that an innumerable number of mixing elements (e.g., rotors, slotted vanes, and blister rings) are available, but that the kneading-type elements account for 90%+ of those used in a corotating TSE.

Another variable in the geometry of mixing elements is the "lobe count." The lobe count refers to the number of screw tips/flights that are wiping the barrel wall. The OD/ID ratio and mode of operation determines the number of lobes that are geometrically possible for a given design. Example bilobal and trilobal TSE screw elements are presented in Figure 1.9. Most corotating intermeshing TSEs are bilobal as, due to interference issues, a corotating intermeshing TSE is limited to two lobes at typical OD/ID ratios (1.4–1.7/1). For low-volume applications a 1.2/1 OD/ID can be specified and three lobes can be used to facilitate low free volumes and high torque for testing 20-g batches or less.

1.4.2   FUNDAMENTALS OF MIXING

There are two main types of mixing: distributive mixing and dispersive mixing. Distributive mixing involves melt division and recombination, while dispersive mixing involves planar and elongational shear. A graphic illustration of two types of mixing is presented in Figure 1.10. Screw designs can be made shear intensive and/or passive, based upon the elements specified in the design. Mixing elements may be dispersive, distributive, or a balance of each/both. Screw elements that accentuate extensional mixing and planar shear effects are dispersive in nature, as compared to elements that facilitate melt divisions/recombinations, which are more distributive and therefore useful for mixing heat- and shear-sensitive materials. Shear-sensitive APIs are often distributed in a melt and then allowed to dissolve into the polymer matrix before exiting the TSE, whereas more severe dispersive mixing is sometimes needed. Other factors that dictate mixing intensity include, but are not limited to, the screw rpm, the gaps between the screws and screw flight/barrel wall, and the "lobe count."

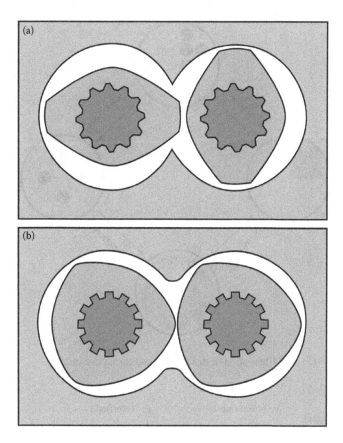

FIGURE 1.9 (a) Example of bilobal TSE screw elements; (b) example of trilobal TSE screw elements.

In a TSE, the materials being processed are bounded by screw flights and barrel walls, often referred to as the melt pool. The materials are separated into small melt pools by screw flights and barrel walls, which is why the TSE is by definition a "small mass" continuous mixer, as compared to the large mass batch mixer described earlier. As shown in Figure 1.11, there are five shear regions in the screws for any TSE, regardless of screw rotation or degree of intermesh. The following is a brief description of each shear region.

Screw channel: A low shear region, highly dependent on the degree of screw fill in a starved TSE; shear is significantly lower as compared to the other shear regions.

Overflight/tip: A high shear region, independent of the degree of screw fill, located between the screw tip and the barrel wall; the material undergoes significant planar shear effects.

Lobal pool: A high shear region, independent of the degree of screw fill; because of the compression/acceleration entering into the overflight region the material experiences a particularly effective extensional mixing effect.

Apex (top/bottom): A high shear region, independent of the degree of screw fill; where the interaction from the second screw results in compression/decompression/

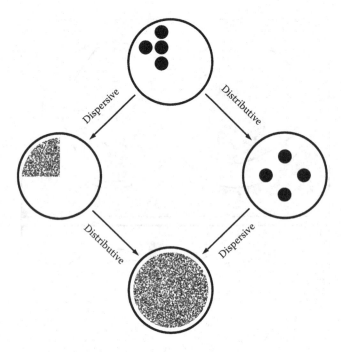

FIGURE 1.10   Graphic illustration of distributive and dispersive mixing.

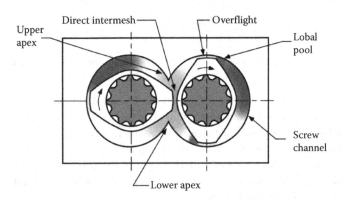

FIGURE 1.11   Cross section view of TSE screw denoting five shear regions.

extensional effects associated with pressure fields and directional flow changes result in increased mixing rates.

Intermesh: A high shear region, independent of the degree of screw fill; it's a high-intensity mixing zone between the screws where the screws "wipe" each other.

As shown in Figure 1.12, each screw, to a degree, wipes the other in a corotating TSE. This is termed "self-wiping." This self-wiping effect sequences unit operations and discharges the small volume of materials in a first-in, first-out sequence with a given residence time distribution (RTD). This results in a uniform deformation/mixing

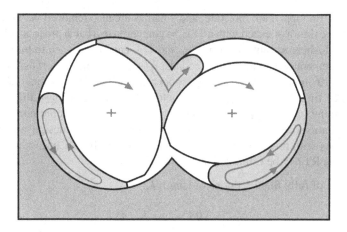

FIGURE 1.12   Self-wiping flow effect in a corotating TSE.

history and, depending on the length and screw design of the TSE, there will be an associated RTD for the process section. The more filled the screws, the tighter the RTD, and the more starved the screws, the wider the RTD. An illustration of the effect of the degree of screw fill on the residence time distribution is presented in Figure 1.13.

For simplicity, the four high mass transfer regions shown in Figure 1.11 can be viewed as independent of the degree of screw fill, which is why, in a starve-fed machine, when rate is decreased at a given screw rpm, more mixing occurs due to a longer residence time in the mixing zones. Alternatively, as rate increases at a given screw rpm, the low shear channel region plays a larger role and the materials pass over the mixing zones quicker. Therefore, there is shorter exposure time to high shear regions and less lobal mixing events.

The intense mixing associated with the short interscrew mass transfer characteristics inherent with a TSE small mass continuous mixer results in highly efficient distributive and/or dispersive mixing that is a more uniform product as compared to large mass

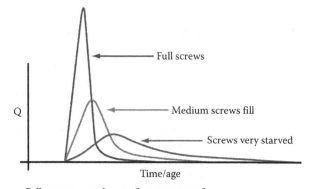

Full screws = good pump/less mass transfer
Empty screws = poor pump/more mass transfer

FIGURE 1.13   Effect of the degree of fill on the residence time distribution in a TSE.

batch mixers. Entrapped air, moisture, and volatiles are also removed via venting. The short residence time associated with a TSE, as compared to a batch process, is beneficial for many heat-/shear-sensitive materials, as the TSE can be designed to limit exposure to elevated temperatures to just a few seconds. RTs range from as short as 5 seconds to as long as 6–10 minutes, with most process operating in the 20–60 second range.

Residence time is a challenging parameter to calculate, because the process in a TSE is a combination of partially and fully filled zones. It is common to use two separate equations making assumptions based on the screw design and processing conditions with regard to filled/unfilled sections. In lieu of access to computer modeling, the RT can be estimated as follows (5):

Residence of fully filled sections of length L_f:

$$\Phi_f = \frac{3.08 \times L_f \times h \times D}{Q}$$

where

Φ_f = residence time in seconds
L_f = length of the section in centimeters
h = overflight gap screw tip to barrel wall in centimeters
D = screw diameter in centimeters
Q = volumetric flow rate in cubic centimeters per second

Residence of starved sections of length L_f:

$$\Phi_s = \frac{2 \times L_s}{ZN}$$

where

Φ_s = residence time in seconds
L_f = length of the section in centimeters
Z = flight pitch in centimeters
N = screw speed in rotations per minute

The residence times for the filled and unfilled sections are then simply added together to estimate the total residence time in the extruder.

Viscosity of the melt also plays a role in mixing. Temperature control, thereby managing the viscosity of the melt, and the staging of elements are also factors. During solid resin melting, viscosity is at its highest so high stress rates are possible, which results in dispersive mixing but can also cause degradation. In the latter stages of the TSE process section, lower viscosities yield lower stress rates that may enable heat and shear APIs to be mixed without degradation.

The following simple formula provides some insight into the different variables impacting peak shear stress. As would be expected, shear-induced heating is highest at the point where the applied shear is highest.

$$\text{Peak shear stress} = \frac{\pi \times D \times n}{h \times 60} \times \text{viscosity}$$

where
   D = screw diameter
   n = screw speed in rpm
   h = overflight gap screw tip to barrel wall

1.4.3 BARREL

The barrel section of a TSE is available in these basic configurations: solid feed, liquid feed, side feed, venting, and closed segments. Each section serves a specific functionality and allows for multiple-unit operations when combined with the desired screw design. Closed barrel zones generally represent the majority of processing length for any TSE and are placed at high-pressure compounding and/or pumping locations. Examples include mixing, kneading, or pumping to the die.

The length of the TSE process section is described in terms of the length to diameter (L/D) ratio and defined by dividing the overall length of the process section by the diameter of the screws. An example of a barrel of 4:1 L/D is presented in Figure 1.14.

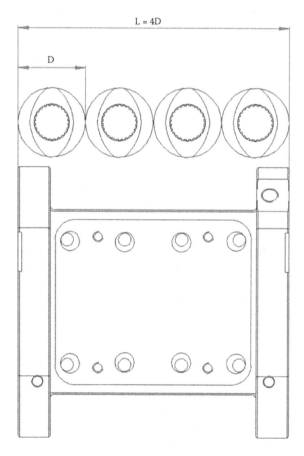

FIGURE 1.14 Length-to-diameter ratio for a TSE barrel section; this barrel section has a 4:1 L/D.

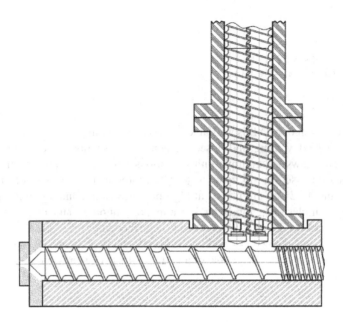

FIGURE 1.15   Pairing up a TSE for high-intensity mixing with a single-screw extruder for cooling and pumping.

For instance, if the OD of a screw is 20 mm and the length of the process section is 800 mm, then the L/D ratio is 800:20, or 40:1 L/D. If the length was 400 mm, the L/D would be 400:20, or 20:1 L/D. Higher L/D values result in a longer process section that can support more unit operations.

The L/D and staging of barrel and screw are dictated based on the number of unit operations to be performed. For example, a system requiring only compounding of drug and polymer with moisture removal and pumping to a die might be conducted in a 20:1 L/D configuration. Comparatively, a 40:1 L/D configuration might be required for a plasticizer injection, compounding of polymer with plasticizer, API addition via side stuffing, or moisture removal and pumping. Multistage venting and/ or foaming processes might even require tandem extrusion systems that link together multiple extruders to string together and resolve conflicting unit operations, such as high-intensity mixing combined with using a second extruder as a heat exchanger to cool the melt. The setup of a TSE for high-intensity mixing mated to a single screw as a cooling and pumping device is presented in Figure 1.15.

1.4.4   FEEDER

The feed system to a TSE typically sets the rate to the TSE and maintains formulation accuracy. Various delivery mechanisms are used, including vibratory trays, single-screw augers, and twin-screw augers. Loss-in-weight (LIW) feeders maintain a constant mass-flow rate to the TSE by adjusting the feed mechanism via a tuning algorithm based on materials usage from the hopper that is situated on a load cell (Figure 1.16). When multiple feed streams are being introduced, the TSE process

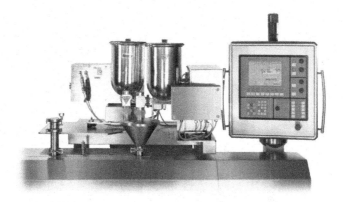

FIGURE 1.16   Setup of multiple loss-in-weight feeders to meter excipients and APIs into a TSE.

section LIW feeders will maintain formulation accuracy. Liquid feed streams use a piston or gear pump, depending upon the viscosity of the liquid. Crammer feeders can also be used for highly filled and/or fluffy materials.

The TSE is starve-fed with the screw rpm being independent from the feed rate and used to optimize process efficiencies. The pressure gradient in the TSE is determined by the selection of screws and operating conditions (rate vs. screw rpm). Flighted elements are strategically placed so that the screw channels are not filled, which results in zero pressure underneath downstream vent/feed sections, which facilitates downstream feeding of materials and prevents vent flooding (Figure 1.17).

The downstream addition of materials into a melt stream is often facilitated by a side stuffer, as shown in Figure 1.18. A side stuffer is a corotating, intermeshing twin-screw auger that "pushes" material into the process melt stream to allow for avoidance of the high shear region associated with melting and also reducing

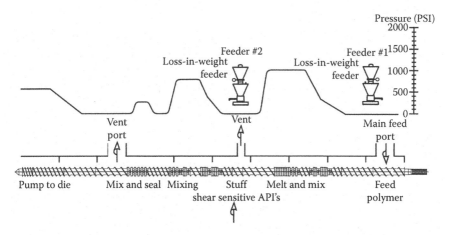

FIGURE 1.17   Pressure gradient in a starve-fed TSE process allows for downstream unit operations.

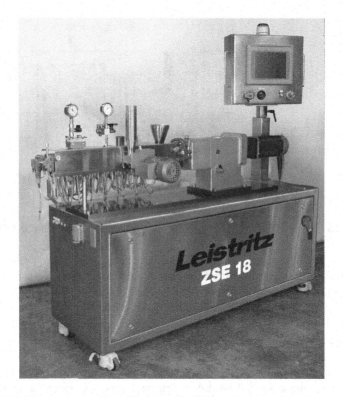

FIGURE 1.18 Downstream side stuffing into the TSE process.

residence time exposure for heat-sensitive materials. Liquid feed points also allow for the introduction of liquids or molten materials downstream in the process. Sequential feeding may also eliminate the need for premixing prior to extrusion.

1.4.5 GEARBOX

The TSE gearbox transmits energy from the motor to the screws and reduces the motor speed to the desired screw rpm while multiplying torque, maintaining angular timing of the screws, and accepting the thrust load from pressure being generated from the process. To avoid damage, a mechanical over-torque coupling connects the motor shaft to the gearbox input shaft that automatically disengages at a designated level.

1.4.6 DEVOLATILIZATION

Another common usage for a TSE is for devolatilization (DV), which is a process to remove various amounts of gases from the process melt, including but not limited to residual solvents, water and other undesirable volatile contaminants. Vent zones facilitate the removal of volatiles from the melt stream. The venting process may also be performed under vacuum and may occur at a series of positions along the length of the TSE process section. Using multiple venting locations, it is possible to remove substantial quantities of volatiles from the melt stream, e.g., 30%+.

Devolatilization efficiencies in a TSE can be improved with a longer residence time under the vents, higher surface area of the melt, higher surface renewal, more nucleation, growth and rupture of bubbles, higher vacuum level, and use of stripping agents to facilitate bubble formation.

1.4.7 PRESSURE GENERATION

Elevated pressure at the die is needed to push polymer melt through the die into various shapes for downstream processing. However, elevated pressure at the die results in temperature rise and is typically detrimental to the process. The following temperature rise formula is meant to be insightful.

$$\Delta T(^\circ C) = \frac{\Delta P(\text{bar})}{2}$$

where
ΔP = pressure rise at die
ΔT = temperature rise at die

Pressure-generating devices can be mated to the TSE to help manage pressures and melt temperature. A positive displacement gear pump or single-screw pump may be attached to the TSE to build and stabilize pressure to the die, and it would be typically used when extruding a transdermal film/patch, multifunctional medical tube, or micropellets. An example setup with a gear pump as the pressure-generating device is presented in Figure 1.19. Downstream systems now size and cool the extrudate with, once again, a multitude of high-tech equipment options available from the plastic and food-processing technologies to make a high-quality, precision-dosage form.

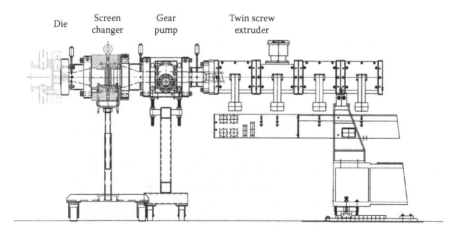

FIGURE 1.19 TSE mated to a gear pump as a positive displacement pumping device.

1.4.8   DOWNSTREAM PROCESSING

The next step is downstream processing. The most commonly used end product shapes for pharmaceutical applications are rods and films that are quenched on conveyors, film belt systems, or chill roll-pin breakers. Pellets can also be produced by a die face pelletizer. In general, strict geometric shaping is not often required because downstream equipment will mill the extruded material into a fine powder for further processing.

Multifunctional medical devices are also possible, such as for antimicrobial medical tubing or implantable drug delivery stents that require precision dies and shaping. Accurate control of part geometry will directly impact final part compliance of target product attributes. Cross-sectional area and internal geometry of the die relative to the mass-flow rate determine the pressure generation requirement, which will directly influence melt temperature and performance for heat-sensitive products.

1.4.9   PROCESS CONTROL PARAMETERS

Process control parameters are screw speed (rpm), feed rate, temperatures, and vacuum levels. Barrels house the screws and are temperature-controlled zones via proportional, integral, derivative (PID) temperature control algorithms. Typical readouts include melt pressure, melt temperature, motor amperage, and vacuum level. Near infrared (NIR), on-line viscosity, formulation imaging, and specialty probes can be integrated into the controls architecture as deemed beneficial. An example of laboratory-scale TSE with provision for probes along the path of the process section is presented in Figure 1.20.

An important TSE parameter to track for any extrusion process is specific energy (SE), which reflects the amount of energy being input into the process and is calculated as follows:

$$\text{Specific energy (kW per kg/hr)} = \frac{\text{kW} \times \% \text{ torque} \times \text{RPM}}{\text{RPM rating} \times 0.97 \times Q \text{ (kg/hr)}}$$

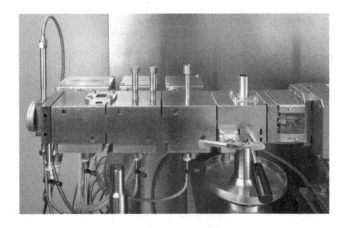

FIGURE 1.20   Lab-scale TSE with provision for probes for process monitoring.

where
  kW = kilowatts (motor rating)
  % torque = % used of the maximum allowable torque
  RPM = screws rotations per minute
  RPM rating = maximum speed of the motor
  0.97 = gearbox efficiency
  Q = feed rate (kg/hr)

In a production setting, tracking SE is important as it is an indicator of any change to the process, whether it's related to hardware or materials. If a TSE processes a given formulation at 0.25 SE and it changes to 0.20 or 0.30, something has changed and therefore the end product may be different too. SE also serves as a helpful scaling factor to determine operating parameters when scaling from a smaller to larger TSE.

1.5 EVOLUTION AND CRITICAL DESIGN FEATURE FOR TSE

1.5.1 CONTROLS AND INSTRUMENTATION

In the 1940s, control systems used manual devices such as hardwired push buttons with analog meters that used electromechanical relays to handle all the logic and interlocks. Direct current (DC) drives and motors were used to vary the speed of the screw rpm and other devices. In the 1990s, alternating current (AC) drives began replacing DC because AC motors were less complicated and maintenance intensive. The usage of AC motors/drives steadily increased and now accounts for 98% of motors/drives below 1000 kW.

Analog temperature controllers were used in early extruders with PID control loops to control the temperature of each heating zone. The analog controller eventually evolved into digital temperature controllers employing microprocessors using software for PID algorithms. Temperature control algorithms are now embedded in the programmable logic controller (PLC) code.

Monitoring gauges have always displayed screw rpm and load to temperature and pressure readings. The analog (dial) gauge has been around for 150 years. In the early 1980s, the new digital gauges were introduced, and today many of the monitoring signals are brought into the PLCs so that logic can be programmed to provide different control features associated with these signals.

The PLC started to replace electromechanical relays in the 1960s and became commonly used on TSEs in the 1980s, when machine interface with graphics began to be used. In the early 2000s, the term *man-machine interface* (MMI) became politically incorrect and evolved into *human-machine interface* (HMI) with alarming, recipes, data logging/trending, and communications to other devices. In the last 10 years, the ability to link/integrate PLCs, referred to as "distributive processing," has become available to integrate multiple subsystems into a fully functioning manufacturing cell (P. Palmer, 2014, personal communication).

TSEs often must adhere to FDA Part 11 of Title 21 of the Code of Federal Regulations, which defines the criteria under which electronic records are deemed trustworthy. Practically speaking, Part 11 requires drug makers to implement controls, audits, and system validation for software and systems involved in processing electronic data. Protocols must be followed with regard to limiting system access to authorized individuals, operational checks, device checks, controls over systems documentation, and a plethora of other guidelines. Strict adherence with regard to copies of records and record retention is part of the guideline.

In the 1990s PLC/HMI controls were avoided by pharmaceutical companies due to perceived validation difficulties. It was often deemed easier to validate a system with 1980s generation controls that more easily conformed to FDA regulations that were composed in the 1950s. Those days have thankfully passed. With a better understanding of the regulations and increased in-house IT acumen, the modern PLC/HMI controls architecture is now common in pharmaceutical environments.

Ironically, a starve-fed TSE is not a "precision device," so state-of-the art controls, although beneficial, will have little effect on mixing performance. That being said, better controls, data acquisition, and communication functionalities only improve performance and insight into the process.

1.5.2 SCREWS: SHAFTS (TORQUE), METALLURGIES, DESIGNS

Rotating screws must be capable of transferring load from the motor to the elements to allow for successful processing. The motor transmits energy to the gearbox and then to shafts, screw elements, and the materials being processed. Screw shafts, upon which the elements are assembled, are typically the torque limiting factor to process materials.

Torque is determined by the cross-sectional area of the shaft, the geometry of the shaft, the metallurgy and hardening of the shaft, and the shaft geometry. Shaft technologies have evolved to allow smaller-diameter shafts to transmit higher torques, facilitating a higher OD/ID ratio and therefore more volume. The following depicts the evolution of shafts used with segmented TSEs:

1. Key-way shaft: industry standard in 1950; used with a 1.25 OD/ID ratio
2. Hexagonal shaft: industry standard in 1960; used with a 1.4 OD/ID ratio
3. Splined shaft: industry standard in 1990; used with a 1.55 OD/ID ratio
4. Asymmetrical splined shafts: invented in 2005; used with a 1.66 OD/ID ratio

A graphic illustration of different shaft designs is presented in Figure 1.21. The current state-of-the-art shaft design is an asymmetrical splined shaft manufactured using 17-4 stainless steel. The geometry of each "tooth" is such that the resulting tangential force vector is isolated, allowing a smaller-diameter shaft to transmit higher torque as compared to previous designs.

One-piece screws (without shafts) are also possible for both corotating and counterrotating TSEs for higher attainable torques. Another plus of one-piece screws in a GMP environment is simplified cleaning, assembly, and validation procedures. A downside, particularly in an R&D setting, is lack of design flexibility inherent with a one-piece design. Just like barrels, metallurgies are matched to the application based on the degree of abrasion and corrosion resistance required.

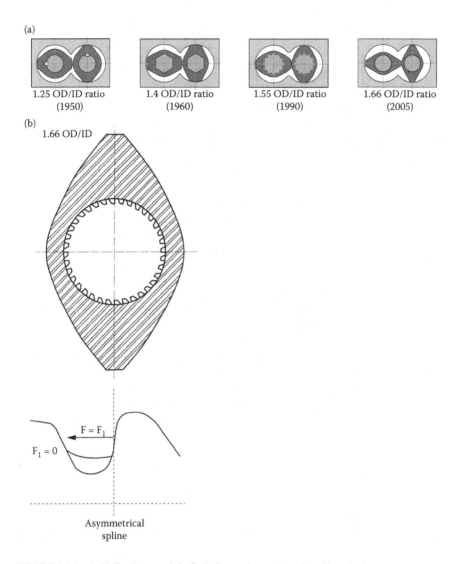

(a)

| 1.25 OD/ID ratio (1950) | 1.4 OD/ID ratio (1960) | 1.55 OD/ID ratio (1990) | 1.66 OD/ID ratio (2005) |

(b) 1.66 OD/ID

$F = F_1$

$F_1 = 0$

Asymmetrical spline

FIGURE 1.21   (a,b) Evolution of shaft design and asymmetric spline shaft.

1.5.3   BARRELS AND HEATING/COOLING

In the 1950s, TSE barrels were generally made from one-piece steel and nitride hardened with a hardened depth ID less than 0.5 mm and external blowers for cooling. During this era, screw rpms were much lower so external cooling blowers were often more than adequate. In the 1970s and 1980s, screw rpm increased and modular barrels, typically 4–5 L/D each, became the accepted industry standard. The following is a brief overview of the evolution of barrel and heating/cooling designs for the modular design:

1. In the 1950s and 1960s, barrels were round with external air cooling via blowers.

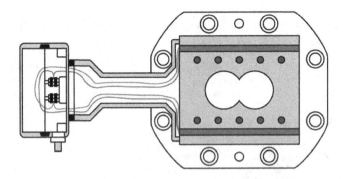

■ Internal cartridge heaters for electric heating
● Longitudinal cooling bores for liquid cooling

FIGURE 1.22   End view of a state-of-the-art TSE barrel.

2. In the 1970s, barrels became segmented in 4 L/D, 5 L/D, and 10 L/D lengths, and barrel liners became available.
3. In the early 1980s, internal cooling bores for liquid cooling became the preferred design with improved heat transfer.
4. In the 1980s, barrels became square with plate heaters, which resulted in better temperature control, and available metallurgies continued to expand, including replaceable barrel inserts/liners.
5. In the 1990s, barrels began to use cartridge heaters that offered higher wattage transference at less cost and improved maintenance.
6. Around 2005, barrels with two (2) cooling inlets/outlets became available that allowed higher flow rates and better heat transfer capabilities.

Modular barrels with internal cartridge heaters and internal cooling bores are deemed state of the art (Figure 1.22). Internal cooling bores are close to the liner for maximum cooling effect. They facilitate higher screw rpms and motor power without overheating. One-piece barrels offer better heat transfer capabilities, whereas barrel liners (Figure 1.23) offer many metallurgical options. Due to the interaction

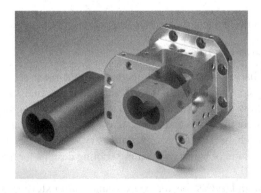

FIGURE 1.23   TSE barrel liner outside and inserted into the barrel housing.

with rotating screws, hardenable stainless steels are required for TSE barrels, as 300 series stainless steels generally have inadequate abrasion resistance. Nickel-based alloys are specified for increased corrosion resistance and powdered metallurgies (PM) for increased abrasion resistance.

1.5.4 GEARBOXES

Historically the gearbox was the weak link in the torque transmission train. A typical 1960s-era extruder ran at much lower screw speeds and could only transmit 25% of the torque compared to what's possible today. Due to the complexity of design and attainable part tolerances, gearbox failures were common. Significant improvements in the fields of metallurgy, heat treating, component design, and tolerances and the use of synthetic gear oil have dramatically improved torques, increased speeds, and decreased failures, making gearboxes essentially "bulletproof." Most failures occur either because of poor maintenance or a catastrophic event, such as a bolt going into the extruder.

1.6 AVAILABLE MODES OF TSEs FOR PHARMACEUTICAL APPLICATIONS

TSEs can be corotating or counterrotating and intermeshing or nonintermeshing. Screw configurations for various TSEs are presented in Figure 1.24. For the purpose of this chapter, these will be defined as low-speed late-fusion (LSLF) TSEs (run up to 50 rpm) and high-speed energy input (HSEI) TSEs (run up to 1200+ rpm). In a low-speed late-fusion process, the materials are not fully melted/fused until the latter part of the TSE process section, as compared to a high-speed energy input process, where materials are melted and significant energy is imparted in the early part of the TSE process section.

The following describes the current market status of each commercially available TSE with comments regarding their current and potential usage for pharmaceutical applications.

1.6.1 COROTATING INTERMESHING TSEs

The most widely used for the plastics and pharmaceutical industries is the HSEI corotating, intermeshing TSE. The screws are termed as "self-wiping," as surface velocities in the intermesh are in opposite directions, which causes the material to be "wiped" from one screw to the other, operate by a first-in/first-out principle, and follow a Figure 1.8 pattern along the length of the screws during processing. In corotation, the rotational clearances limit the lobe count to two for standard flight depths, which are in the 1.5–1.8 OD/ID range.

Corotating intermeshing TSEs may utilize the latest splined shafts and/or one-piece screw designs for the highest torque transmittal possible. State-of-the-art models integrate modular barrels with electric heating via cartridge heaters and internal cooling bores. Gearboxes also reflect the latest technologies available and facilitate screw rpms of 1200+ and short process residence times—even five seconds or less

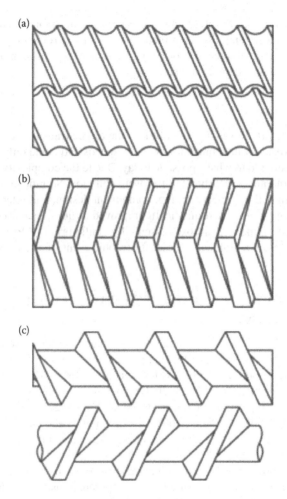

FIGURE 1.24 Commercially available screw configurations for TSEs: (a) intermeshing corotating; (b) intermeshing counterrotating; (c) nonintermeshing counterrotating.

is possible. The residence time distributions generally have much sharper tails than other extruder modes, which is beneficial because all the materials experience an equivalent processing history.

For a variety of technical and marketing reasons, the HSEI corotating TSE dominates the plastics, food, and pharmaceutical industries for mixing/mass transfer intensive processes. Controlled pumping and wiping of the screws in combination with a modular design make this model an extremely versatile engineering tool, which is why this mode was embraced in the 1990s by plastics compounders, effectively ending early forays using single-screw extrusion for this application. Since the corotating intermeshing TSE is a semi-drag-flow device with limited pumping/pressurization capabilities, a gear pump front-end attachment may be required for shape extrusion. It is expected that the corotating intermeshing mode will continue to lead the way for twin-screw technology, which is not to say it's always the best choice.

1.6.2 COUNTERROTATING INTERMESHING TSEs

Counterrotating intermeshing twin screw extruders are available in either the high-speed energy input configuration or in a low-speed late-fusing format. The LSLF intermeshing counterrotating mode of operation dominates the plastics industry for polyvinyl chloride shape extrusion of profiles with tens of thousands of worldwide installations. Interestingly, the HSEI intermeshing counterrotating TSE mode has proven superior for a number of pharmaceutical applications, as evidenced by an interesting 2014 study that compared corotation and counterrotation by Justin Keene and others for compounding of a poorly soluble API. As shown in Figure 1.25, the counterrotating extruder was observed to form amorphous solid dispersions with a narrower residence time distribution.

A side-by-side comparison of the screw design for corotating and counterrotating TSE is presented in Figure 1.26. A counterrotating intermeshing TSE shares many of the features/attributes of its corotating intermeshing TSE cousin, except the screws rotate in opposite directions and it feeds on two screws instead of one for corotation. Screws can be modular or one piece and the OD/ID ratios are typically in the 1.5/1 OD/ID range. Barrels can be modular with internal coring for liquid cooling and also can use a one-piece design with blower air cooling, especially for low-rpm versions. Screw rpm are generally lower as compared to corotation, with a maximum of approximately 600 rpm for the high-speed version and less than 50 rpm for the LSLF counterrotating TSE. In counterrotation, in contrast to corotation, the surface velocities in the intermesh are in the same direction, which results in materials being forced up and through the screws, referred to as the "calendar gap," where a very effective extensional mixing effect occurs. A top and end view of the calendar gap is presented in Figure 1.27. At higher screw speeds, the associated screw deflection effects result in metal-to-metal contact and wear, and this is what limits the attainable screw rpms compared to corotation.

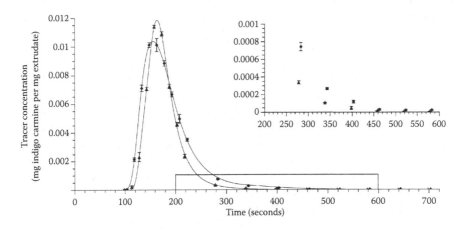

FIGURE 1.25 Mean residence time and variance were all reduced in counterrotation when compared to the corotating TSE.

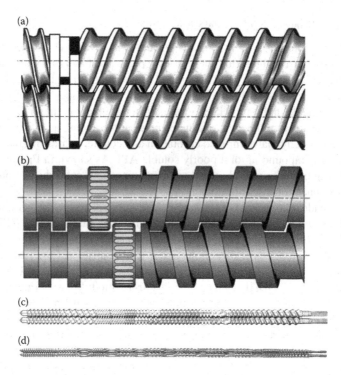

FIGURE 1.26 Co- and counterrotating TSE screw elements: (a) corotating; (b) counterrotating; (c) corotating; (d) counterrotating.

In addition to the calendar gap mixing effect, a wide variety of elements are available to facilitate mixing. Because the elements mesh similar to a gear, up to six lobes are possible at the same flight depth as bilobal corotating TSEs, which translates into more mixing events for each screw rpm. An example of a hexalobal mixing element for counterrotating intermeshing TSE is presented in Figure 1.28. Also by displacing the mixing requirement exclusively from the calendar gap to a more balanced mixing effect, higher screw rpms (600+) are possible.

In this TSE mode, positive displacement discharge elements may be specified to build and stabilize pressure to the die. Screw-to-screw flights are slanted in the same direction with minimal clearances/leakage in the nip region to facilitate a positive conveying. Only the counterrotating, intermeshing TSE provides these closed "C-shaped" chambers (Figure 1.29), which essentially function as a positive displacement pump to the die and can eliminate the need for a gear pump.

In addition to the parallel design, conical LSLF counterrotating intermeshing TSEs (Figure 1.30) are manufactured where a large-diameter feed zone has a continuous taper to the discharge end (or tips) of the screws. The small discharge diameter provides a low volume area with a positive pumping effect against die head pressures, and also minimizes rotational shear and heat generation as the screws pump the material through the die. Conical LSLF counterrotating TSEs are currently not commercially available for pharmaceutical production applications.

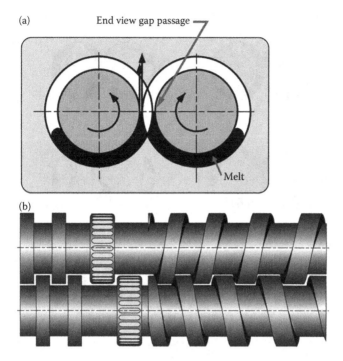

FIGURE 1.27 (a) Top and (b) end view of a calendar gap of a counterrotating intermeshing TSE.

The extensive worldwide usage of counterrotating intermeshing TSEs (probably 50%+ for plastics) suggests that this mode should be considered more frequently for pharmaceutical products. Possible benefits include better mixing at lower screw rpms, processing formulations with a tighter RTD, and improved pumping to the die. To date, most of the research activities have focused exclusively on the corotating TSE; however, the counterrotating TSE might prove to be a viable/preferred alternative.

1.6.3 COUNTERROTATING NONINTERMESHING TSEs

The counterrotating, nonintermeshing TSE utilizes side-by-side screws where the flight of one screw doesn't penetrate the fight depth of the second screw, which allows for unique design capabilities that can be mirrored or dissimilar. A small root diameter (and larger flight depth) may also be specified in the feed area for low bulk density feed stocks. Similar to a single-screw extruder, the root diameter can be tapered up after the feed section to compress and melt the polymer. Screw elements include forward or reverse flights, different helix angles, thick or thin flight thicknesses, multiple screw starts, and other single-screw design features. Screw elements can be matched or staggered at different points along the process length to facilitate pumping and/or mixing. Various screw configurations for counterrotating nonintermeshing TSEs are presented in Figure 1.31.

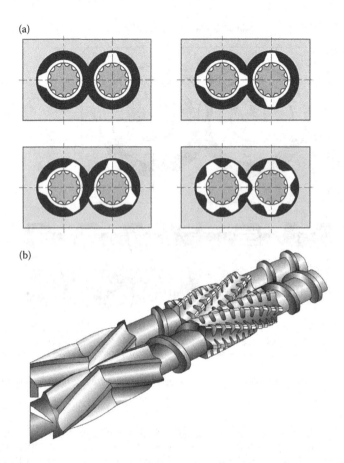

FIGURE 1.28   (a,b) Examples of hexalobal mixing elements for counterrotating intermeshing TSE.

A typical process length for this TSE mode is 30–60:1 L/D with screw rpms up to 500. Due to the absence of an intermesh and the associated geometric limitations, the nonintermeshing mode may be specified at 100+:1 L/D, which allows for long RTs, which may be beneficial for some processes, e.g., high-level devolatilization processes. The lack of an intermesh is problematic for dispersive mixing applications as intermesh and apex zones are gentler than in the intermeshing designs, and the self-wiping effects inherent with intermeshing geometries are also somewhat lacking.

The geometric freedom inherent with nonintermeshing screws has been largely untapped. Into the early 1990s, the nonintermeshing counterrotating TSE was still deemed viable for many plastic products, but due to a lack of development efforts for hardware (e.g., screws segmented via triple start threads), process research, and marketing efforts, this mode has faded from commercial acceptance. That being said, the HSEI counterrotating nonintermeshing TSE is still preferred for some niche applications. Pharmaceutical class GMP models are currently not available, although its attributes might offer benefits for atypical processes.

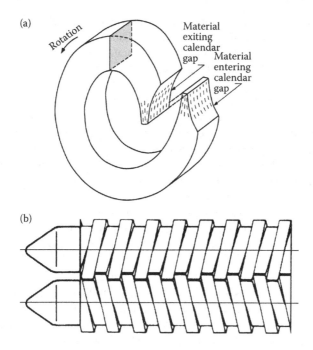

FIGURE 1.29   (a,b) C-locked counterrotating discharge screws and the associated melt flow effect for counterrotating intermeshing TSE.

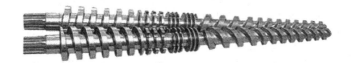

FIGURE 1.30   Processing section of a conical intermeshing counterrotating TSE.

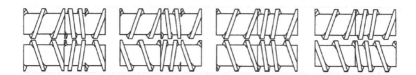

FIGURE 1.31   Different screw configurations for counterrotating nonintermeshing TSE.

1.7   CONCLUSION

Before the TSE was deemed the best continuous mixer by the plastics community, other devices (e.g., single-screw extruders) were utilized. The superior mixing characteristics inherent with a TSE allowed this device to dominate other continuous mixers and spurred intensive development efforts and experimentation that spawned highly engineered formulations for the commodity and high-tech plastic products we use every day. Today, twin-screw extrusion is a battle-hardened, well-proven manufacturing process that has been validated in 24-hour/day industrial settings for more than half a century. What would our lives be like without plastics that were compounded on TSEs?

The evolution of melt extrusion in the pharmaceutical industry resembles what has occurred for plastics. TSE designs for pharmaceutical applications replicate the staging of unit operations and mixing mechanisms used for plastics, and the extensive development of long-standing production principles learned by the plastics industry has allowed quick implementation of proven technologies to pharmaceutical processes, e.g., Rezulin™. The TSE process is a well-known entity.

New extrusion technologies applied to advanced drug delivery systems have risen to the forefront of pharmaceutical products. They allow targeted and alternative delivery systems. In the design of such systems, melt extrusion and the supporting downstream systems can make almost any shape to facilitate unique dissolution profiles.

TSE suppliers have now downsized and redesigned equipment for GMP environments, and additional efforts have been made to design TSE systems to test early-stage materials available only in limited quantities. Coextruded products utilizing multiple extruders and integration with in-line molding represent the next generation of development efforts. These efforts will also be based upon proven technologies that have been used for decades in the plastics industry.

With so many drug candidates having solubility issues, it is clear that melt extrusion will continue to play a significant role in producing amorphous molecular dispersions of these new chemical entities. The plastics industry embraced continuous processing to make better, more consistent products at lower cost. Now pharmaceutical companies are doing the same and reaping the benefit of 100+ years of those efforts. As pharmaceutical scientists become more familiar with this technology and the equipment, we will continue to see an expanding number of extrusion-related publications, patents, and new products.

Led by the TSE, the "extrusion evolution" will continue. The best indication of the future is the past. The future is bright and the path is well proven. It's déjà vu all over again.

BIBLIOGRAPHY

1. White JL, Bumm SH. Perspectives on the transition from batch to continuous mixing technologies in the compounding industry. In: *Polymer Processing XXV*. Munich, Carl Hanser Verlag; 2010. pp. 322–326.
2. 2014 Year-end Machinery Reports. Society of Plastics Industry (SPI). Compiled by Veris Consulting. [cited 2015 Jan].
3. Martin C. Processing thermoplastics urethanes via twin screw extrusion. In: Szycher M, editor. *Szycher's Handbook of Polyurethanes, Second Edition*. Boca Raton, FL: CRC Press; 2013. pp. 865–888.
4. Thiele W. Twin screw extrusion and screw design. In: Ghebre-Sellassie I, Martin C, editors. *Pharmaceutical Extrusion Technology*. Boca Raton, FL: CRC Press; 2003. pp. 69–98.

5. DiNunzio J, Martin C, McGinity J, Zhang F. Melt extrusion. In: Miller DA, Watts AB, Williams III RO, editors. *Formulating Poorly Water Soluble Drugs*. New York: Springer; 2012. pp. 311–362.
6. Jerman R. Devolatilization of polymers via twin screw extrusion. *Proceedings of the Leistritz Twin Screw Extrusion Workshop*; 2006 Nov 29–30; Bridgewater, NJ.
7. Szycher M. Intelligent antimicrobial products via twin screw extrusion. *Proceedings of the Leistritz Pharmaceutical Extrusion Seminar*; 2015 Jun 17–18; Clinton, NJ.
8. Todd D, Zhu L. Polymer devolatilization. *Proceedings of the Leistritz Twin Screw Extrusion Workshop*; 2013 Jun 12–13; Clinton, NJ.
9. FDA Process Analytical Technology Initiative, (2004).
10. Ghebre-Sellassie I, Martin C. Future trends. In: Ghebre-Sellassie I, Martin C, editors. *Pharmaceutical Extrusion Technology*. Boca Raton, FL: CRC Press; 2003. pp. 383–392.
11. Thummer M. Dispersive mixing in co-rotating twin screws—principles & examples. *Proceedings of the Leistritz Twin Screw Extrusion Workshop*; 2011 Nov 30–Dec 1; Clinton, NJ.
12. Martin C. Devolatilization via twin screw extrusion: theory, tips and test results. *Proceedings of 30th International Conference of the Polymer Processing Society*; 2014 Jun 8–12; Cleveland, OH.
13. Keen JM, Martin C, Machado A, Sandhu H, McGinity JW, DiNunzio JC. Investigation of process temperature and screw speed on properties of a pharmaceutical solid dispersion using corotating and counter-rotating twin-screw extruders. *The Journal of pharmacy and pharmacology*. 66(2); 204–217: 2014.
14. Thiele W. Counterrotating intermeshing twin-screw extruders. In: Todd DB, editor. *Plastics Compounding Equipment and Processing*. Cincinnati, OH: Hanser/Gardner Publications; 1998. pp. 47–70.
15. Martin C. Twin screw extruders. In: Vlachopoulos J, Wagner JR, editors. *SPE Guide on Extrusion Technology and Troubleshooting*. Brookfield, CT: The Society of Plastics Engineers; 2001. pp. [2–1]–[2–26].
16. White JL. Flow mechanisms and modeling of non-intermeshing counter-rotating twin screw extruders. In: *Twin Screw Extrusion, Technology and Principles*. New York, NY: Oxford University Press; 1991. pp. 110–130.
17. FDA Process Analytical Technology Initiative, (2004).
18. DiNunzio C, Martin C, Zhang F. Melt extrusion—Shaping Drug Delivery in the 21st Century. In: *Drug Delivery Magazine*. Iselin, NJ: Pharmaceutical Technology; 2010. pp. 30–37.
19. Gray M. British Patent 5056; 1879.
20. Breitenbach J. Melt extrusion can bring new benefits to HIV therapy. *Am J Drug Deliv* 4(2); 61–64: 2006. https://doi.org/10.2165/00137696-200604020-00001.

2 Extruder Design

Richard Steiner and Brian Haight

CONTENTS

2.1 INTRODUCTION

Pharmaceutical-class extruders are evolving as continuous processing devices to mix drugs with carriers for solid dosage forms and transdermal films, as well as to produce wet granulations. In melt extrusion, which has been used for many years in the plastics industry, the carrier is melted and mixed with an active ingredient, devolatilized, and pumped through a die. In contrast, wet granulation refers to the process of fine powdered materials being mixed with liquids to impart morphological and other specific characteristics to facilitate the production and the performance of tablets and other solid dosage forms. The focus of the discussion will be primarily aimed at melt extrusion, the more common application and, to a lesser extent, at the wet granulation process.

2.2   GENERAL CHARACTERISTICS OF VARIOUS EXTRUDERS

Inside any extruder, a number of basic process functions are performed, which include feeding, melting, mixing, venting, and developing die and localized pressure. The motor facilitates the extrusion process via the rotation of the screw(s) that impart shear and energy into the extrudate. Variable-speed alternating current (a.c.) drives are typically used. The gearing reduces the motor speed to the desired screw rotations per minute (rpm) while multiplying torque. In the case of a twin-screw extruder, the distribution gear maintains the angular timing of the two screws and absorbs the thrust load from the screw set.

Extruders process materials that are bounded by screw flights and barrel walls (1). Process control parameters include screw speed (rpm), feed rate, temperatures along the barrel and the die, and the vacuum level for devolatilization. Typical read-outs include melt pressure, melt temperature, motor amperage, viscosity, and specific energy consumption (see Figure 2.1).

A common term used in extrusion is length-to-diameter ratio, or L/D. This is the length of the screw divided by the diameter. For instance, an extruder that is 1000 mm long with a 25-mm screw diameter has a 40:1 L/D. Typical extrusion process lengths are in the 24:1–40:1 L/D range. Single-screw extruders are generally 36:1 L/D or shorter. Intermeshing twin-screw extruders may be configured for up to a 60:1 L/D. The nonintermeshing twin-screw extruder can be specified at 100:1 L/D or longer, due to the absence of intermesh clearance constraints. Extruder residence times are generally between 10 sec and 10 min.

Other common terms include the outer diameter of the screw, or OD. For instance, when referring to a 20-mm extruder, this refers to the outer diameter of the screw for a single-screw device or the diameter of each screw for a twin-screw machine. The inner diameter, or ID, is the OD minus the depth of the flight. The comparative OD/ID ratios determine the available free volume in any extruder. There are also various "gaps" in the extruder, either between the screw OD and the barrel wall (overflight gap) or, in the case of twin-screw extruders, between the screws (intermesh gap).

An important design factor in any extruder is the channel or flight depth. A deeper channel depth increases the free volume in the machine. It must be recognized that a deeper flight depth in the feed zone area decreases the screw shaft cross section and limits the possible torque transmittal. In the design of any extruder, it is important to find the optimum balance between free volume and torque, as this directly impacts

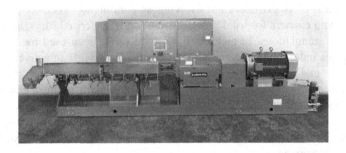

FIGURE 2.1   A typical extruder system.

attainable throughput rates, as well as the mass transfer energy that is imparted into the materials.

Barrels for extruders (single or twin) can be either one-piece or modular. The cross section of the barrel for a single-screw extruder reveals a circular hole for the screw, whereas the twin-screw extruder is characterized by a barrel opening in the shape of a "figure 8." The inner surface of the barrel is tempered and honed. The barrel housing is made of high-strength steel, whereas the liner is manufactured from a wear-resistant and corrosion-resistant material as warranted by the intended service.

The screw is generally deemed to be the most important part of any extruder. The screw design distinguishes the processes that the extruder can fulfill and, therefore, determines the quality of the extruded material. Similar to barrels, screws can be either one-piece or segmented. If segmented, the screws are assembled on shafts, usually either keyed or splined. Segmented screws allow for extreme process versatility, but may present cleaning issues in a good manufacturing practice (GMP) environment. One-piece screws can be selected to minimize cleaning issues associated with the disassembly of segmented screw elements from the shafts.

A fundamental condition for material viscosity and the chemical reactions that occur inside the process section are temperatures and mass transfer rates. The extruder barrel is typically heated, which can be accomplished by various methods. Conventional barrel heating is electrical, either by external heater bands or angular plates, or by internal electrical cartridge heaters. Barrels can also be heated by a liquid, such as treated water or oil, as dictated by the process and manufacturing environment.

The extruder barrel(s) are cooled via air or liquid, either externally or internally. The most effective heat transfer design uses axial cooling bores inside the barrel and close to the process melt stream. For certain applications, the number of cooling bores in the barrel may be increased to ensure better energy absorption. It is worth noting that twin-screw extruders dissipate up to two-thirds of the drive capacity into the product; therefore, it is essential to absorb this additional energy in a controlled way. Barrel cooling helps prevent material degradation and maintains the desired melt viscosity within the process section (see Figure 2.2).

Wear is caused by three mechanisms: corrosion, abrasion, and adhesion, often referred to as part of the "tribological system." The following is a brief description of each:

- Corrosion is mainly based on reaction processes between the barrel/screw surfaces and the processed material, but can also result from high humidity and/or acidic atmospheres.
- Abrasive wear occurs when screw metal rubs on barrel metal and/or when the processed material between the screw and the barrel gap is abrasive. The process melt allows the screw(s) to "float" in the barrel to help prevent this type of wear from occurring. The more lubricating that material is, the more freely the screws may rotate and the lower the abrasive wear. Abrasive wear usually appears smooth.
- Adhesive wear may occur when there is a loss of material presence between the screw and the barrel. Instead of abrading each other, interface pressures

form tiny metallic fusion bridges, which then are almost immediately broken during the screw's rotation. For instance, this will occur if the identical stainless steels are specified with the same hardness. The result is a rough-looking circumferential surface. If these same materials are treated so that the hardness of the screw is slightly lower than that of the barrel, adhesive wear is prevented. Selecting different metals for screws and barrels is another common solution.

Specific energy is an important factor in troubleshooting any extrusion process because it indicates the amount of energy that is required to perform a process. Heater energy is usually not factored into this calculation. Specific energy is also an excellent troubleshooting indicator to determine if something in the process has changed. The formula for specific energy (SE) is as follows (2):

$$SE = \frac{K_{wm} \times EG\% \times TS\% \times (RPM_{run}/RPM_{max})}{Q_h}$$

SE is the specific energy (kW hr/kg).
K_{wm} is the kW rating of the motor being used (kW = HP/1.3405).
EG% is the efficiency of the gear system (0.954 is a reasonable estimate).
TS% is the torque used versus the maximum torque.
TS% = amperes running/amperes maximum rating.
RPM_{run} is the running screw speed (rotations per minute).
RPM_{max} is the highest screw speed.
Q_h is the output rate (kg/hr).

The specific energy of the extruder can readily indicate whether something has changed with the machinery or the formulation. Higher or lower specific energy might identify a material problem or an electrical, mechanical, or processing parameter that has malfunctioned or has been modified.

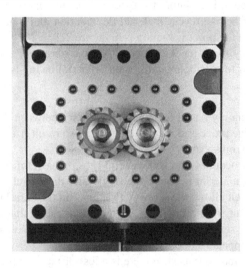

FIGURE 2.2   An end-view twin-screw barrel with internal cooling bores.

2.3 VARIOUS EXTRUSION DEVICES AVAILABLE FOR PHARMACEUTICAL PROCESSING

There are various types of extruders that can be utilized to process pharmaceutical products. Each type has attributes and has been successful in demanding production applications for many years in markets such as medical devices, electronics, packaging, and construction, among others. Because other chapters are dedicated to the specific types, only a brief description is provided.

2.3.1 SINGLE-SCREW EXTRUDER

The single-screw extruder (SSE) is the simplest and most widely utilized type of extruder in the world (3). The SSE is most typically used as a high-pressure pump and to extrude shapes or parts, such as a catheter tube or thin film. A screw rotates inside the barrel, with wide-ranging processes possible with various screw designs to allow for feeding, melting, devolatilizing (sometimes), and pumping (see Figure 2.3). Mixing is often a secondary process goal, as compared to building and stabilizing pressure (pumping) to the die. Mixing, distributive and dispersive, is accomplished for less demanding applications via various mixing designs. The process section (barrel and screw) usually has three or more heating zones to raise the barrel and screw to the required process temperature with barrel cooling via air blowers or liquid. Screw rpms are often below 100 and discharge pressures are possible for 5000+ psi.

Typically, single-screw extruders for pharmaceutical applications are between 20/1 and 50/1 L/D (length divided by diameter) and are between 6 to 30 mm in diameter. The output of the extruder is a function of screw diameter more than any other variable. The extrusion of pharmaceutical materials, however, is more challenging than the extrusion of typical plastics because the material sometimes lacks the ability to flow.

Single-screw extruders are generally "flood-fed" with a hopper over the screw (see Figure 2.4) that dispenses material into the screw by gravity and is conveyed forward. Comparatively, twin-screw extruders are "starve-fed," where the feeder(s) set the rate and the screw rpm is used to optimize compounding efficiencies.

The feed section of the barrel is a distinct section that is typically water cooled to prevent heat from prematurely melting material and stopping transportation. After the feedstock has been transported through the solids-conveying zone and is preheated, there is enough energy available for melting. The decreasing channel volume compresses the material as it moves through the decreasing space of the melting zone. This forces the material against the barrel where melting occurs. Melting takes place as the metal barrel conducts energy into the polymer, forming a melted layer. The advancing flight then scrapes the polymer into a rotating pool on the leading edge of the flight.

Once the material is melted, it can be pumped via drag flow through a filled/pressurized mixing element on the screw for homogenization of the melt. There are

Material flow

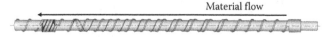

FIGURE 2.3 SSE processing section. (From Baird J. Screw theory & SSE for medical applications. *Leistritz Pharmaceutical Extrusion Seminar.* Holiday Inn, Clinton, NJ. 7 June 2017 (4).)

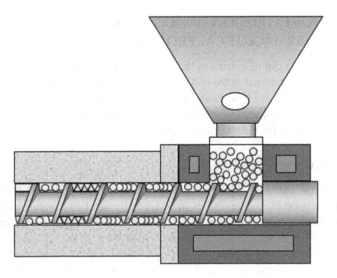

FIGURE 2.4   Flood-fed feed zone of a SSE. (From Baird J. Screw theory & SSE for medical applications. *Leistritz Pharmaceutical Extrusion Seminar.* Holiday Inn, Clinton, NJ. 7 June 2017.)

unlimited mixing designs for SSEs. Two common distributive-type mixers are mixing pins, which are placed at the end of the screw as a series of pins that act as obstructions to the spiral flow of the metering section, where the flow is split and recombined, and slotted flight mixers, one or more flights that are made discontinuously. Fluted mixers are comparatively more dispersive than distributive. Material is forced down an inlet channel that dead-ends at a radial barrier, where elevated shear forces occur (see Figure 2.5), and is then forced through an outlet channel.

After melting and mixing, material can be pumped into a decompression zone and processed through a second screw section to allow the extraction of volatiles such as water, entrapped air, and residual monomers from the extruder. The screw sections are designed so that the output of the first stage is less than the second, ensuring zero pressure and allowing the extraction of gases. Finally, after the material has been melted, mixed, and vented, it fills the metering channel, which builds enough pressure to overcome the die resistance. Longer metering sections produce proportionally higher pressures and make the SSE ideal for producing dimensionally stable shapes and parts.

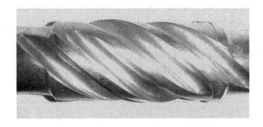

FIGURE 2.5   Helical mixing head. (From Baird J. Screw theory & SSE for medical applications. *Leistritz Pharmaceutical Extrusion Seminar.* Holiday Inn, Clinton, NJ. 7 June 2017.)

2.3.2 Co-kneader

The co-kneader is a single-screw continuous compounding system that differs significantly as compared to a conventional single-screw extruder, due mainly to the axially oscillating movement of the screw. The screw is designed as a discontinuous flight with up to three equidistant interruptions or gaps per revolution. For example, in conveying sections, there is only a single interruption, while in mixing sections there are three gaps per revolution. Correspondingly, there are rows of fixed pins mounted along the barrel wall at equivalent spacing as on the screw flights. To avoid interference between screws and pins, there is a complete forward and reverse stroke per revolution. The pins intermesh with the flights at the mixing elements so that the front and the back of each screw flight are wiped by the stationary pin. The kneading pins work like a static screw and are the counterpart to the rotating screw. Co-kneaders utilize a split-barrels design and segmented screws. These devices are typically starve-fed and use a discharge device, either screw pump or gear pump, to pressurize the die (see Figures 2.6 through 2.8).

2.3.3 High-Speed Twin-Screw Extruders

High-speed twin-screw extruders are mass transfer devices that are primarily used for compounding, devolatilization, and reactive extrusion. Corotating and counter-rotating types are available. High-speed machines are defined as those that have a top end of 300–1200 screw rpm capability and are starve-fed with the output rate determined by the feeder(s). The screw rpm is independent from feed rate and is used to optimize compounding efficiencies. These devices typically utilize modular screws/barrels, which offer extreme process flexibility.

High-speed twin-screw extruders are primarily specified in the corotating mode. One of the characteristics of corotating extruders is their ability to mix the material longitudinally as well as transversely. Consequently, the material is

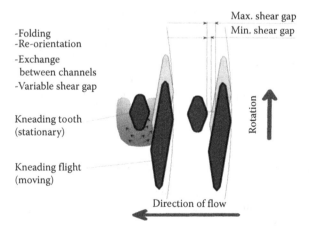

FIGURE 2.6 A co-kneader mixing mechanism. (From Anderson P. Improved design and performance characteristics of the reciprocating single screw extruder. *Performance Compounding Conference*, San Antonio, TX, April 10–12, 2002.)

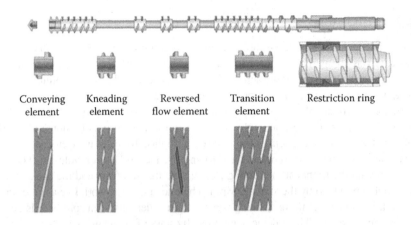

FIGURE 2.7   A co-kneader segmented screw system.

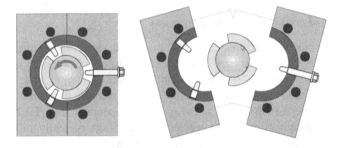

FIGURE 2.8   A co-kneader split-barrel design. (From Anderson P. Improved design and performance characteristics of the reciprocating single screw extruder. *Performance Compounding Conference*, San Antonio, TX, April 10–12, 2002.)

transported from one chamber of the screw to the other, which results in excellent mixing. Figure 2.9 shows various numbers of flights in the screw elements [(a) two flighted, (b) three flighted]. The self-wiping of the two screws during rotation helps assure that intermeshing twin-screw extruders are self-cleaning. The intermesh of the screws also supports the zoning of unit operations. Mixing primarily occurs in the kneading elements. Specialty high-speed counterrotating twin-screw extruders are available with up to six lobes for mixing, while tangential (nonintermeshing) designs are utilized for specialty applications (see Figure 2.10).

2.3.4   Low-Speed, Late-Fusion Twin-Screw Extruders

The low-speed, late-fusion counterrotating intermeshing mode is characterized by a gentle melting and mixing effect that ensures a narrow residence time in conjunction with a high-pressure buildup, as compared to the high-speed twin-screw extruder that is specified for energy-intensive applications. The screw flights converge in the same direction in the nip region, causing the open spaces between the flights to be small, minimizing leakage from one screw channel to the next. This device can be

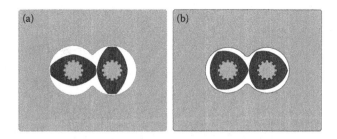

FIGURE 2.9 (a) Two- and (b) three-lobe twin-screw flight designs. (From Schuler W. Auslegung und Ausführung der Verfahrenszonen von gleichsinnig drehenden Zweischneckenextrudern. In: *Der Doppelschnecken Extruder.* VDI-K Verlag, 1995.)

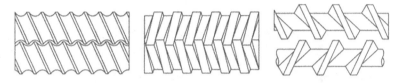

FIGURE 2.10 High-speed intermeshing and nonintermeshing twin-screw modes of operation—corotating/counterrotating.

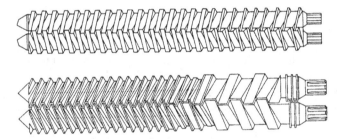

FIGURE 2.11 Late-fusion counterrotating screw sets.

used for applications where shear-sensitive or temperature-sensitive materials are being processed, where high head pressures are desired, and/or where the materials do not convey well by drag flow. Corotating designs can be made to operate similarly through the use of nontraditional screw geometries (see Figure 2.11).

2.4   WHAT IS THE DIFFERENCE BETWEEN A STANDARD AND A GMP EXTRUDER DESIGN?

The general process requirements and throughputs for the pharmaceutical industry are oftentimes less stringent than the demands of plastics processing.

A "pharmaceutical class" extruder is characterized not just by barrels/screws metallurgies, but also by special fittings and increased documentation, which are part of the "GMP philosophy." High degrees of sanitation, process reproducibility, and stringent documentation are typically important goals. Modifications, as compared to a plastics extruder, often include the following:

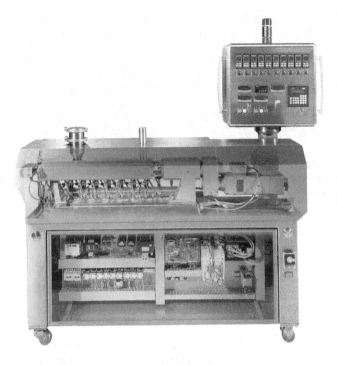

FIGURE 2.12   A GMP twin-screw extruder design superimposed over a standard machine.

- A polished, detailed design for all components with respect to cleaning
- Machine frame and barrel cover in stainless steel
- Ground and polished welding seams
- Complete calibration and documentation of all process parameters
- Quick-release couplings for cooling and heating system
- The use of gear oils and lubricants approved by the Food and Drug Administration (FDA)
- Mercury-free pressure sensors
- Materials in contact with products of stainless steel or nickel-based alloys
- FDA-approved paints for parts that cannot be manufactured in stainless steel, such as the extruder gearbox
- Validated programmable logic control (PLC) and computer-based controls

Metallurgies for screws, barrels, and other parts that contact the materials being processed are typically a hardened stainless steel or nickel-based steel, which are specified for FDA service so as not to be reactive, additive, or absorptive. The machine system should be configured for GMP cleanability and validation (see Figure 2.12).

2.5   CLEANING THE GMP EXTRUDER

There are two overall strategies for cleaning: the so-called clean-in-place (CIP) method and a complete disassembly of the process section.

2.5.1 CLEAN-IN-PLACE

Clean-in-place in the case of the extruder is not truly clean-in-place, because in all cases, the screw set must be removed from the extruder, but does not require a complete machine disassembly. Clean-in-place usually begins by purging the extruder with the screws turning at a low speed, typically 50 rpm or so. If the processed material softens or melts at an elevated temperature, the temperature setting in the process section should be above this temperature by several degrees.

The choice of purging material is dependent on the normally processed material, but many times a natural "solvent" can be found that will have a cleaning effect, and it may be a liquid, such as a simple solution of water and detergent. The extruder is purged for several minutes with the discharge flange completely open, and the exiting material is collected in a container.

After purging, the extruder is stopped and the screw(s) are removed from the barrel. Normally the screw set is placed on a workbench for further manual cleaning. A set of two plastic "U" blocks made to fit the screws is helpful to keep the screw(s) from rolling off the workbench and allows access underneath the screw(s). Depending on the residual material left on the surface of the screw(s), further cleaning may involve brushing with stainless-steel wire brushes, wiping them with clean rags, and washing with more water/detergent. When the material residue is cleaned from the surfaces, the final step is to wipe down the screws with alcohol.

The first step in cleaning the barrels is to unbolt and to remove all the inserts for manual cleaning. A round wire brush attached to a long piece of stainless-steel pipe is run up and down the barrel bore. If stubborn material deposits there, the brush pipe may be attached to an electrical drill and run up and down the bores while rotating. After this step, the bores are cleaned further using cloth swabs. After the bores are free of all residues, the last step is to swab up and down the bores with a clean cloth soaked in alcohol.

If the machine is to be run again within a day or so, it can be left in this state for the next run. If it is to be stored for more than a few days, the screw and the barrel surfaces should be sprayed with an FDA-compliant anticorrosion coating. This is necessary because the intensive cleaning leaves the stainless-steel surface vulnerable to corrosion, even in a humidity-controlled room.

Clean-in-place is designed to be able to prove that the machine is clean, but it is not as rigorous as a complete disassembly because there is the possibility of very small particles residing in the junctures. For this reason, most pharmaceutical companies have a policy of using CIP for perhaps three cleanings in between production runs, and at the fourth cleaning, a full disassembly of the process section is done.

2.5.2 COMPLETE DISASSEMBLY/CLEANING OF THE EXTRUDER PROCESS SECTION

Before a full disassembly, the purging procedure as described above is still recommended to remove most of the material and to make the screw(s) easier to remove and clean. Prior to the teardown, the main electrical disconnect switch for the extruder should be turned off and locked out. A full disassembly involves unbolting all the barrel sections. For segmented screws, the elements are removed from the screw

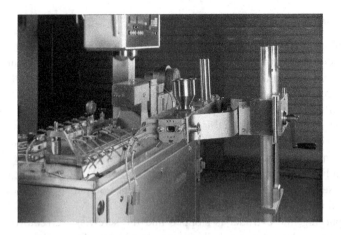

FIGURE 2.13   A barrel removal device.

shafts. With a small laboratory-sized extruder, it may be easier to remove the entire barrel section from the machine as a unit, and disassemble the barrels on a bench. With a larger extruder, the barrel sections must be removed one at a time, starting at the discharge end. Once all the parts are on a workbench, all the surfaces are much easier to access.

Depending on the difficulty of cleaning the particular process material, the barrel(s) may be simply manually cleaned on the workbench with the heaters still attached. The heaters have to be removed if it is necessary to submerse the barrels in a bath of water/detergent or some other liquid. Ultrasonic baths for barrels and screw elements have also been used to facilitate cleaning. As with the CIP method, the last step is to wipe all the surfaces with alcohol and to apply a corrosion-inhibitor spray (see Figure 2.13).

2.6   SCALE-UP FOR PHARMACEUTICAL EXTRUSION SYSTEMS

Many applications involve scale-up from a few grams in the laboratory mixed in small batches to a continuous extrusion process. The basic challenge is to properly choose those batch unit laboratory-scale operations that are best suited for use with the continuous extruder and its accessories.

It is extremely useful to have a laboratory extruder to benchmark very small batch subprocesses. From this starting point, dedicated processes can be configured for production at rates of 5, 10, 20, and 200+ kg/hr. It is difficult to generalize this translation due to the widely differing variables involved between products. However, a few rough guidelines follow (5):

- Simple reactions are a product of time, temperature, and mass transfer to produce the same result. This is experimentally, scientifically, and intuitively determined.
- Distributive mixing requires the same number of same divisions per kilogram. This can be empirically calculated.

- Dispersive mixing requires that the same product of stress rate and time per kilogram above the threshold level be created. This is calculated with some assumptions and empirical help.
- Coarse devolatilization requires the same heat of vaporization with an adequate surface area. This is calculated.
- Fine devolatilization requires the establishment of proportional surface renewal. This is a combination of calculation and empirical data.

Factors that affect scale-up include volume, heat transfer, and mass transfer. Different processes are factored differently based upon which issue dominates. GMP extruder applications are generally more oriented to process precision rather than raw maximum output. However, execution and scale-up from batch processes and benchtop extruders remain governed by the same basic scale-up technology for other technical applications.

2.7   PHARMACEUTICAL PROCESS EXAMPLES

Extrusion technology is an increasingly accepted method for the continuous process-ing of pharmaceutical materials and often offers significant advantages as compared to batch processes. Upstream materials handling and downstream systems work in conjunction with the chosen extruder to perform the intended manufacturing opera-tion. The following are a few examples of systems that have been successfully uti-lized in this capacity.

2.7.1   WETTING OF A POWDER MATRIX WITH A FLUID

In this application, a powder is mixed with a liquid in a multifunctional feed port of a corotating extruder. The purpose of the fluid may be to lubricate, to become absorbed, or to facilitate a reaction. The feed port may be cooled to control the vaporization loss of the liquid. The powder, or another material, may also be added shortly downstream. After mixing is complete to the target morphological, rheo-logical, or chemical condition, the material is discharged to downstream drying, compacting, or other equipment. Many of these materials cannot flow through dies. Discharge may be from protruding screws. Special features include the following:

- Early liquid injection and powder wetting
- Small pitch screws in the feeding section so that fluid does not move back-ward toward the gearbox
- Mostly conveying elements combined with some distributive mixing elements
- Screws protrude from the barrels to facilitate discharge to a downstream dryer

2.7.2   COMPOUNDING OF A THERMOPLASTIC URETHANE PREMIX

A thermoplastic urethane (TPU) premix is dried in a dessicant hopper/dryer and fed into a twin-screw extruder to extrude a product with antibacterial effects. Because atmospheric humidity causes the TPU to transform into a carcinogenic substance, an inert gas is introduced at the feed throat. Low-energy input pumping elements are specified for the second half of the process length to facilitate the removal of heat from the melt via barrel cooling for the heat-sensitive TPU. The mixing must be extremely homogeneous to optimize the antibacterial effect. Special features include the following:

- Inert gas atmosphere (N_2) for the feeder hopper and feed throat
- Extensive low-energy distributive mixing
- Intensive barrel cooling via internal bores to maintain a desirable melt temperature

2.7.3   DEVOLATILIZATION OF A CELLULOSE MATRIX

High levels of water vapor can be removed from a cellulose solution by means of a corotating extruder (6). Effective devolatilization is based upon the surface area of the melt pool, the surface renewal of the melt, and the residence time under the vent(s). Multiple-stage degassing units along the extrusion process length are used. It is possible to remove 50%+ of volatiles via the extrusion process. Special features include the following:

- A screw design that incorporates multiple melt seals for vacuum and zero pressure under the vents
- Multiple vacuum pumps to facilitate volatile removal
- A gravimetric twin-screw feeder to meter moist cellulosic feedstock

2.7.4   INCORPORATION OF A PHARMACEUTICAL PREPARATION INTO A CELLULOSE MATRIX

The materials are mixed and devolatilized in a twin-screw extruder and mated to an air quench micropelletizing system (7). The in-line die minimizes stagnation in the machine front end and a self-adjusting cutter reduces the need for operator adjustment. Cold air nozzles can facilitate the cutting of materials that tend to smear at the die face. The microgranulate can be used to directly fill capsules without further size reduction. Special features include the following:

- A twin-screw extruder with extra process length to cool the melt prior to the die
- An air pelletizer with a cold air gun and a die assembly for micropelletization

2.7.5   INCORPORATION OF AN ACTIVE SUBSTANCE AND FLUID INTO A CARRIER MATERIAL

The materials are added in the following order: carrier material, fluid, and active substances. The active substance is fed into the extruder at a very late stage of the process to minimize the residence time in the machine to prevent thermal damage. Special features include the following:

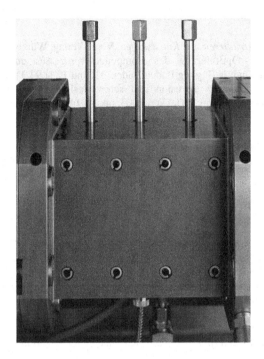

FIGURE 2.14   A liquid injection barrel.

- Multistage liquid injection with mass flow meters (see Figure 2.14)
- Air quench strand pelletizing system with a conveyor

2.7.6   CONVEYING AND COMPACTION OF A TABLET PREMIX

In contrast to melt extrusion, the screw geometry has minimal shear-inducing elements. It is designed with conveying elements with different pitches, which facilitates the conveying and the compaction of the powdered premix. Special features include the following:

- A screw design that primarily conveys elements (except at discharge)
- A special screw discharge to reduce stagnation before a die or a sanitary open release

2.8   CONCLUSION

Single- and twin-screw extruders are replacing traditional batch processes because of the consistent and repeatable nature of continuous extrusion. Without addressing the specific application, it is impossible to state which type of extruder is best for the job. Fortunately, as evidenced by this text, there are many design options from which to choose. It is important to also recognize that the extruder is just another tool, albeit a powerful and versatile one, in the design of a continuous processing system for various drug delivery products.

REFERENCES

1. Ebeling F-W. *Extrudieren von Kunststoffen.* Vogel-Verlag, Würzburg, 1974.
2. VDI K, Hrsg. Optimierung des Compoundierprozesses durch Rezeptur- und Verfahrensverständnis. Tagung Baden-Baden, 11. und 12.11.97, Düsseldorf, 1997.
3. Luker K. Single-Screw extrusion and screw design. *Pharmaceutical Extrusion Technology,* vol. 133, Marcel Dekker, 2003, pp. 39–68. Drugs and the Pharmaceutical Sciences.
4. Baird J. Screw theory & SSE for medical applications. *Leistritz Pharmaceutical Extrusion Seminar.* Holiday Inn, Clinton, NJ. 7 June 2017.
5. Anderson P. Improved design and performance characteristics of the reciprocating single screw extruder. *Performance Compounding Conference,* San Antonio, TX, April 10–12, 2002.
6. Schuler W. Auslegung und Ausführung der Verfahrenszonen von gleichsinnig drehenden Zweischneckenextrudern. In: *Der Doppelschnecken Extruder.* VDI-K Verlag, 1995.
7. Reimker M. Wärmezu- und Wärmeabfuhr. In: *VDI, Hrsg. Grundlegende Aufbereitungsschritte von thermoplastischen Kunststoffen. Bericht vom Symposium am 21. und 22.4.98, München.*
8. Thiele WC. *Trends and Guidelines in Devolatilization and Reactive Extrusion.* Chicago, IL: National Plastics Exposition, Society of the Plastics Industry, June 18, 1997.
9. Martin C. Continuous Mixing/Devolatilizing Via Twin Screw Extruders for Drug Delivery Systems. *Interphex Conference,* Philadelphia, PA, March 20, 2001.

3 Control Strategy Considerations for Continuous Manufacturing Using Hot Melt Extrusion*

*Celia N. Cruz, Rapti Madurawe,
Naresh Pavurala, and Sharmista Chatterjee*

CONTENTS

3.1 INTRODUCTION

Hot melt extrusion (HME) is a continuous process operation that has been successfully applied to the manufacture of quality drug products over the last decade [1–4].

---

* This chapter reflects the views of the author and should not be construed to represent the FDA's views or policies.

HME achieves the molecular mixing of active pharmaceutical ingredients (API) and excipients at temperatures above their glass transition temperatures (T_g) and/or melting temperatures (T_m) [5,6]. The excipients in HME can be broadly classified as matrix carriers, release-modifying agents, fillers, thermal lubricants, stabilizing agents, plasticizers, antioxidants, and miscellaneous additives. Most commonly, the objective of the HME process is to enhance the dissolution profile of poorly water-soluble drugs by converting the formulation components into a single-phase amorphous product with uniform content, size, and shape. Several other applications of HME include taste masking [5,6]; microencapsulation [7]; films [8,9]; abuse deterrence [10,11]; implants for drug delivery via oral [12], transdermal, and transmucosal routes [9]; and nanoparticulate systems [2]. Additionally, HME is a solvent-free process with high throughput, which is an advantage over other processes used to achieve the same products and dosage properties. Several research articles and patents have been reported based on HME technology in pharmaceutical applications [2,13–18]. Some of the commercially available products based on HME (Table 3.1) show how the technology can enable versatility in product design and quality attributes.

There is increasing interest in the pharmaceutical industry and encouragement from the FDA to implement continuous manufacturing processes for pharmaceutical manufacture [22,23]. Continuous manufacturing has the potential to offer several advantages such as flexible operation, lower capital and operational costs, rapid process development, and elimination of scale-up problems [24]. Continuous manufacturing can be defined as the process where the material(s) and product are continuously charged into and discharged from the system, respectively, throughout the duration of the process. Further, in continuous manufacturing, materials produced during each process step are sent directly and continuously to the next step for further processing. In an end-to-end continuous pharmaceutical manufacturing process, different process steps are sequenced together to form a continuous production line where product removal occurs concurrently at the same rate as input of raw materials. While the HME process is a continuous operation, in current pharmaceutical manufacture the hot melt extrudate is typically collected after a predetermined time interval and further processed in a series of downstream batch processes such as milling and blending to form the finished dosage form. However, HME process trains are capable of integrating material feeding, processing, monitoring, and rejection/removal continuously, and can be incorporated with typical pharmaceutical process steps downstream (e.g., milling, blending, dosing), which also have options for continuous manufacturing. In addition, the material transformations and typical rate of manufacture in HME allow for in-process monitoring and characterization of material during operation, which can be linked to process performance and product quality. Therefore, the application of end-to-end continuous manufacturing principles to HME is technically feasible and can be considered as a natural progression of this technology for the manufacture of pharmaceuticals [23,25]. This chapter focuses on the scientific considerations when developing and defining the control strategy for continuous manufacture of pharmaceuticals using hot melt extrusion.

TABLE 3.1

Some Marketed HME Products with Indication, Route of Administration, Polymers Used as Matrix, and Final Product Size and Shape

Name, Company (Drug)	Indication—Route of Administration[a]	Polymer[a]	Product Size and Shape[a]
Lacrisert®, Valeant (hydroxypropyl cellulose)	Dry eye syndrome— Ocular insertion	HPC	Rod-shaped implant 1.27 mm × 3.5 mm
Ozurdex®, Allergan (dexamethasone)	Macular edema; uveitis—Ocular insertion	PLGA	Rod-shaped implant 0.46 mm × 6 mm
Zoladex®, AstraZeneca (goserelin acetate)	Prostate cancer— Subcutaneous insertion in the anterior abdominal wall below the navel line	PLGA	Rod-shaped implant 1.2 mm × 10–12 mm or 1.5 mm × 16–18 mm
Implanon®, Merck (etonogestrel)	Contraceptive— Subcutaneous implantation in the inner side of the upper arm	EVA	Rod-shaped implant 2 mm × 40 mm
NuvaRing®, Merck (etonogestrel/ethinyl estradiol)	Contraceptive— Intravaginal ring	EVA	A ring with an outer diameter of 54 mm and a cross-sectional diameter of 4 mm
Belsomra®, Merck (suvorexant)	Insomnia—Oral tablet	PVP/PVA	Round tablet
Noxafil, Merck (posaconazole)	Fungal infection—Oral tablet	HPMC-AS	Oval tablet
Norvir®, Abbott (ritonavir)	Viral infection (HIV)— Oral tablet	PEG—glyceride	Ovaloid tablet
Kaletra®, Abbott (lopinavir/ritonavir)	Viral infection (HIV)— Oral tablet	PVP/PVA	Oval tablet
Onmel®, Merz (itraconazole)	Onychomycosis—Oral tablet	HPMC	Oval tablet
Gris-PEG®, Pedinol (griseofulvin)	Onychomycosis—Oral tablet	PEG	Oval tablet
Covera-HS®, Pfizer (verapamil HCL)	Hypertension and angina pectoris—Oral tablet	HPC	Round tablet
Nurofen (Meltlets lemon®), Reckitt Benckiser Healthcare (ibuprofen)	Analgesic—Oral tablet	HPMC	Round tablet
Eucreas®, Novartis (vildagliptin/metformin HCL)	Diabetes type 2—Oral tablet	HPC	Oval coated tablet

(Continued)

TABLE 3.1 (*Continued*)

Some Marketed HME Products with Indication, Route of Administration, Polymers Used as Matrix, and Final Product Size and Shape

Name, Company (Drug)	Indication—Route of Administration[a]	Polymer[a]	Product Size and Shape[a]
Zithromax®, Pfizer (azithromycin enteric-coated multiparticulate prepared by HME and melt congealing)	Bacterial infection—Oral tablet	Pregelatinized starch	Oval tablet
Palladone (hydromorphone HCl), Purdue Pharma	Pain Management—Oral capsule	Ammonio methacrylate copolymer type B	Capsule
Nucynta (tapentadol), Depomed Inc.	Pain Management—Oral tablet	Microcrystalline cellulose	Round tablet
Opana ER (oxymorphone HCl), Endo Pharmaceuticals	Pain Management—Oral tablet	PEO/PEG/PVA	Round tablet
Viekira Pak (ombitasvir, paritaprevir, ritonavir, dasabuvir), AbbVie	Chronic hepatitis C virus (HCV)—Oral tablet	Copovidone/PEG/PVA	Oval tablet
Venclexta (venetoclax), AbbVie	Chronic lymphocytic leukemia (CLL)—Oral tablet	PVA/PEG	Oval tablet

Source: Stanković, M., H.W. Frijlink, and W.L. Hinrichs, *Drug Discovery Today*, 2015. 20(7): pp. 812–823; Kesisoglou, F. et al., *Journal of Pharmaceutical Sciences*, 2015. 104(9): pp. 2913–2922 [19]; Meyer, R., C. Neu, and B. Smith-Goettler, *FDA-AIChE Workshop on Adopting Continuous Manufacturing*. 2016. San Francisco [20]; Chen, B. et al., *Developing Solid Oral Dosage Forms* (Second Edition). 2017, Academic Press: Boston. pp. 821–868 [21].

[a] Refer to prescribing information.

3.2 HME PROCESS

HME is a process in which heat and shear are applied to melt the feed (containing a mixture of polymer, API, and other additives) and force it though an orifice. A typical HME setup consists of an extruder, which is segmented barrels containing one or two rotating screws. These rotating screws are used to transport the material down the barrel section. Figure 3.1 shows a simplified model extruder containing a hopper, transport section, and die. The hopper is used to continuously supply material to the extruder. The barrel and screws in the transport section simultaneously mix and convey the material. The die at the end of the extruder gives a desired shape to the extrudate [18,26]. This extrudate is subjected to further downstream processing such as cooling and cutting.

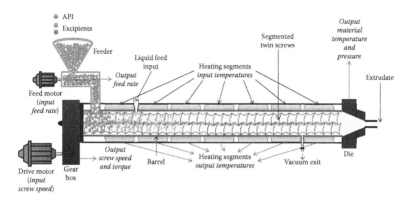

FIGURE 3.1   A typical hot melt extruder assembly with input and output process parameters.

The assembly consists of a drive motor that has the capability to rotate the screw at a given operational speed while accounting for the torque and shear generated. Heat is generated in the extruder due to frictional heating within the barrel, and shearing between the rotating screws and between the screws and the wall of the barrel in the case of twin-screw extruders. Heaters are mounted on the barrel, and water is used for cooling to maintain the desired temperature. The temperatures in the barrel are maintained such that the melt viscosity allows for proper conveying and mixing, without thermally degrading the materials. The equipment consists of a central electronic control unit that controls the various process parameters such as screw speed (rpm), feed rate, temperatures along the barrel and the die, and the vacuum level for devolatilization. The central electronic control unit also contains information about other parameters such as melt pressure and temperature, motor amperage, viscosity, and specific energy consumption. Downstream processing equipment can be used to process the extrudate, such as water baths and air knives for cooling, strand-cutters and pelletizers for cutting the extrudate, and spoolers for extrudate collection.

3.3 DEVELOPMENT: CRITICAL QUALITY ATTRIBUTES AND PROCESS RISK FACTORS

The critical quality attributes (CQA) of a product are defined as "a physical, chemical, biological, or microbiological property or characteristic that should be within an appropriate limit, range, or distribution to ensure the desired product quality" (ICH Q8). In the hot melt extrusion process, the goal is to generate a product of uniform solid dispersion (or solution) from individual materials, with a specified content and physical state. The solid dispersion can then be incorporated into a final dosage form in a variety of ways. A simplified example of an HME-based manufacturing process for solid oral dosage form is shown in Figure 3.2. The process flow diagram is meant to be a depiction of a candidate process for the purposes of discussion of process risks in relation to critical quality attributes; HME processes can vary based on product.

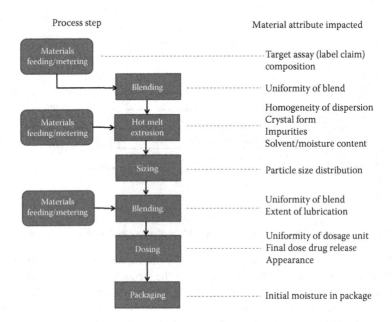

Process step   Material attribute impacted

FIGURE 3.2 Example process flow diagram of a drug product continuous process using HME for solid oral dosage form.

Establishing the drug product CQA and identifying potential process risks is an important first step for developing a control strategy [27]. The CQA for a drug product manufactured through hot melt extrusion typically include identity, potency, content uniformity, purity, and quality attributes related to bioavailability such as form and drug release. Product usage and formulation attributes such as color, odor, and taste can also be impacted by the hot melt extrusion process and should be considered based on the intended use of the product.

The following section includes brief descriptions of the process risks to consider when developing a control strategy for a continuous hot melt extrusion process.

3.3.1 INCOMING MATERIALS

Incoming materials for HME typically include a fixed ratio of polymer and API, with the addition of functional excipients, such as surfactants and plasticizers, and processing aids such as glidants. Other excipients such as flavorants can also be incorporated. Whether a dispersion or solution is generated by HME depends on the solubility of the materials in the solid state, which can be elucidated through prior bench-top characterization of the formulation materials [28–30]. Due diligence on the potential for thermal properties and thermal degradation on the API is critical for establishing the feasibility of HME. Also important is the understanding of the incoming impurity profile, solvent content, and physical properties of the API and excipients with regard to material processability. Table 3.2 is a summary of potential process risks related to incoming material properties. Though not an exhaustive list, it presents some process risks that may be specific to a continuous HME process.

TABLE 3.2

Identification of Potential Risks from Incoming Materials and Process Parameters in a Hot Melt Extrusion Process

Product Critical Quality Attribute	Ingredient Properties	Potential Process Risk	Related Process Parameters
Assay	API physical properties[a] Excipient physical properties	Improper continuous feeding	Feeder limits and controls, minimum fill
Content uniformity	API physical properties Excipient physical properties	Improper continuous blending or segregation	Feeder limits and controls, minimum fill Screw configuration, screw speed, material throughput Blender speed and feed rate (degree of fill) Sizing parameters (e.g., mill speed, material throughput, mill type/ screen)
Bioavailability/drug release/form	Glass transition or melting temperature of materials Solubility of materials in the solid state (e.g., max ratio of API:polymer) Melt viscosity of polymer	Ability to form an amorphous dispersion	Barrel temperature profile Screw configuration Screw speed Material throughput Quench time/cooling time
	Recrystallization potential of API at stressed conditions	Ability to maintain an amorphous dispersion	Room temperature and RH Storage/processing/ annealing time
Purity	API and excipient solvent content Temperature ranges for triggering degradation (thermal properties) Hygroscopicity	Insufficient removal of water or solvent that may destabilize the amorphous dispersion Formation or growth of thermal impurities Absorption of moisture	Vacuum for extrusion Maximum temperature of the melt Room temperature and RH

[a] For example, particle size, solid cohesion, liquid viscosity.

From a control strategy development perspective, excipient and API attributes such as moisture/solvent content, particle size and flow properties, impurities, and thermal properties can be used to inform HME ranges for processing temperature, solvent removal, and feed rates. Similarly, studies varying the composition for key functional ingredients (e.g., API-polymer-surfactant ratios via melt quenching or solvent casting) can be very informative in establishing acceptable ranges for content variation and understanding risk factors for physical stability failures. Therefore, understanding incoming material attributes for API and excipient can inform formulation properties and help set limits for processing in HME.

3.3.2 Process Parameters

Identifying HME and downstream process parameters that can impact the critical quality attributes is also important in the development of a control strategy. Table 3.2 is an example of potential process risk in continuous HME manufacturing and related process parameters.

Whether fed continuously into the extruder as individual metered quantities or as a blend from a continuous blender, material feeding capabilities and variations due to feeder performance (solid or liquid) will always be an important risk factor to evaluate with respect to variability in assay. Feeder capabilities at the intended manufacturing throughput rates will be important to understand as part of control strategy development.

Typically, the materials entering the extruder undergo conveying, melting, mixing, and quenching to be transformed into a solid solution. The concepts for HME development and scale-up are discussed in the literature [31,32]. For any given formulation, the processing parameters of feed rate, screw speed, barrel temperature profile, and screw configuration impact degree of fill, the residence time, and specific energy. The screw configuration, for example, will impact the degree of mixing and therefore uniformity of the solid dispersion. Also, the energy contributions from the heated barrel and from the number of mixing screw elements combined with the residence time distribution will impact the maximum temperature of the melted phase and any thermally related attributes (e.g., impurities). Because of the multifactor nature of HME process, multivariate analysis of effects is a feasible and effective way to understand process risks. Coupled with the continuous and fast response of the process to factor changes, design of experiments can be an efficient way to increase process understanding: define a process operating range and establish a comprehensive control strategy for HME. Whether developed via intentional variation of process variables or within a fixed operating range, a risk-based approach for establishing HME parameters can be informed by the observed changes in material properties potentially impacted by the process steps (Figure 3.2).

Downstream continuous processing for HME usually includes a sizing step, which can include cutting, multistage milling, and/or particle size selection. The milling properties of a glassy amorphous dispersion can be challenging; therefore, milling parameters or sizing equipment may be important process variables to consider in a risk-based approach to HME development.

Continuous blending parameters, whether used for preblending or postblending in the HME process, may impact content uniformity of the solid dispersion (extrudate) or of the final dose and therefore could be considered as a process risk factor during development.

Overall, it is important to evaluate and assess process parameters that can vary during a continuous manufacturing run for potential to CQA variation. This is coupled with the understanding that the HME process may have significant interactions of process parameters within extrusion and that downstream processing and storage requirements of the extrudate can limit the properties of the solid dispersion suitable for final dosing.

3.3.3 CONTINUOUS OPERATION

One of the aspects of process development specific to continuous manufacturing is the understanding of residence time distribution through the processing steps and the understanding of the degree of intermixing between processing steps. Characterization of residence time distribution in the extruder, continuous blenders, particle sizing, and any material transfer units is important for evaluation of material traceability and removal or segregation of nonconforming material (i.e., of unacceptable quality). There are several approaches in the literature to characterize residence time distributions in these processing steps [33–35]. The techniques used for tracing, accounting for, and separating unwanted material consumed or produced during a continuous process may vary depending on equipment and operational considerations; however, understanding the characteristics of the process during development enables the development of control strategies for successful continuous operation. Another key aspect of developing and scaling up a continuous HME process is establishing an overall manufacturing throughput or line rate. A manufacturing rate can determine process requirements for feeder capabilities, sampling frequency, process analytics response time, and material sampling and segregation capabilities. Manufacturing throughput changes can have fundamental changes in shear, mixing, and heating that can impact material quality attributes during extrusion, blending, and other processing. HME can also have special limitations on throughput for a configuration, such as having adequate quenching and cooling of the extrudate at higher manufacturing throughput. Therefore, the definition of manufacturing throughput ranges in continuous operation of the HME process is an important part of development and definition of the overall control strategy.

Finally, for development of a continuous manufacturing process it is important to understand startup and shutdown requirements, where the rapid changes in process parameters and degree of fill of equipment may impact critical quality attributes. For HME, characterization of typical times to adjust each feeder and to achieve the barrel temperature profile, as well as the determination of an acceptable strategy to ramp up and ramp down the extruder during startup and shutdown, can be important for designing a robust control strategy.

3.4 CONTROL STRATEGY

When developing a control strategy for a continuous process, it is important to consider the unique aspects of continuous operation and to include elements that control the variation of the process over time. As material continuously flows through the HME process, variation in process, materials, or environmental conditions has the potential to impact product quality over a determined period of time. HME variation considerations can include short-term factors (e.g., feeding disturbances or material lot changes) and long-term factors (e.g., temperature drifting or equipment wear and tear). These can be incorporated in the overall risk assessment and control strategy of the process.

Therefore, a robust control strategy is essential to ensure that consistent quality of product is formed over the total operation time. The key elements and concepts that can be included in the control strategy for HME continuous manufacturing are addressed below.

3.4.1 STATE OF CONTROL

The objective in establishing a state of control for a continuous manufacturing process is to provide assurance that desired product quality is being consistently manufactured and nonconforming materials are appropriately segregated. Although a continuous process might not be in a state of control during process startup and shutdown or during a process disruption, the process is expected to reach and maintain a state of control after some time. One of the main functions of the control strategy is the ability to detect and remove nonconforming material that may be formed during startup, shutdown, or process upsets. The first step is to establish criteria for what is conforming material. For an HME operation, some metrics for establishing conforming material can include active content of the extrudate within acceptable limits, amount of crystallinity in the extrudate, and limits on degradation. The establishment of appropriate limits is typically based on product performance understanding, such as bioavailability considerations, qualification of impurities, and physical stability limitations, to name a few. Establishing appropriate limits also includes selecting an in-process measurement system that is capable of measuring material attributes or process parameters, manipulating independent variables in a feed-forward or feedback manner as necessary, and diverting nonconforming material. Examples of variables or attributes that can be monitored in real time for HME processes include barrel temperature; extrudate properties such as temperature, amount of crystallinity, and active content; screw speed; torque; and drive amperage. Monitoring devices can be placed throughout the length of the HME or at the point of the extrudate to enable these measurements. Additionally, when selecting a monitoring strategy for continuous operation, it is important to select a monitoring frequency that would be capable of detecting process upsets. Planned disturbances such as feeder refills and how those disturbances propagate through the system may be important in determining sampling frequency. Furthermore, techniques such as multivariate modeling can be used to support the control strategy [36]. Multivariate modeling allows the option to leverage information from multiple input measurements for verification of process consistency during routine operation.

The U.S. FDA has encouraged the implementation of quality by design (QbD) and process analytical technology (PAT), which are essential tools in the development of an HME process, to enhance product and process understanding [37]. As a continuous process, HME fits well within this framework. Critical quality attributes typically monitored via PAT in real time are drug content, impurities, extrudate temperature, and crystallinity/form. The implementation of PAT for critical in-process controls of extrudate quality are often accompanied with visual checks of extrudate clarity and the process monitoring of critical process parameters (e.g., screw speed, feed rates, and barrel temperatures), for a holistic approach to control strategy. PAT tools including Raman and near-infrared (NIR) spectroscopy play an important role in real-time quality evaluation and understanding of the extrusion process in the production pharmaceutical dosage form [38–48].

3.4.2   COLLECTION/DIVERSION/REJECTION

The ability of the HME process to divert or reject material that is nonconforming based on prespecified quality criteria is a key element of the continuous manufacturing control strategy. During planned startup and shutdown of the HME process train, there will be periods of time when the desired material attributes might not be achieved and when criteria for initiating and stopping collection of product could be implemented. During normal operation, there may be temporary process upsets or disturbances over the total operation time. There may be situations where product made during the disturbance could be removed while the remainder of the product is retained; other situations could warrant rejection of the entire batch instead of a portion of a batch. These scenarios rely on the ability to isolate nonconforming material at some point in the process.

Physical separation of nonconforming material can occur immediately at the point of the detected failure or downstream if justified by time-based traceability. For HME, the ability to isolate material of undesirable quality typically includes consideration of (a) the state of the material, i.e., hot melt, cool extrudate, powder mixtures, or final dose; (b) the minimum amount to be diverted to include the nonconforming material; and (c) the required time delay from the failure event to an isolation point. Physical and timing limitations of the system on sampling and isolation of the material can be considered in the control strategy development. Also, the understanding and demonstration of when quality is achieved during startup, lost during shutdown, and recovered during process upsets may be important in designing the material diversion system.

Establishing *a priori* criteria for product collection, product rejection, or rejection of an entire batch and indicating how to make or who makes those decisions will be important for a continuous manufacturing process, given that response times and decision times may be limited. The establishment of process-monitoring criteria (e.g., alarms, adjust limits, and isolation limits) can prevent *ad hoc* decisions and ensure the desired quality and consistency of the collected product. Consideration of the disposition strategy of product obtained when the process is not under control (e.g., during startup, shutdown, and process upsets) is an important component to assure quality during the manufacturing run.

3.4.3   UNIFORM QUALITY AND CHARACTER OF PRODUCT

The development of limits for process operating parameters, incoming materials, and in-process material attributes for the HME continuous manufacturing process, combined with the ability to isolate material not conforming to those limits, will help establish that the manufactured product is of uniform quality and character. However, for a continuous process, a determination of uniformity within the quantity of material manufactured under the given conditions could involve some analysis of product quality and process parameter variation over time. The sampling frequency and application of statistical methods for determining the uniformity of quality measurements (in process or final product) could be different than traditional end product testing for batch mode processing. For example, the establishment of uniform quality and character for the CQA of amorphous content of an HME product could involve process parameter limits with adequate controls for the extruder (e.g., temperature, screw speed, material feeds); in-process limits for extrusion process response (e.g., torque); in-line process sampling of the extrudate and/or final product at an established frequency (e.g., temperature of the melt or spectroscopic detection of crystallinity); and a final analysis of the variability of such measures over the time of manufacture, within appropriate limits, representative of the batch. Limits for adjusting parameters to remain in a state of control (e.g., in-line blending settings) and allowable deviations (e.g., content variation) could be important to consider when justifying uniformity of an attribute across a manufacturing run. Statistical multivariate models (e.g., a principal component analysis–based model) could also help in developing linkages between process parameters and intermediate material attributes, to establish a fingerprint for the continuous process. Furthermore, sophisticated supervisory controls (e.g., model predictive controls) can be implemented that include monitoring the process, detecting deviations from a stable process state, and acting on possible deviations. This involves integration and interaction between several different analyzers, actuators, and statistical models associated with the unit operation (e.g., HME) via a central data acquisition system [e.g., supervisory control and data acquisition (SCADA)] [36].

Additionally, if using different lots of raw materials for a continuous run, it is important to understand the impact of interface between different lots. One can consider identifying raw material properties that have a potential to impact quality (e.g., Table 3.2) due to continuous processing and including appropriate incoming material specifications.

3.4.4 TRACEABILITY OF PRODUCT

As with any drug product, material traceability for continuous HME includes knowledge of the specific lots of input materials (excipient and actives) present in the final product. This requires knowledge of how materials or products move through the continuous process line. Since these materials are fed over time in an HME continuous manufacturing process, material traceability also involves understanding the history of the process parameters during the time the final product was manufactured. This is important for many quality control aspects, including potential recalls and quality investigations and is fundamental to good manufacturing practice. A process failure or deviation at a point in the process could impact downstream quality. Therefore, understanding the flow of materials through the system (e.g., residence time distribution in each processing step) is key for establishing traceability. Extruders and other pharmaceutical equipment have the capacity for back mixing, which may help achieve homogeneity, but represents a physical limitation to traceability. Experiments determining residence time distribution vs.

extruders processing parameters are described in the literature [49]. However, for a fully continuous manufacturing process, understanding of material traceability and characterization of material flow should consider all processing steps, transitions, and buffers that could induce material holdup. Overall, the capability to establish material traceability by monitoring process time and tracking of material consumption and flow through the system will be another key element of the control strategy for continuous HME.

3.5 SCALE-UP

HME, being a continuous process, is much easier to scale up compared to a batch process. The technology transfer for scale-up requires a thorough characterization of the HME process. According to Patil et al., process parameters such as melt temperature, melt viscosity, mechanical strength of die, distribution of melt within the device, and geometry of the die could be used to determine the precise replication of the HME process during scale-up [50]. For continuous HME, scale-up can be achieved in several ways that include running for a longer time, increasing material throughput in the same equipment, increasing barrel size and screw diameter, or adding parallel units [51]. The risks to quality associated with each type of scale-up strategy can be considered based on the product and process understanding during development of the control strategy [32,52–54]. For example, increasing throughput in fixed-size units could impact residence time distributions and time constants, thus affecting homogeneity. Additionally, effectiveness of the sampling strategy and response to process upsets could be affected when increasing throughputs. When increasing manufacturing or run time, physicochemical conditions may be affected. For example, due to heating/cooling capabilities of the system, equipment parts may experience additional wear and tear or material could build up over time. Changes in physiochemical conditions could impact finished product quality and stability. Finally, there may be operational considerations when increasing manufacturing or run time, which could include failure modes due to personnel, materials, or equipment switchovers during the run time. Overall, the risks due to scale-up can be addressed by the evaluation of process parameters and throughputs during development and the consideration of processing time as an additional factor in the control strategy's robustness.

3.6 STABILITY

The quality of an HME drug product could vary over time due to environmental factors such as light, humidity, and temperature. Critical quality attributes of the drug product that are at risk of changing over time are evaluated under a stability testing program to determine the shelf life of a drug product in which the product is demonstrated to be of acceptable quality. Stability attributes such as description, assay, degradation products, water content, and dissolution are applicable to most drug products and are not discussed here; only stability attributes that are of special interest to hot melt extrudate (i.e., solid dispersions) are discussed below.

For drug products made with hot melt extrusion, a change of amorphous content over shelf life could adversely affect dissolution or in vitro release and could potentially lead to decreased bioavailability and/or efficacy. During product development, characterization of the failure modes for recrystallization, such as relative humidity, temperature, excipient interaction, glass transition temperature, and water content, can facilitate the development of an appropriate control strategy for amorphous/crystalline content [55]. This knowledge can be leveraged into the appropriate selection of excipient quality, process and environmental conditions, and design of the container-closure system in order to maximize the shelf life. Measurement of the crystalline content in intermediates and/or drug product could be obtained through in-line or on-line physical measurements during the continuous manufacturing process and stability evaluations [42,56,57]. A discriminating off-line dissolution method for crystalline content of the drug product could also be considered [58]. During the initial stability studies, measurement of the amorphous or crystalline content of the drug product through the end of shelf life could help determine the overall risk to recrystallization and whether a test for crystallinity should be considered as part of routine stability testing.

Hot melt extrusion can also impact the odor and taste of the drug product. Depending on the use of the drug product, these attributes may also need to be considered for evaluation over stability.

3.7   BRIDGING FROM BATCH TO FULLY CONTINUOUS

When instituting a change from running a HME in a batch mode to a fully continuous manufacturing process, the control strategy should be reexamined and modified as appropriate to assure that a state of control and product quality can be maintained over time. The control strategy employed for a batch HME process may not be appropriate for a fully continuous HME as potential variability introduced is not averaged out by subsequent batch mixing steps. Of particular importance is the control strategy for maintaining the uniform character and quality of the amorphous/crystallinity and active content of the extrudate. Careful identification and evaluation of the risks of specific changes would help determine the need for new control strategy elements (e.g., sampling, in-process controls, and operational changes). The risk analysis could also include additional factors such as the complexity of the product (e.g., highly potent, low dose, etc.), drug release characteristics, and stability profile. As in other process changes, a comparative analysis of product quality between the batch operation and continuous operation can inform the impact to the drug product. The comparability of the quality data in the event of a change in measurement system (e.g., in-line vs. off-line testing) may need to consider intermediate material properties and stability, critical quality attributes of the final drug product, and the bridging of analytical methods.

3.8   REGULATORY REFERENCES

Currently there is nothing in U.S. regulations or guidance that prohibits implementation of continuous manufacturing. The regulatory expectations for the assurance of reliable and predictive processing and product quality in a commercial setting are considered to be the same for batch and continuous processing. Regulatory authorities across the globe are emphasizing the adoption of science- and risk-based approaches to assure product quality. These concepts are captured in the International Council on Harmonisation (ICH) Q8(R2), Q9, Q10, and Q11 [59–61] guidance; the FDA Guidance for Industry, PAT-A Framework for Innovative Pharmaceutical Development, Manufacturing, and Quality Assurance [37]; and by QbD paradigm. The process analytical technology (PAT) guidance specifically states that the introduction of continuous processing may be one of the outcomes from the adoption of a scientific risk-based approach to process design. These guidance documents and the QbD framework could be used to develop and implement a fully continuous HME process.

The definition of a batch or lot has significant regulatory implications, particularly with respect to current good manufacturing practices (CGMPs), product recalls, and other regulatory or enforcement actions. 21 Code of Federal Regulations (CFR) 210.3 defines a batch as "a specific quantity of a drug or other material that is intended to have uniform character and quality, within specified limits and is produced according to a single manufacturing order during the same cycle of manufacture." Additionally, a lot is defined as "a batch, or a specific identified portion of a batch, that has uniform character and quality within specified limits; or, in the case of a drug product produced by continuous process, it is a specific identified amount produced in a unit of time or quantity in a manner that assures its having uniform character and quality within specified limits." While 21 CFR 210.3 allows flexibility in the definition of a batch or lot, the underlying regulatory expectation for implementing continuous manufacturing is that the batch or lot is of "uniform character and quality within specified limits." For a continuous HME process, a batch or lot can be defined considering production time period, an amount of material processed, or production variation (e.g., different lots of incoming raw material). A priori delineation of a batch or lot facilitates design of an optimal control strategy during process development.

3.9 CONCLUSION

A fully continuous HME process is feasible from both a technical and regulatory perspective. A control strategy that addresses unique aspects of continuous processing, such as material traceability, and elements that control process variability over time reduces risk to product quality. The ability to maintain a state of control and to assure the uniform character and quality within specified limits may be the key to justifying and achieving operational benefits for continuous manufacturing. A scientifically sound, risk-based, and robust control strategy is intrinsic to achieving this objective.

REFERENCES

1. Breitenbach, J., Melt extrusion can bring new benefits to HIV therapy. *American Journal of Drug Delivery*, 2006. 4(2): pp. 61–64.
2. Crowley, M.M. et al., Pharmaceutical applications of hot-melt extrusion: Part I. *Drug Development and Industrial Pharmacy*, 2007. 33(9): pp. 909–926.
3. Repka, M.A. et al., Pharmaceutical applications of hot-melt extrusion: Part II. *Drug Development and Industrial Pharmacy*, 2007. 33(10): pp. 1043–1057.

4. Shah, S. et al., Melt extrusion with poorly soluble drugs. *International Journal of Pharmaceutics*, 2013. 453(1): pp. 233–252.
5. Dreiblatt, A., Process design. *Drugs and the Pharmaceutical Sciences*, 2003. 133: pp. 153–170.
6. McGinity, J.W. et al., Hot-melt extrusion as a pharmaceutical process. *American Pharmaceutical Review*, 2001. 4: pp. 25–37.
7. Patil, H., R.V. Tiwari, and M.A. Repka, *11 Encapsulation via Hot-Melt Extrusion*. 2016.
8. Repka, M.A. et al., Influence of plasticizers and drugs on the physical-mechanical properties of hydroxypropylcellulose films prepared by hot melt extrusion. *Drug Development and Industrial Pharmacy*, 1999. 25(5): pp. 625–633.
9. Repka, M.A., S.L. Repka, and J.W. McGinity, Bioadhesive hot-melt extruded film for topical and mucosal adhesion applications and drug delivery and process for preparation thereof. 2002, Google Patents.
10. Kraus, A. et al., Expanding hot-melt extrusion based abuse-deterrent formulation technology from extended release (ER) to immediate release (IR) application. Aachen, Germany: Grünenthal GmbH. 2016.
11. Maddineni, S. et al., Formulation optimization of hot melt extruded abuse deterrent pellet dosage form utilizing design of experiments (DOE). *The Journal of Pharmacy and Pharmacology*, 2014. 66(2): pp. 309–322.
12. Stanković, M., H.W. Frijlink, and W.L. Hinrichs, Polymeric formulations for drug release prepared by hot melt extrusion: Application and characterization. *Drug Discovery Today*, 2015. 20(7): pp. 812–823.
13. Patil, H. et al., Formulation and development of pH-independent/dependent sustained release matrix tablets of ondansetron HCl by a continuous twin-screw melt granulation process. *International Journal of Pharmaceutics*, 2015. 496(1): pp. 33–41.
14. Shah, S., and M.A. Repka, Melt extrusion in drug delivery: Three decades of progress, in *Melt extrusion*. 2013, Springer: New York. pp. 3–46.
15. Repka, M.A. et al., Melt extrusion: Process to product. *Expert Opinion on Drug Delivery*, 2012. 9(1): pp. 105–125.
16. Repka, M.A. et al., Applications of hot-melt extrusion for drug delivery. *Expert Opinion on Drug Delivery*, 2008. 5(12): pp. 1357–1376.
17. Patil, H. et al., Continuous manufacturing of solid lipid nanoparticles by hot melt extrusion. *International Journal of Pharmaceutics*, 2014. 471(1): pp. 153–156.
18. Breitenbach, J., Melt extrusion: From process to drug delivery technology. *European Journal of Pharmaceutics and Biopharmaceutics*, 2002. 54(2): pp. 107–117.
19. Kesisoglou, F. et al., Development of in vitro-in vivo correlation for amorphous solid dispersion immediate-release suvorexant tablets and application to clinically relevant dissolution specifications and in-process controls. *Journal of Pharmaceutical Sciences*, 2015. 104(9): pp. 2913–2922.
20. Meyer, R., C. Neu, and B. Smith-Goettler, A decade's experience delivering clinical and commercial supplies using fully continuous hot melt extrusion. In *FDA-AIChE Workshop on Adopting Continuous Manufacturing*. 2016. San Francisco.
21. Chen, B. et al. Chapter 31—Process Development and scale-up: Twin-screw extrusion. In *Developing Solid Oral Dosage Forms* (Second Edition). 2017, Academic Press: Boston. pp. 821–868.
22. Lee, S.L. et al., Modernizing pharmaceutical manufacturing: From batch to continuous production. *Journal of Pharmaceutical Innovation*, 2015. 10(3): pp. 191–199.
23. Byrn, S. et al., Achieving continuous manufacturing for final dosage formation: Challenges and how to meet them. May 20–21, 2014 Continuous Manufacturing Symposium. *Journal of Pharmaceutical Sciences*, 2015. 104(3): pp. 792–802.
24. Hurter, P. et al., Implementing continuous manufacturing to streamline and accelerate drug development. *AAPS Newsmagazine*, 2013. 16: pp. 15–19.

25. Mascia, S. et al., End-to-end continuous manufacturing of pharmaceuticals: Integrated synthesis, purification, and final dosage formation. *Angewandte Chemie-International Edition*, 2013. 52(47): pp. 12359–12363.

26. Maniruzzaman, M. et al., A review of hot-melt extrusion: Process technology to pharmaceutical products. *ISRN Pharmaceutics*, 2012. 2012.

27. ICH, *Pharmaceutical Development. Q8 (R2)*. As revised in August, 2009.

28. Yoo, S.u. et al., Miscibility/stability considerations in binary solid dispersion systems composed of functional excipients towards the design of multi-component amorphous systems. *Journal of Pharmaceutical Sciences*, 2009. 98(12): pp. 4711–4723.

29. Baird, J.A., B. Van Eerdenbrugh, and L.S. Taylor, A classification system to assess the crystallization tendency of organic molecules from undercooled melts. *Journal of Pharmaceutical Sciences*, 2010. 99(9): pp. 3787–3806.

30. Rumondor, A.C. et al., Evaluation of drug-polymer miscibility in amorphous solid dispersion systems. *Pharmaceutical Research*, 2009. 26(11): pp. 2523–2534.

31. Keen, J.M. et al., Investigation of process temperature and screw speed on properties of a pharmaceutical solid dispersion using corotating and counter-rotating twin-screw extruders. *Journal of Pharmacy and Pharmacology*, 2014. 66(2): pp. 204–217.

32. Rauwendaal, C., *Polymer Extrusion*. Carl Hanser Verlag GmbH Co KG: Los Altos Hills, CA. 2014.

33. Reitz, E. et al., Residence time modeling of hot melt extrusion processes. *European Journal of Pharmaceutics and Biopharmaceutics*, 2013. 85(3): pp. 1200–1205.

34. Ganjyal, G. and M. Hanna, A review on residence time distribution (RTD) in food extruders and study on the potential of neural networks in RTD modeling. *Journal of Food Science*, 2002. 67(6): pp. 1996–2002.

35. Todd, D.B., Residence time distribution in twin-screw extruders. *Polymer Engineering & Science*, 1975. 15(6): pp. 437–443.

36. Markl, D. et al., Supervisory control system for monitoring a pharmaceutical hot melt extrusion process. *AAPS Pharm Sci Tech*, 2013. 14(3): pp. 1034–1044.

37. FDA, *Guidance for Industry: PAT—A Framework for Innovative Pharmaceutical Development, Manufacturing, and Quality Assurance*. DHHS, Rockville, MD, 2004.

38. Wahl, P.R. et al., Inline monitoring and a PAT strategy for pharmaceutical hot melt extrusion. *International Journal of Pharmaceutics*, 2013. 455(1): pp. 159–168.

39. Krier, F. et al., PAT tools for the control of co-extrusion implants manufacturing process. *International Journal of Pharmaceutics*, 2013. 458(1): pp. 15–24.

40. Saerens, L. et al., In-line NIR spectroscopy for the understanding of polymer–drug interaction during pharmaceutical hot-melt extrusion. *European Journal of Pharmaceutics and Biopharmaceutics*, 2012. 81(1): pp. 230–237.

41. Saerens, L. et al., Raman spectroscopy for the in-line polymer–drug quantification and solid state characterization during a pharmaceutical hot-melt extrusion process. *European Journal of Pharmaceutics and Biopharmaceutics*, 2011. 77(1): pp. 158–163.

42. De Beer, T. et al., Near infrared and Raman spectroscopy for the in-process monitoring of pharmaceutical production processes. *International Journal of Pharmaceutics*, 2011. 417(1): pp. 32–47.

43. Gendrin, C., Y. Roggo, and C. Collet, Pharmaceutical applications of vibrational chemical imaging and chemometrics: A review. *Journal of Pharmaceutical and Biomedical Analysis*, 2008. 48(3): pp. 533–553.

44. Roggo, Y. et al., A review of near infrared spectroscopy and chemometrics in pharmaceutical technologies. *Journal of Pharmaceutical and Biomedical Analysis*, 2007. 44(3): pp. 683–700.

45. Barnes, S. et al., Vibrational spectroscopic and ultrasound analysis for the in-process monitoring of poly (ethylene vinyl acetate) copolymer composition during melt extrusion. *Analyst*, 2005. 130(3): pp. 286–292.

46. Tumuluri, S.V.S. et al., The use of near-infrared spectroscopy for the quantitation of a drug in hot-melt extruded films. *Drug Development and Industrial Pharmacy*, 2004. 30(5): pp. 505–511.
47. Coates, P. et al., In-process vibrational spectroscopy and ultrasound measurements in polymer melt extrusion. *Polymer*, 2003. 44(19): pp. 5937–5949.
48. Vankeirsbilck, T. et al., Applications of Raman spectroscopy in pharmaceutical analysis. *TrAC Trends in Analytical Chemistry*, 2002. 21(12): pp. 869–877.
49. Zhang, X.M. et al., Local residence time, residence revolution, and residence volume distributions in twin-screw extruders. *Polymer Engineering & Science*, 2008. 48(1): pp. 19–28.
50. Patil, H., R.V. Tiwari, and M.A. Repka, Hot-melt extrusion: From theory to application in pharmaceutical formulation. *AAPS Pharm Sci Tech*, 2016. 17(1): pp. 20–42.
51. Dreiblatt, A., Technological considerations related to scale-up of hot-melt extrusion processes. *Hot-Melt Extrusion: Pharmaceutical Applications*, 2012: pp. 285–300.
52. Almeida, A. et al., Upscaling and in-line process monitoring via spectroscopic techniques of ethylene vinyl acetate hot-melt extruded formulations. *International Journal of Pharmaceutics*, 2012. 439(1): pp. 223–229.
53. Guns, S. et al., Upscaling of the hot-melt extrusion process: Comparison between laboratory scale and pilot scale production of solid dispersions with miconazole and Kollicoat® IR. *European Journal of Pharmaceutics and Biopharmaceutics*, 2012. 81(3): pp. 674–682.
54. Potente, H., Existing scale-up rules for single-screw plasticating extruders. *International Polymer Processing*, 1991. 6(4): pp. 267–278.
55. Shibata, Y. et al., Effect of characteristics of compounds on maintenance of an amorphous state in solid dispersion with crospovidone. *Journal of Pharmaceutical Sciences*, 2007. 96(6): pp. 1537–1547.
56. Breitenbach, J., W. Schrof, and J. Neumann, Confocal Raman-spectroscopy: Analytical approach to solid dispersions and mapping of drugs. *Pharmaceutical Research*, 1999. 16(7): pp. 1109–1113.
57. Tumuluri, V.S. et al., Off-line and on-line measurements of drug-loaded hot-melt extruded films using Raman spectroscopy. *International Journal of Pharmaceutics*, 2008. 357(1): pp. 77–84.
58. Albers, J. et al., Mechanism of drug release from polymethacrylate-based extrudates and milled strands prepared by hot-melt extrusion. *European Journal of Pharmaceutics and Biopharmaceutics*, 2009. 71(2): pp. 387–394.
59. ICH, *Development and Manufacture of Drug Substances (Chemical Entities and Biotechnological/Biological Entities) Q11*. 2012.
60. ICH, *Pharmaceutical quality system Q10*. Current Step, 2009. 4.
61. ICH, *Quality risk management Q9*. Current Step, 2005. 4.

4 Twin-Screw Extrusion and Screw Design

William Thiele

CONTENTS

4.1   INTRODUCTION

For those unacquainted with twin-screw extruders (TSEs), there is cause for cautious optimism in knowing that the use of this well-proven and versatile tool is within grasp to make a better, more repeatable, "good-manufacturing-practice" (GMP) product. However, given the peculiar nature of pharmaceutical-grade materials and processes, potential users should also exercise caution about importing solutions that worked for plastics and rubber, which served as the preamble for most of this work.

4.2   BASIC PROPERTIES

This discussion will begin with the most basic properties of the key process elements for a twin-screw extruder, namely, the barrels, the screw elements, and the shafts on which they are staged and driven (1). Whether corotating or counterrotating, intermeshing or nonintermeshing, some basic statements may be made about these continuous, longitudinal, small-mass mixing devices (see Figure 4.1). Characteristics inherent with a twin-screw extruder include

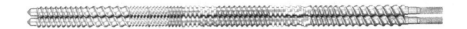

FIGURE 4.1 Continuous nature of twin-screw extruders.

TSEs are "sanitary." Designs can ensure that material is continuously exchanged on metal surfaces of the extruder to avoid stagnation.

TSEs are "continuous." A production run may continue uninterrupted until completion. This facilitates process stability and reproducibility.

TSEs are "small mass." The localized bounded domain of a mass of material is contained by the screw shapes and the barrel walls. Short, local, mass-transfer distances promote accurate distribution of small formulation constituents. In contrast, high-shear batch-mixer devices are often large mass because the processed material is bounded by the whole volume of the device. The transport distances to the moving elements and to the walls are comparatively large, causing accurate distribution of components to take more time. The short mass-transfer distances within screw sections promote both mixing accuracy and speed. Also, the heat-transfer surface area in extruders tends to be about six times greater than that of batch mixers. This, plus the ability to engineer favorable heat-transfer coefficients, helps to maintain critical temperature control. In general, "small mass" is a favorable property to maintain process control.

TSEs are "longitudinal." Over the length of the process section, consisting of barrels and screws, subprocesses (unit operations) may be sequenced as necessary to perform many of the manufacturing steps for the product. In fact, unit operations may be added and/or existing operations may be expanded until some boundary condition finally limits the system. Boundaries may include shaft torque, heat transfer, vent velocity, minimum dwell time, or several other limitations.

TSEs have "screw interaction." Both distributive and dispersive mixing may be enhanced by the flow patterns in the "apex region" where the two screws come together in the "intermesh" or "proximity" region where the screws most intimately mesh and approach each other. Screw interaction is also used to enhance pumping, to separate subprocesses (zoning), and to make twin screws more sanitary (self-cleaning).

TSE processes receive "power through two screws." As a result of modern technology, shafts transmit high torque and can power a substantial length of screws, long enough for significant numbers of unit operations.

4.3   COMMERCIAL TWIN-SCREW EXTRUDERS

Medical/pharmaceutical extruders have been adapted from the food and plastic industries. The strongest, most widely disseminated, and versatile come from the latter. A brief summary of the available types of twin-screw extruders appears in Table 4.1.

TABLE 4.1
Commercial Twin-Screw Extruders

Generic Type and Origin		Sample Builders
Counterrotating, intermeshing		
Slow speed	Profile heritage	Cincinnati-Milacron, Krauss-Maffei, etc.
High speed	Compounding heritage	Leistritz
Counterrotating, nonintermeshing (sometimes called "tangential")		
High speed	Compounding heritage	Welding Engineers, JSW
Corotating, intermeshing		
Low speed	Profile heritage	L.P. (Colombo), Windsor
High speed	Compounding heritage	Leistritz, Coperion etc.

Nonintermeshing twin-screw extruders are less common for mixing applications because of weaker screw interaction and less self-cleaning ability. Low-speed, late-fusion, counterrotating twin-screw extruders often use on-piece barrels and screws. Lower screw speeds and shorter process lengths support the execution of fewer unit operations. Therefore, the most likely candidates for pharmaceutical reacting, compounding, devolatilizing, granulating, and purifying tend to be adaptations of the higher-speed intermeshing machines in both corotation and counterrotation.

Regardless of extruder type, the machine must be validation friendly, with certifiable GMP construction, i.e., stainless steel and easily cleanable, and documentation that will support the validation process.

4.4 TWIN-SCREW ELEMENTS—CLASSICAL AND NOVEL TYPES

The most common twin-screw element shapes that are described in the literature are generally old, with the last core patents filed circa 1950 (2) (see Figure 4.2). For these original patents, the mathematical cross-sectional profiles were designed for

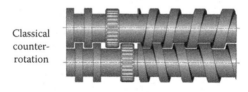

Classical counter-rotation

Rotational intermesh tracking + power through two shafts

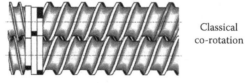

Classical co-rotation

FIGURE 4.2 Classical intermeshing corotating and counterrotating screws.

close, constant, intermesh tracking of the screws into each other during rotation (3). In the case of the most widely used mode, intermeshing corotation, that intermesh is called "self-wiping." This tracking property entirely determined the mathematics that shaped the classical cross-sectional profiles used for corotating extruders. Therefore, the cross-sectional profile shape had nothing to do with mixing, but rather with self-wiping.

The property of self-wiping was supposed to produce "self-cleaning." It usually does, but the primary jobs of extruders involve unit operations such as feeding, melting, mixing, draining, venting, and pumping, all of which were undertaken in classical twin-screw extruders under the constraints that the screw elements had to obey this intermesh tracking formula discipline. This is one of several reasons why technology that has proven acceptable for plastics may not be acceptable for executing unit operations in pharmaceutical processes, which may require different heat and mass transfer, and for which strong intermesh tracking may be undesirable.

Classical, tightly meshing screws, corotating or counterrotating, are preferred for many pharmaceutical processes, even though this use was never envisioned. These devices can enhance pumping and subprocess separation, and they can maximize process sanitation by being self-wiping. However, it is important to note that even open meshing screws, which do not self-wipe, have higher mixing rates on their metal surfaces to maintain sanitation than mixing bowls, for example.

Sanitation, the continuous exchange of material present on a metal surface, is primarily a matter of achieving threshold levels of mass transfer for each material. At or above the critical threshold level, the extruder (or even the batch-mixing bowl) will operate in a sanitary manner. Therefore, one need not be constrained to classical screw types whose self-wiping may be excessive and may demand unnecessarily high energy from the screw shafts, at the expense of producing excessive mass or localized viscous heating.

Usually the optimum screw design will consist of a mixture of classical self-wiping screw types and new designs, which might not meet the threshold of being termed self-wiping (see Figure 4.3). Some of the "new" types are merely modifications of classical elements. Others are conceived solely to perform specific heat and mass-transfer operations (see Figure 4.4). The short residence time (RT) associated with a TSE (typically in the 15 sec to 3 min range) is particularly beneficial for heat/shear-sensitive formulations, as the TSE can be designed to limit exposure

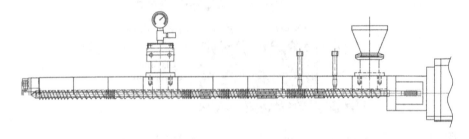

FIGURE 4.3   Mixed classical and newer screws.

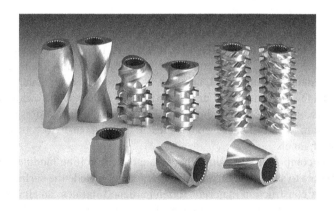

FIGURE 4.4   Typical, nontraditional, corotating screws.

to elevated temperatures to just a few seconds (8). In any case, screw types are chosen and sequenced along the screw shafts to perform the specific unit operations along the process length of the barrels/screws. Specific screw types will be discussed later.

4.5   DETERMINING SANITATION THRESHOLD LEVELS

In the plastics industry, the traditional market for twin-screw extruders, engineers tend to speak about "shear rate." This is unfortunate for two reasons. Strain rate usually consists of both shear and extensional components. Extensional mixing is often the most critical component, particularly for mixing low- and high-viscosity components together, which is frequently a requirement for pharmaceutical materials. Also, shear rate is not relevant to the resistance to straining. At the same shear rate, much more energy will be expended straining a higher-viscosity material, like tar, as compared to a lower-viscosity material, like water.

The sanitation threshold will, as implied above, be influenced by applied "stress rate." This stress rate is the product of the strain rate times the controlling modulus. The expression for this is as follows:

$$\frac{ds}{dt} = E_c * \frac{de}{dt}$$

Units: $(ds/dt) =$ stress rate $= [(kg/m^2)/sec]; E_c =$ composite viscosity $= (Pa\ sec)$; $(de/dt) =$ strain rate $= (1/sec)$

Applied: $[(kg/m^2)/sec] = (Pa\ sec) * (1/sec) * 0.102$
(*Divide by 1000 if your composite viscosity is in centipoise.)

There are a couple of important issues to note. Strain rate in extruder screw channels may be about $100\ sec^{-1}$ ($+200/-90\ sec^{-1}$). Dispersive mixers can be thought of as about $1000\ sec^{-1}$ ($+2000\ sec^{-1}, -700\ sec^{-1}$). Of course, the strain rate may be in shear or it may be in elongation.

The E_c ("controlling modulus") is the apparent viscosity of all the components together in their good or poor state of mix at that point in the extruder. For example, for compatible materials with viscosities that are different by perhaps a factor of three or less, the resulting E_c might be determined by their individual viscosities as proportioned in the formulation. If, however, a very low-viscosity material is present at more than a few percent, it will disproportionately influence the overall E_c.

Taking these guidelines, water in screw channels would have a stress rate of only about 0.01 (kg/m²)/sec. Polymeric composites might be about 10 to 1000 (kg/m²)/sec in the screw channels.

Interacting component viscosities that create the controlling modulus are not the sole contributors to sanitation threshold. Other factors include the surface chemistry of the extruder construction materials (often hardened stainless steel) (8) in combination with the resulting interactions with the processed materials. Materials that "stick" to the screw surfaces have elevated threshold levels. However, for any material there is a stress-rate threshold for achieving process sanitation.

Generally, "sticky" materials have higher sanitation thresholds than "watery" ones. Again, for materials in any given morphological state, it is generally possible to determine a stress rate that makes the operation function in a sanitary manner. Should that stress rate be too high, solutions may include modifying the process sequencing, adjusting the formulation, changing the screws' and barrels' construction materials, and/or a variety of other possible solutions (see Figure 4.5).

There are greater problems in maintaining sanitation in output adapters, and dies vs. screws, because of the screws' higher stress rates. In adapters and connections, the self-cleaning screw properties do not apply. The design in this aspect of the installation is critical to maintain self-cleaning and sanitation. Cleaning is also an issue with wiped mixing bowls, but the relatively poor sanitation of bowls and other batch mixers makes the contrast with delivery and exit hardware seem less pronounced than with extruders.

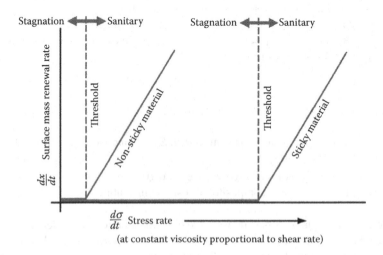

FIGURE 4.5   Sanitation stress-rate threshold for material types.

4.6 GETTING STARTED

What is important in screw and barrel discipline for pharmaceutical applications is to

Define the unit operations that need to be performed in the extruder to identify the candidate barrel configurations.

Take into account the required mass-transfer regions inside the extruder barrel profile for each unit operation, which relates to how screws behave inside the barrels.

Define, at least conceptually, the basic screw types.

Identify heat- and mass-transfer requirements and boundaries for the unit operations.

Expect that a few iterations might be necessary and that solutions and modeling for plastics applications may not completely apply. Most pharmaceutical applications involve customization of the extruder (4).

4.7 BASIC SCREW TYPES

Rather than describing screw element types as either classical by their common names or by special case, it seems useful to reduce the selection available to three basic functional types. Screw elements may be broadly classified as forwarding, mixing, and zoning (see Figure 4.6). It is not uncommon for a screw piece to have more than one of these attributes, and sometimes all three. Generally, however, a screw element will be mainly one of these basic types.

Forwarding elements perform the task that the classification implies and are used wherever there is an opening in the process, including at barrel holes to forward material away from feed openings [i.e., either the main feed or downstream feeding of heat- and shear-sensitive active pharmaceutical ingredients (APIs) to minimize exposure to shear forces and dwell time (8)], at vent openings to maintain a zero

 1. Forwarding: Almost always flighted
feeding, pumping, driving mixers

 2. Mixing: Great variety of geometries
dispersive and distributive mixing
(Kneader shown)

 3. Zoning: Restrictive mixers and flighted elements
*separates unit operations, assists
mixers to function.*
(Reverse mixer shown)

FIGURE 4.6 Basic screw element types.

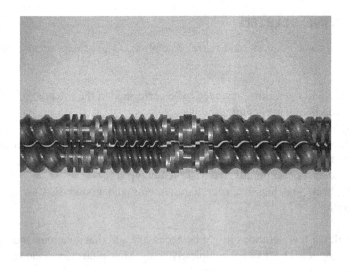

FIGURE 4.7   Driver-mixing sequence.

pressure, drain openings to positively convey materials, and at the discharge end of the extruder to pressurize the die. Forwarding is generally directly proportional to rotational velocity and pitch angle (7). There can be exceptions, such as some injection holes to inject liquids or gases immediately prior to mixers.

Forwarding elements also serve as drivers to provide forwarding pressure to supply material into mixers. Some mixers are not self-centering in the extruder barrels and rely upon flighted elements and self-centering mixers and zoning elements to keep them properly centered. Forwarding elements usually perform this centering task (see Figure 4.7).

Forwarding elements are almost always flighted. The classical types are close meshing and self-wiping. The newer energy-focused elements are often open meshing, and not self-wiping in the traditional sense.

Mixing elements can be dispersive or distributive. Dispersive mixers are used to break down morphological units such as phase domains, droplets, and agglomerates. Distributive mixers, on the other hand, space the morphological units without altering them. Similar to the case of sanitation stress-rate threshold, a stress-rate threshold exists for dispersive mixing (see Figure 4.8). Theoretically, no basic stress-rate threshold exists for distributive mixing (see Figure 4.9). Mixers may also be used to multiply surface area in devolatilizing and draining and often serve to isolate unit operations from each as a "zoning" function (see Figure 4.10).

Besides being dispersive or distributive, a further subclassification may be added. Mixers may be forwarding, neutral, or reversing (see Figure 4.11). Forwarding mixers are capable of transporting material and may exhibit a small positive or negative pressure drop across the element. Neutral mixers have sections that push material neither forward nor backward and may exhibit small to substantial pressure drops. Reversing mixers have elements that tend to push material backward and may exhibit moderate to large pressure drops. To most rules there are exceptions. For example, a forward-vaned gear or combing mixer may be productively paired with a

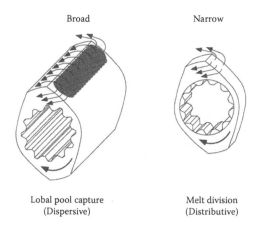

Lobal pool capture   Melt division
(Dispersive)   (Distributive)

FIGURE 4.8   Basic kneading section for dispersive and distributive mixing.

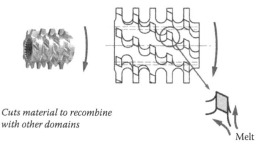

*Cuts material to recombine
with other domains*

Melt

FIGURE 4.9   Combing distributive mixer.

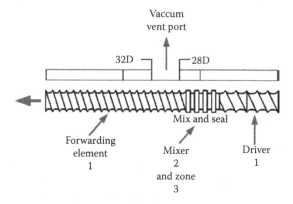

FIGURE 4.10   Mixer as a vent zoning element.

reverse-vaned one to constitute a mixer pair that is both forwarding and reversing to perform more longitudinal homogenization (see Figure 4.12).

Dispersive mixers tend to capture material domains in pressure traps that cause the material to become squeezed, sheared, and elongated. The shapes of these

Kneading blocks—co-rotation

30° Forward   90° Neutral   30° Reverse

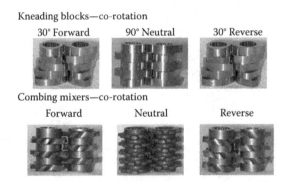

Combing mixers—co-rotation

Forward   Neutral   Reverse

FIGURE 4.11   Forward, neutral, and reverse combing elements and kneading blocks.

Combing mixer Vanes opposed	Combing mixer Vanes aligned left	Combing mixer Vanes aligned right

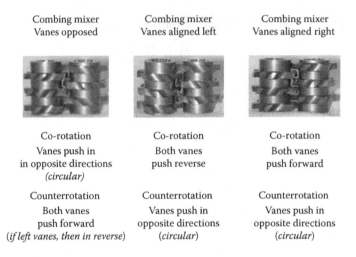

Co-rotation	Co-rotation	Co-rotation
Vanes push in in opposite directions *(circular)*	Both vanes push reverse	Both vanes push forward
Counterrotation	Counterrotation	Counterrotation
Both vanes push forward *(if left vanes, then in reverse)*	Vanes push in opposite directions *(circular)*	Vanes push in opposite directions *(circular)*

FIGURE 4.12   Opposing-flow distributive mixers.

mixers individually, and usually in interaction with the second screw, cause the processed material to become captured, deformed, and stressed when the screws turn (see Figure 4.13). Wide-section kneaders, lobal accelerators, and shearing discs are examples of dispersive mixing elements.

Distributive mixers tend to divide and recombine the material and ideally they do not capture locally pressurized domains like dispersive mixers do, but rather form easy paths for the dividing and recombining process to facilitate low energy and stress rate per division within the process section. Narrow section kneaders, gear elements, vane mixers, combing mixers, pin mixers, and interrupted screw flight elements are all examples of distributive mixing elements.

Many common mixing elements have evolved to balance dispersive and distributive mixing (see Figure 4.14). Kneaders utilize the width of the sections and the angular advance or decline of the progressive stacked elements to set the strength of lobal capture and dispersive mixing by allowing controlled leakage paths for domain division and distributive mixing. For most pharmaceutical applications, the

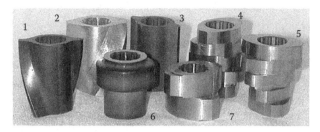

1. Lobal capture element with acceleration shape
2. Lobal capture element with traditional shape
3. 0° Pitch lobal capture elements
4. 30° Forward close staged kneader
5. 30° Reverse close staged kneader
6. Shearing disc
7. 90° kneader with wide lobes

FIGURE 4.13   Lobal capture and shearing elements for dispersive mixing.

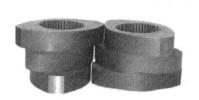 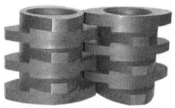

	More dispersive	More distributive
Width:	Wider lobes	Narrower lobes
Staging:	30° angles between lobes	90° angles between lobes
Leakage:	Little bypass possibilities around lobes	Many bypass possibilities around lobes
	Much lobal capture	Reduced lobal capture
Type:	Dispersive with distributive component	Distributive with dispersive component

FIGURE 4.14   Dispersive elements with distributive leakage paths.

maximum number of kneading segments will not exceed two four-paddle sequences due to the shear-sensitive nature of the materials used in compounding and the limited residence time requirements to achieve target product properties (7).

Table 4.2 provides some basic generalizations for kneading sections with dispersive and distributive mixing. Zoning elements separate unit operations, e.g., to provide a pressure seal so that vacuum at a vent does not reach upstream or downstream to disturb other operations. Similarly, a zoning element might set the boundaries of an injected liquid or force a drain to release liquid (see Figure 4.15). Other zoning elements may block large particles from continuing down the screws following a melting or mixing zone. A restrictive zoning element might also be used to enhance

TABLE 4.2
Generalized Mixing Behavior of Kneading Blocks

Factor	Dispersive	Distributive
Section width	Wide	Narrow
Advance angle between sections	Small	Large
Direction of advance angle	Reverse	Forward

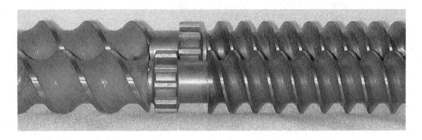

FIGURE 4.15   Zoning elements before vacuum vent.

the operation of a mixer, usually downstream of that mixer to ensure that it will be entirely full of material to best perform its mixing.

A pure zoning element provides no mixing itself, but rather serves a support function. A reverse-flighted screw element can be fairly pure by that definition as it is usually a poor mixer. Often mixers themselves serve "double duty" when zoning is needed.

Examples of zoning elements include reverse-flighted elements, shearing discs, multisection neutral or reversing kneaders, and neutral/reversing distributive mixers. As a group, these screw elements serve a barrier function. Like with mixers, simple reasoning about the unit operations to be performed will provide a starting point for choosing zoning elements.

4.8   MASS-TRANSFER REGIONS

One way to describe how a twin-screw extruder operates within barrels is to visualize the cross-sectional activity regions and the related effects inside the twin-screw extruder. Process designs may be created to promote or suppress activity in the five basic screw regions: channels, lobes, tips, apexes, and intermesh (see Figure 4.16).

Channels in a twin-screw extruder are comparatively gentle, mainly because the process melt is not captured and pressurized domains for heavy mixing do not occur. Most twin-screw extruders are starve-fed, where the feeders set the rate to the machine, and extruder rpm is independent. Therefore, the channels are not full, resulting in zero-pressure regions. In reality, 100% fill of the extruder will not be achieved across the length of the process section. Screw elements will often be starved, with only 100% fill achieved in the higher-pressure regions, i.e., leading to kneading/mixing elements and before the die (7). While channel regions are generally associated with forwarding elements, they may also be designated in mixing and zoning elements. Processes dominated by channels tend to be less shear intensive relative to the other regions described below.

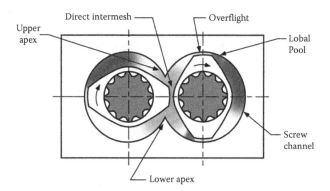

FIGURE 4.16 Five mass-transfer regions.

The lobal regions capture and pressurize material in "lobal pools," which are relieved up and over the screw tips to facilitate extensional and shear-strain rate components. Lobal capture powers most dispersive mixing processes. Typical kneading blocks are called "bilobal" because they capture two lobal pools. Deep-flighted counterrotating machines may be up to hexalobal. Distributive processes avoid lobal events.

Screw tips, the overflight, usually provide shear and an exit for lobal pools with very high shear. For processes that cannot use shear stress for mixing, the shearing length and intensity should be minimized. Some lobal capture elements can be made to perform better as compared to the traditional kneaders. Extensional mixing is difficult to estimate, but a reality.

Apexes are where the barrels join in lower and upper peninsulas of metal. These are screw regions that provide some moderate extensional and shear mixing. In corotation, the upper and lower apexes host a productive material direction change as the material transfers from screw to screw. Mild to moderate apex stress rates occur to support distributive mixing and dispersive mixing of a low stress-rate threshold. For the intermeshing, counterrotating twin-screw extruders, the lower apex provides a powerful lobal-like capture.

The intermesh is where the screws come together. While this region is often ignored in corotation, it hosts higher stress rates than the apexes, particularly with "sticky" materials. In counterrotation, it provides strong extensional and shear mixing components. For an intuitive understanding of the twin screw, the screw regions as described above are summarized in Table 4.3 below. It is important to note that the feeding devices in twin-screw extruders set the rate, whereas the screw speed, screw design, and temperatures are used to control process severity in the unit. If the feeders are kept at a constant rate, raising the screw speed will cause remastication in the high-stress regions, which will also occur at proportionately higher strain rates (see Table 4.4).

The OD/ID ratio of a TSE is defined by dividing the outside diameter (OD) by the inside diameter (ID) of each screw. For instance, a TSE with an OD of 50 mm and an ID of 30 mm would have an OD/ID ratio of 1.66 (50/30). A higher OD/ID ratio (i.e., 1.66/1 vs. 1.55/1 OD/ID) results in both a deeper channel and narrower kneader crest (see Figure 4.17). The materials that pass over the kneader tip experience less RT in planar shear. Both factors contribute to a lower average shear rate inherent

TABLE 4.3
Generalized Processing Effects Within the Twin-Screw Five Mass-Transfer Regions

Region	Mode	Extensional Mixing	Shear Mixing
Channels	Co- and counterrotation	Weak	Weak
Lobes	Co- and counterrotation	Strong	Strong
Tips	Co- and counterrotation	Weak	Strong
Apexes	Corotation	Moderate	Moderate
	Classical counterrotation	Moderate++	Moderate
Intermesh	Corotation	Moderate to strong	Moderate to strong
	Classical counterrotation	Strong	Strong

with a deeper-flighted TSE, which is often beneficial for processing shear-sensitive formulations (8).

4.9 MIXING

In this chapter so far, we have addressed dispersive and distributive mixing, as well as shear-stress rate and extensional-stress rate. This was in the context of screw element types, of mass-transfer regions formed by screws and barrels, and of achieving

TABLE 4.4
General adjustment for gentle and strong mixing intensity

Type of Processing	Gentle	Strong
Screws' speed	Low	High
Mixing rate in each of the five mass-transfer regions at each point along the screws is proportional to screws' RPM		
Screws' fill	High	Low
Starving the feed increases remastication and time in mixers to increase process intensity.		
Temperature	High	Low
Lowering the temperature increases the controlling modulus in dispersive stress rate = $E_c \times$ strain rate		
Screws' lobality	Low	High
Increasing the number of lobal events and their intensity increases process severity. Within its boundary conditions the same is true of planar shear.		
Sequential feed	Depends	Depends
Sequential feed may be employed to either capture or avoid high stress rate exposure.		

Note: In twin-screw extruder compounders, reactors, and devolatilizers, the balance between the rate determining feeders and the screws' speed is critical, not just screw speed, rate, temperature, and screw design by themselves.

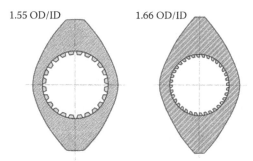

1.55 OD/ID   1.66 OD/ID

FIGURE 4.17 OD/ID ratio comparison.

sanitation stress-rate level. However, the issues of pharmaceutical unit operations and mixing mechanisms to achieve target morphologies have not yet been discussed.

Pharmaceutical processes may also involve solids reduction, phase separations, precision distributions, reaction and purification operations, and validated reproducibility in a way more stringent manner than the world of plastics and food processing common to twin-screw extruders.

The basic model for distributive mixing is dividing and recombining material without disturbing the individual morphological components (see Figure 4.18). There is no stress-rate threshold, as no agglomerate, droplet, or the like will be reduced. The divisions, therefore, should be made as efficiently as possible. Using sharp leading edges to cut the processed material tends to be more efficient than dull cutting edges inherent with kneading elements, which require additional energy and cause viscous heating in the material and load on the screw shafts. Distributive divisions may be extended to cause ever more precise equal distribution of morphological components. In practice, twin-screw extruders homogenize distributions rapidly. This is

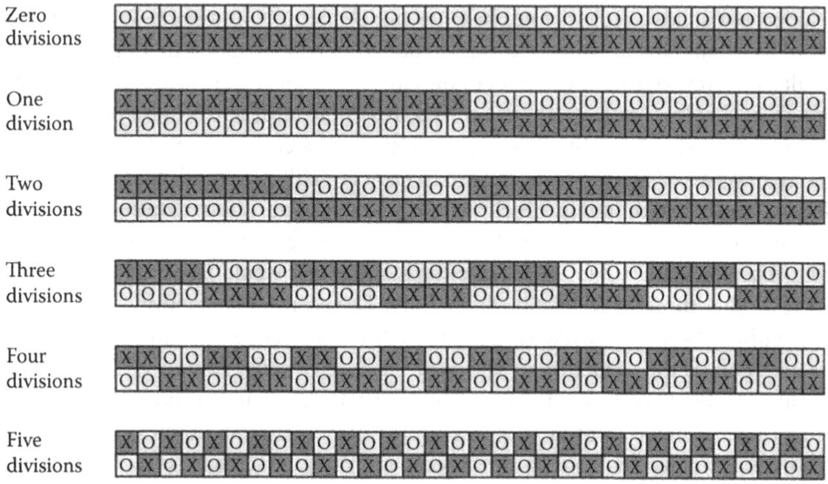

Zero divisions

One division

Two divisions

Three divisions

Four divisions

Five divisions

FIGURE 4.18 Distributive mixing model.

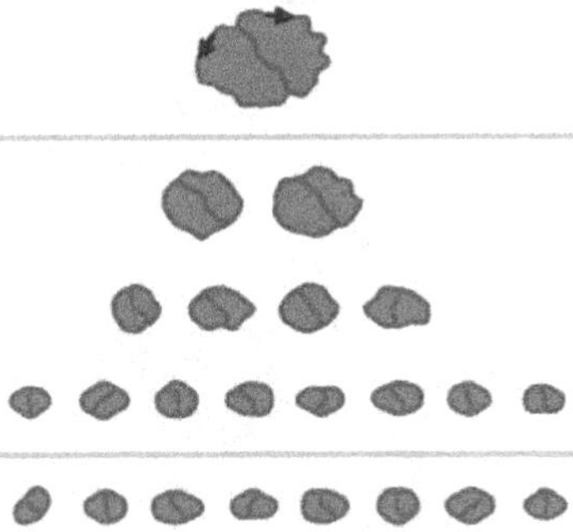

Division number	Shear rate req'd	End pieces	
1st	60	2	
2nd	240	4	
3rd	960	8	
4th	3840	8	
5th	15360	8	Beyond available shear rate
5th	61440	8	

FIGURE 4.19 Shear mixing model.

partly the product of being a small-mass device with short transport distances. Often distributive mixers alter morphological units and are effectively dispersive mixers, particularly when the material has a low threshold level for dispersive stress rate.

When the morphological components are to be reduced, dispersive mixing is required. Extruders, mixing bowls, and most other mixers produce more shear strain, and therefore shear stress, than extensional strain and extensional stress. Very much like the sanitation threshold, a certain critical stress rate must be achieved before the reduction process begins.

Most commonly, "shear" is thought of in connection to dispersive mixing (see Figure 4.19). In a shear field, the differential forces of the carrier acting upon a particle tend to cause a fissure in it.

Suppose a solids' agglomerate, in a mixing element, is in a shear-strain rate field of 1000 sec^{-1} and the agglomerate is low enough in concentration that the controlling modulus is governed by the viscosity of the carrier, which at that shear rate and temperature, from rheology data, is 100 Pa sec. The resultant shear-stress rate would be about 10,000 (kg/m^2)/sec. Actually, that agglomerate only needed, say, 5000 (kg/m^2)/sec to fracture into two or more pieces, so that division is easily accomplished. However, the half-sized particle remaining, which may still be too large, might require roughly four times the stress rate to break again because, in its reduced size, it is about four times as strong. Therefore, a 20,000 (kg/m^2)/sec shear-stress rate would be needed.

A few other things may also be happening. The carrier may be thinning from viscous heating. As higher screw speeds are attempted in hopes of a higher stress rate, the result can be the reduction of viscosity because of shear thinning. The nature of the materials being processed must be considered relative to this point.

In practice, shear is used to successfully disperse agglomerates and droplets, often through many divisions. And for some morphologies, such as stacked platelets, it is the most productive mode, but with each size reduction, the smaller particles are significantly more difficult to break, and there are limitations.

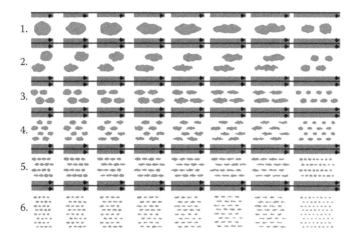

FIGURE 4.20 Extensional mixing model.

Fortunately, extensional strain rates may also be generated in twin-screw extruders (5) (see Figure 4.20). As in shear-based strain rate, there is a threshold level for particle reduction. However, the reduced particles, and droplets in particular, do not seem to become as difficult to divide with decreasing mass, but respond to issues of surface chemistry, carrier viscosity, and other values determining the ability of the particle to respond to the percent elongation of the field in which it is present during extensional mixing. What is known is that divisions of particles and droplets often may continue in extensional fields long after divisions would have stopped in shear fields.

When the stress rate, whether in shear or in elongation, falls below the necessary threshold level, dispersive mixing stops while distributive mixing and viscous heating continue. In order to recover dispersive activity, the strain rate and/or the controlling modulus must be increased to raise the stress rate above the threshold for reducing the target morphological domain.

Screw elements with higher strain rates and running the screws at higher speeds might be beneficial. But these factors may also cause shear thinning and heating, which would reduce E_c, perhaps more than offsetting the higher strain rate (see Figure 4.21). Several possibilities exist to solve the problem. Using screws conducive to removing heat from the process via barrel cooling could decrease the temperature of the material, stiffening it, before mixing again. A formulation component with a lower, typically ambient temperature could be fed downstream into a melt to increase viscosity before mixing. Likewise, a liquid could be added and vented, carrying with it the heat of vaporization. Stronger mixers could be separated to mitigate viscous heating effects. The materials being processed determine the optimum approach.

There are cases where the threshold level is not a minimum, but rather a maximum, over which some unwanted action occurs. In such cases, some component might need protection from mechanical or molecular degradation caused by heat or stress. Gentle screws, downstream feeding where E_c has become very small, lubrication of the component, and special heat-transfer barrels and screw elements are among the candidate solutions to these problems.

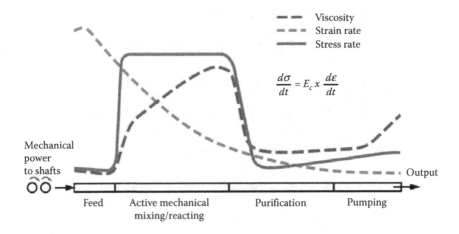

FIGURE 4.21   Stress-rate profiles down the length of the extruder.

The differing demands of pharmaceutical processes preclude generalized solutions to screw and barrel design. Fortunately, twin-screw extruders can be modular so that customization of these devices is practical.

4.10   SCALE-UP AND SCALE-DOWN

Many pharmaceutical products are initially developed via small batch processes, which might be impractical when scaled up as larger batch processes. By plastics industry standards, pharmaceutical processes are small, making scale-up easier. Some boundary conditions and scale-up rules follow.

Volume is a boundary value. Each unit operation will use some of that volume. Extruders tend to scale volumetrically to about the cube of their screw diameters, provided their screw diameter-to-centerline spacing ratios are the same. Volume in each unit operation determines dwell time at a given rate. Many unit operations are greatly accelerated in the twin-screw vs. batch mixers.

Heat transfer is a boundary value. Each unit operation will need heat input or dissipation. Modern twin-screw extruders tend to scale thermally to about the square of the screw diameter. Twin-screw extruders may have about six times the heat transfer area to volume as compared to mixing bowls, and they have more favorable overall heat-transfer coefficients per unit area of barrels. In many processes, most heat input originates from the main drive motor, through the gearbox, and from the screw shafts and screws, with rather nominal temperature-control requirements.

Mechanical energy is a boundary value. It originates at the motor and is applied through the gears to the screw shafts. Both small and large twin-screw extruders have similar power available to power each unit volume per rotation of their screws. It is this energy that primarily powers all the unit operations performed on the twin-screw extruder.

These and other boundary values generally determine the basic size of the extruder to produce a given output. Some expansion or contraction will be made according to specific scale-up situations. Most often, however, similar twin-screw extruders scale between the square and the cube of their screw sizes, depending upon whether the processes are more thermally or volumetrically dependent.

Distributive mixing is a direct scale-up value. The same divisions per kilogram in Process A generally equal the same divisions per kilogram in Process B. Even if the division rate of a mixer in a smaller machine is miscalculated, when it is miscalculated in the same way in the larger machine the result is usually valid.

Dispersive mixing is a direct scale-up value. The same product of time and stress rate at the same level over the threshold level in Process A generally equals Process B. Dispersive element groups in larger extruders can "look different" than in smaller machines. Scale-up values between sizes may require some empirical adjustments. Kneaders and other lobal capture elements dominate this group of mixers.

Coarse devolatilization is a direct scale-up value. Supply the same heat of vaporization per weight of volatile in Process A as in B and the results will generally be equivalent, having boiled off the same relative moles of volatile. Boundary conditions may include critical barrels' area per mole of volatile and vent velocity. Channels of simple flighted elements dominate this screw element type, which are sometimes supported by viscous-heating mixers.

Fine devolatilization is a direct scale-up value. Equivalent surface renewal with or without matched stripping yields scale-up. A variety of mixers and flighted screw elements are used.

Reaction dwell is a direct scale-up value. Given the same balance of activity in the mass-transfer regions and temperature, or trade-off balancing, scale-up is achieved. Almost all screw types and mass-transfer regions are used (see Figure 4.22).

Generalizations fail with nonstandard materials and processes. But if the process is divided into its unit operations within the extruder, it is generally possible to choose modular parts to service each subprocess, especially if that product is already running in a batch device or another continuous-mixing device.

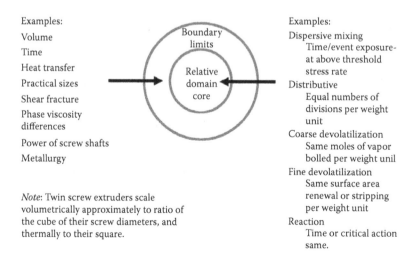

Examples:

Volume
Time
Heat transfer
Practical sizes
Shear fracture
Phase viscosity differences
Power of screw shafts
Metallurgy

Note: Twin screw extruders scale volumetrically approximately to ratio of the cube of their screw diameters, and thermally to their square.

Boundary limits

Relative domain core

Examples:

Dispersive mixing
    Time/event exposure-
    at above threshold
    stress rate
Distributive
    Equal numbers of
    divisions per weight
    unit
Coarse devolatilization
    Same moles of vapor
    bolled per weight unil
Fine devolatilization
    Same surface area
    renewal or stripping
    per weight unit
Reaction
    Time or critical action
    same.

FIGURE 4.22 Basic scale-up small vs. long machine.

4.11   UNIT OPERATIONS

The unit operations in a typical plastics twin-screw extruder are feeding, melting, mixing, venting, and pumping (6) (see Figure 4.23). While some pharmaceutical processes are simple, some are not. Pharmaceutical twin-screw process designs tend to be considered proprietary and confidential. Therefore, the unit operations concept will be described with a merely hypothetical configuration.

The process could be simple mixing and pumping, or alternatively could be reaction steps, among other applications. This sample unit operation as described below involves preparation of a carrier, to which active and inert components are added; a normal devolatilization step; a purification step; and sanitary discharge (see Figure 4.24, Table 4.5). The length of the barrel process section is frequently described in terms of the length to diameter (L/D) ratio, with greater L/D values indicating a longer process section. The L/D ratio is defined by dividing the overall length of the process section by the diameter of the screws.

For most pharmaceutical compounding operations, L/D values ≤40 are used, while reactive and devolatilization extrusion operations may utilize longer values, such as 60/1 L/D process sections. Heat- and shear-sensitive products often use shorter process sections, such as a 20/1 L/D process length. It becomes obvious that the longer the L/D, the more unit operations can be performed along the length of the process section. For instance, if the OD of a screw is 20 mm and the length of the process section is 800 mm, then the L/D ratio is 800/20 or 40/1. If the length is 400 mm, the L/D would be 400/20 or 20/1 (8).

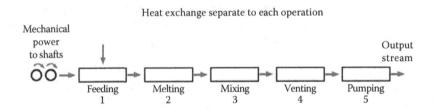

FIGURE 4.23   Unit operations of a simple plastic's compounding extruder.

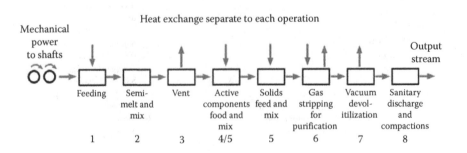

FIGURE 4.24   Unit operations of a hypothetical pharmaceutical process.

TABLE 4.5

Example of Possible Staging of Subprocesses in a Pharmaceutical Extruder

Unit Operation	Barrels/screws
1. Solids feeding of carrier components.	#1 Feeding, with nitrogen purge.
2. Semimelting and mixing of carrier components.	Forwarding close meshing.
	#2 Solid barrel section.
3. Near atmospheric venting of volatiles.	Distributive/dispersive mixers.
	#3 Vent. Light draw-off and condenser.
4. Feeding active and inert solids.	Forwarding close meshing.
	#4 Side-stuffed feed barrel.
5. Mixing solids into carrier.	Zoning and forward close meshing.
(Liquid could be injected here.)	#5, #6 Solid barrel sections.
6. Gas stripping for purification.	Distributive then dispersive.
	#7 Solid barrel with gas injector.
	Zoning, inject to distributive mixers.
	#8 Vent. Vacuum, vent gas/impurities.
	Distributive mixers, forward close mesh.
7. High vacuum devolatilization	#9 Vent. High vacuum. Condenser.
	Zoning seal. Forward close meshing.
	#10 Solid.
8. Sanitary discharge and compactions.	Forward open meshing to zoning seal.
	#11 Solid.
	Forward open meshing to compaction.
	Material exits from divider/distributors.

4.12 SCREW AND BARREL DESIGNS FOR TOTAL SYSTEMS

Extruders may be surrounded by support devices such as feeders, prereactors, driers, pumps, condensers, bulk premixers, mills, and many other pieces of equipment. Tandem extruders, where a primary extruder melt feeds a secondary extruder of a different design, are also possible. Multiple extruders can be linked in a system to make layered products by coextrusion. Other than the common stainless-steel GMP constructions, equipment configurations and applications differ greatly between pharmaceutical projects. Other chapters describe these variations.

If the total system has the minimum number of necessary devices running well, then process validation, operation, and clean-downs will be simplified. Part of this strategy may often include consolidating as many unit operations as possible on continuous, sanitary, twin-screw extruders. By analyzing the unit operations, process streamlining is often possible.

4.13 COROTATION OR COUNTERROTATION?

Corotating twin-screw extruders are generally the extruder of choice because they are available in the newest high-strength and heat-transfer configurations. Additionally, corotators are excellent feeding devices for powders, pellets, and fibers. In this

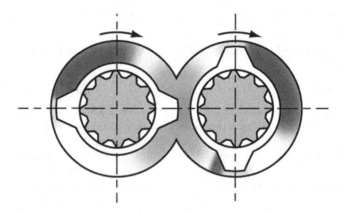

FIGURE 4.25   Cross section of bilobal mixer.

design, the intermesh wiping rate with close-meshing screws can be the highest of any extruder or batch device. This is important only when the sanitation stress-rate threshold is very high.

Corotators suffer in two areas: pumping is via drag flow, like single-screw extruders, and in "typical" flight depths, the lobe count of the screws is limited to two (see Figure 4.25).

Counterrotators solve these two problems. Only ram extruders and close-meshing counterrotating extruders are non-drag-flow pumping. This is useful for managing high-percentage, low-viscosity phases. Because of a common intermesh movement direction in counterrotators, lobe counts of six and even eight may be incorporated to accelerate dispersive mixing (see Figure 4.26). State-of-the-art counterrotators need not rely upon intermesh mixing as their classical versions did, but rather upon lobal mixing to achieve mixing, just as in corotation (1).

Screw and barrel designs in corotation and counterrotation are basically the same. However, commercial realities heavily encourage opting for corotation for many applications.

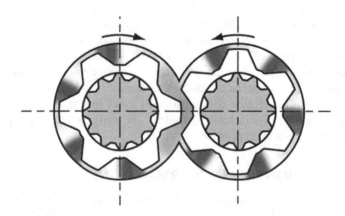

FIGURE 4.26   Hexalobal mixer cross section, counterrotation only.

4.14 SUMMARY

A generalized approach has been given to screw and barrel designs for pharmaceutical applications. Twin-screw extruders are sanitary, reproducible, continuous, small mass, and longitudinal, and they can utilize modular platforms upon which unit operations may be sequenced.

Pharmaceuticals are different than plastics so it is not surprising that different barrel configurations and screw types are used. Twin-screw components are chosen to perform unit operations of the total process. Efficiency is important to maximize productivity and inclusiveness of unit operations.

Twin screws are scale-up friendly between each other and from most batch processes. As with any process, boundary conditions and scale-up values must be observed.

REFERENCES

1. Todd DB, ed. *Plastics Compounding Equipment and Processing*, Chapter 3. New York: Hanser, 1998.
2. Erdmenger R. German patents 815,641 and 813,154, filed Sept 1949.
3. Booy ML. Geometry of fully wiped twin-screw equipment. *Polym Eng Sci* 1978; 18:973.
4. Martin C. Continuous mixing/devolatilizing via twin screw extruders for drug delivery systems. *Interphex Conference*, Philadelphia, PA, March 20, 2001.
5. Utracki LA, Abdellah A. *Compatibilization of Polymer Blends*. Boucherville, PQ: Canadian National Research Council, May 1995.
6. Thiele WC. Trends and guidelines in devolatilization and reactive extrusion. National Plastics Exposition, Society of the Plastics Industry, Chicago, IL, June 18, 1997.
7. Di Nunzio J et al. Melt extrusion. *Formulating Poorly Water Soluble Drugs*, vol. 3, Springer, 2012, pp. 311–362. AAPS Advances in the Pharmaceutical Sciences Series 3.
8. Martin C. Twin screw extrusion for pharmaceutical processes. *Melt Extrusion: Materials, Technology and Drug Product Design*, American Association of Pharmaceutical Scientists, 2013, pp. 47–79. AAPS Advances in the Pharmaceutical Sciences Series 9.

5 Die Design

John Perdikoulias and Tom Dobbie

CONTENTS

Extrusion is a reasonably mature technology. The most demanding applications historically lie within the plastics industry in which great advancements have been made and from which pharmaceutical extrusion technology has evolved. The main job of the die is to give shape to the final product. Some extrusion processes are easy and the dies are simple, and some are not. Extrusion technology covers a variety of machine types, dies, and an even bigger multitude of materials. One of the most common problems is the mismatch among material, die, and machine. By reviewing some of the techniques in extrusion die design and supplying a few insights, it is possible to design dies to produce quality products.

The die, the material, and the machine are all involved. At any stage (see Table 5.1) in the extrusion process, there is more than one flow type. (For example, at the entrance to the die system there is constrained flow, mixing flow, and bulk deformation. During a coextrusion there is also a free surface between the materials.) Because of the historical difficulties with calculation, most engineers have focused any quantitative analysis of pressures and flow rates based on simple formulae. With the evolution of computer-aided engineering (CAE), software, and computer models, detailed calculations can be made to see the fine details that lead to quality products.

The ram extruder is one of the simplest machines and provides good insights into what actually happens during the extrusion through a cylindrical die.

The material to be extruded is packed into a metal barrel with a cylindrical channel leading to a die. The metal barrel is heated. The barrel is set to some temperature. The material comes to thermal equilibrium with the barrel. (The thermal gradient across the barrel is typically less than 0.5°C.) The material is forced through a capillary die with a rate or pressure controlled plunger. The material exits the die and swells slightly (see Figure 5.1).

This technique is well suited to the precision extrusion of very high value materials. The material temperature can be controlled very precisely. The ram exerts modest

TABLE 5.1

The Four Distinct Stages and Five Flow Processes in an Extrusion Process

The four distinct stages in an extrusion process	
Melting and mixing	The material is made homogeneous in composition and temperature.
Transporting	The material is moved to the next process stage.
Shaping	Deformation of the melt into the final shape and orientation.
Finishing	Mainly the removal of heat but also shape control.
The five flow processes	
Low flow	Low stresses, e.g., surface tension, gravity, and stress relaxation.
Mixing flow	Dispersion, distribution, homogeneity, and work.
Constrained flow	Pressure driven and moving surface driven.
Free surface flow	Bulk deformation and surface deformation.
Bulk deformation	Variation with melting, solidifying, and pressure.

and repeatable pressure on the material. This leads to minimal degradation of the extrudate as well as a very consistent extrudate diameter. Various improvements can be implemented to increase the efficiency of this simple batch process. Also, detailed understanding of material changes can be found through the use of simulation.

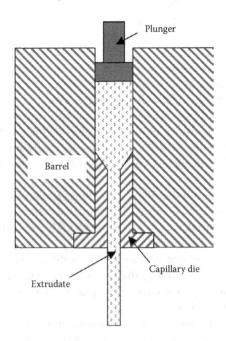

FIGURE 5.1   Simple ram extrusion using a capillary die.

5.1   FLAT DIES

For the production of flat sheets or tape, as would typically be used for transdermal drug delivery systems, the material must be converted from the circular shape into a thin and wide sheet. If the sheet is not too wide (i.e., more like a tape) then the transition can be fairly simple as shown in Figure 5.2.

The balancing in this type of die needs to account for the shorter material path along the centerline versus the sides.

If some correction is not applied, the sheet will end up being thicker in the middle than at the sides. One method of correcting the shape is to enlarge the opening at the sides versus the middle, giving the cross section a "bow tie" appearance. Another method would be to make the land section in the middle longer than at the edges. These correction methods are demonstrated in Figure 5.3.

If much wider sheets are required, the die takes on a more traditional, flat die shape shown in Figure 5.4. The various components for this type of flat die system are comprised of a manifold, restrictor, relaxation chamber, and die lips. These sections of the die are designed so as to achieve a uniform distribution of material across the width with the shortest length of die.

In general, the design of the manifold and preland area is much more important for uniform distribution than the lip gap adjustment. The manifold and preland shape is what actually governs how well the die creates a uniform melt curtain. If this area is not properly sized and shaped (engineered) for the material properties and throughput rate, a nonuniform flow will result, and the operator may not be able to "fix" it using the lip adjustments. However, thanks to available CAE tools for simulating the flow in these types of dies, the flow channels can be engineered to achieve a uniform distribution.

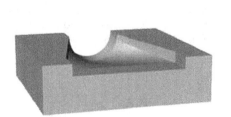 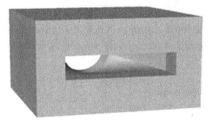

FIGURE 5.2   A simple circular to slit transition.

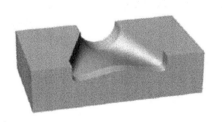 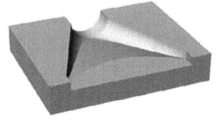

FIGURE 5.3   A slit die with a bow tie flow correction (left) and land correction (right).

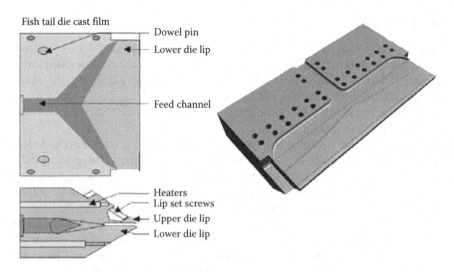

FIGURE 5.4 A typical "coat hanger" flat die (left) and an "epoch" style (right). (Courtesy of Cloeren Inc.)

The die lip adjustment capability should be thought of as being intended only for making very small changes to the material gauge thickness. Just as the take-off rolls are too late in the process to fix a nonuniform melt curtain, the die lips are too late in the die to fix a flow-distribution problem. This is a result of materials having a persistent "memory" effect.

5.2 ANNULAR DIES

The most common types of annular dies used in medical device applications for tubing are of a relatively simple "spider" type construction. Figure 5.5 shows a typical

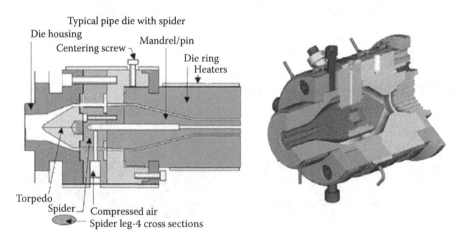

FIGURE 5.5 A typical spider die (left) and a 3-D view (right). (Courtesy of Genca.)

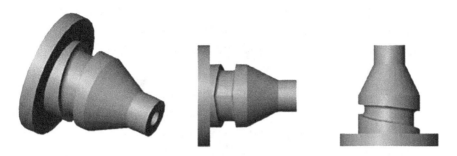

FIGURE 5.6 A typical side-fed die.

"spider" type annular die. The name comes from supports extending from the central mandrel to keep it centered to the body. The dies basically consist of a mandrel and body that form the main annular section and a set of die lips or tooling that form the final annular section near the exit of the die. These are also referred to as a central pin and outer bushing. The die lips are designed to form the material to the desired size prior to exiting the die.

Additional types of annular dies include "side fed" (or "cross-head") and "spiral mandrel." Examples of each of these are shown in Figures 5.6 and 5.7, respectively.

Side-fed dies are normally used in applications where a substrate needs to be coated because they allow a straight path through the axis of the die. Spiral mandrel dies generally provide improved product uniformity because of the mixing/layering effect of the helical flow distribution channels, if engineered correctly, and are

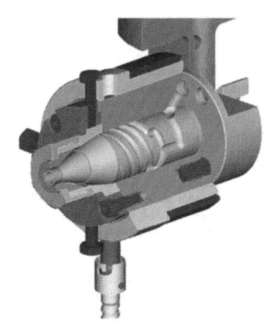

FIGURE 5.7 A spiral mandrel type die. (Courtesy of Genca.)

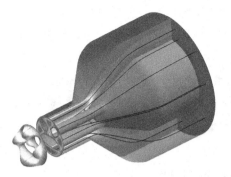

FIGURE 5.8 Multilumen tubing die.

commonly used in the production of polymer films. The majority of annular dies incorporate some sort of centering adjustments of the exit lips in order to adjust the thickness uniformity of the product.

Annular dies are often also used to create the initial flow distribution for dies used to produce multilumen tubing such as shown in Figure 5.8.

More detailed information on extrusion dies can be found in textbooks by Michaeli (1) and Rauwendaal (2).

5.3 DESIGN CRITERIA

In the description of the geometry of the various dies in the previous sections, the main design criterion that was described was the thickness uniformity. However, it must be emphasized that there are other equally important criteria that define the performance of an extrusion die. Probably the next most important criterion is residence time and residence time distribution. Simply put, this is the amount of time that the material spends within the extrusion system. This is especially important in pharmaceutical applications, as the materials are generally more prone to degradation when exposed to processing temperature for a prolonged time. The main reason that a spiral mandrel type of die may not be well suited for pharmaceutical material extrusion is that it is prone to imparting a large residence time distribution to the material.

There are basically two aspects to residence time with respect to die design: mechanical and rheological. From a mechanical aspect, the residence time is affected by how well the components that make up the die are machined and polished. Mating surfaces must match precisely and, where possible, should be machined and polished together. Any mismatch in mating surfaces can provide a "ledge" where material can stagnate and degrade. The mechanical aspect is relatively easy to observe and control, but the rheological aspect to residence time is more difficult to control. This is because the residence time distribution depends on how the material flows within the channels and what shear stress is exerted on the flow channel walls. In order to emphasize this point, consider the flow of 1 cm³/s of material in a tube with a 100-mm-diameter channel. This will result in an average velocity of about 0.127 mm/s. This is, of course, an uncommon and extreme condition as the channel is much too large for this small flow rate, but it will help to demonstrate the point. It is relatively easy to imagine that no matter how smoothly polished the internal surface of the channel is, the average velocity of the material will be too slow, resulting in excessive residence time. Furthermore, the material will tend to define its own smaller flow channel in the center of the large channel, leaving a large portion of essentially stagnant material near the walls. This condition is referred to as "channeling" and must be avoided.

Channeling occurs when the channel is essentially too large for the required flow rate. It is also affected by the rheological properties of the materials. What this means is that the flow channel needs to be sized so as to achieve sufficient shear stress on the wall to keep the material moving. The actual value of the shear stress depends on the material but can, usually, be easily determined from some simple experiments.

The next criterion that also needs to be considered is the overall resistance or pressure drop through the system. The pressure drop is related to the residence time in that a lower pressure drop or resistance generally implies a larger residence time (all other parameters being constant). In fact, the pressure drop is the sum of the shear stress over the entire flow channel, which means that the higher the shear stress, the higher the pressure drop through the system.

However, generally the designer's goal is to limit the maximum pressure drops through a die because the pressure drop energy is converted to heat within the die. This is referred to as viscous dissipation or shear heating. An estimate of the bulk temperature rise that results from the conversion of pressure drop to heat can be obtained from the following formula:

$$\Delta T = \frac{\Delta P}{\rho * C_p}$$

where ΔT is the temperature rise, ΔP is the pressure drop, ρ is the melt density, and C_p is the heat capacity. However, the problem with the above formula is that it gives the theoretical, steady-state, bulk temperature rise. Because of the low thermal conductivity of polymer melts, viscous heating is generally confined to the areas of high, local shear rate (near the wall). Since it is difficult to measure this effect precisely, engineers rely on CAE analysis tools to avoid these problems. This is demonstrated with the following example using the commercially available Virtual Extrusion Laboratory™ CAE software (3).

Consider the flow in a simple capillary die shown in Figure 5.1 with a reservoir diameter of 10 mm and a capillary of 1 mm. The material temperature in the barrel is usually precisely controlled and in this example, it will be assumed that the required temperature is 95°C. Some typical material properties are selected ($C_p = 2000$, $k = 0.15$) and the flow conditions are simulated at a piston speed of 0.5 mm/s. Figure 5.9 shows the development of the temperature along the capillary.

It can be seen that the temperature is not uniform and that the material is hotter near the wall. Figure 5.10 is a graph of the temperature vs. radial position in the

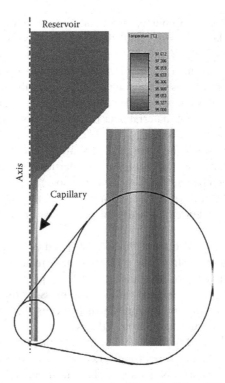

FIGURE 5.9 Temperature development in a capillary die (Virtual Extrusion Laboratory™).

capillary near the exit. Figure 5.9 show that there is a maximum in the temperature a short distance from the wall, which is controlled at the desired temperature. The heat generation takes place at the high shear region near the wall and because of the low thermal conductivity of the material, the heat is not easily transferred away. This is an important issue in all extrusion processes and die design but it is especially

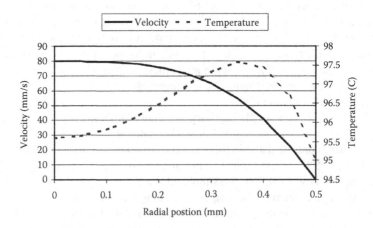

FIGURE 5.10 Velocity and temperature profiles near the capillary exit.

important in medical device and pharmaceutical applications where the processing range (or window) of the materials is often much smaller.

5.4 MATERIALS OF CONSTRUCTION

The materials for construction of a die for pharmaceutical applications need to be very stable and inert. For this reason, high-grade stainless steels that are resistant to corrosion are usually specified. The most resistant to corrosion are the 300 series, with 316 stainless being the most common. The drawback to this material is that it is relatively soft and can be damaged easily. Most die manufacturers prefer to use a 420 or a 17-4PH stainless steel, which have slightly less corrosion resistance but are harder and more durable materials. The higher-temperature materials can also withstand oven cleaning; however, when doing so, care should be taken not to exceed the hardening temperature, which will result in annealing of the material. Capillary dies are often made out of tungsten carbide to ensure dimensional stability during cleaning in an oven.

Surface coatings like chrome or nickel plating are not generally used in pharmaceutical applications because the base steels are generally corrosion resistant and there is a possibility that the coatings may flake off and contaminate the product. Records of material specification and quality assurance (QA) test should be maintained and are generally supplied with the dies.

5.5 MANUFACTURING

Dies for medical device and pharmaceutical applications tend to be very small and so the material costs are relatively low in comparison with the manufacturing cost. The materials may be stress relieved before and after machining and generally hardened after machining and polishing. Standard turning and milling equipment can be used for most dies, but some very small components and high precision may require more specialized techniques. One of these is the electrical discharge machining (EDM) method.

EDM uses a high voltage discharge to essentially vaporize the metal at the surface of the electrodes and thus form the desired shape by controlled erosion of the metal. The electrode can take the male form of the cavity that is desired and then plunged into the steel, or the electrode can take the form of a wire that cuts through a plate in a similar fashion to a typical band saw, but much more precisely.

5.6 SUMMARY

Almost every pharmaceutical extrusion system uses some type of forming die that results in the desired end product shape prior to sizing and cooling of the extrudate. This aspect of the extrusion system is no less critical than the material formulation, extruder type, or downstream system. A working knowledge of the properties of the material being processed, in combination with computer-aided design and working experience in "fine tuning" the internal flow geometry, are all important factors for producing a successful pharmaceutical extrusion die.

REFERENCES

1. Michaeli W. *Extrusion Dies for Plastics and Rubber.* Hanser Gardiner, Cincinnati, OH, 1992.
2. Rauwendaal C. *Polymer Extrusion.* Hanser Gardiner, Cincinnati, OH, 1994.
3. Virtual Extrusion Laboratory™, Compuplast International, Zlin, Czech Republic, 2003.

6 Feeding Technology and Material Handling for Pharmaceutical Extrusion

Sharon Nowak

CONTENTS

6.1 INTRODUCTION

In both hot melt extrusion and extrusion granulation, the constant delivery of the formulation to the extruder is critical to its overall uniform output. This delivery can include a premix of the ingredients or can involve separate deliveries of the active pharmaceutical ingredient (API), polymer, and/or excipients. The selection of the proper bulk solids feeder technology in pharmaceutical extrusion is a critical step in resultant process efficiency and product quality. In the extrusion process, feeders are used in a variety of unit operations, including feeding of the API to a mill or micronizer, batch dispensing of the individual ingredients to the blender for a preblend mix, or feeding individual components to a continuous blender or extruder (Figure 6.1).

Extruder feed streams can be configured using two separate methods. Feed streams can be introduced via a starve-fed manner, whereby the rate is set by the

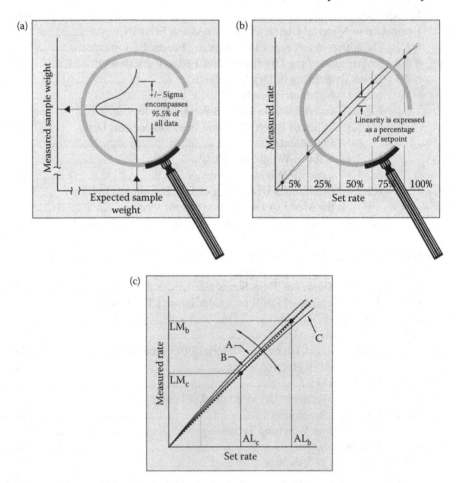

FIGURE 6.1   (a) Repeatability, (b) linearity, and (c) stability.

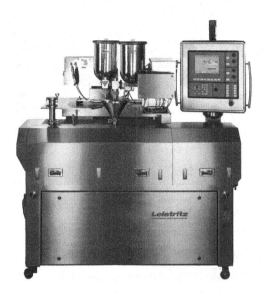

FIGURE 6.2   Loss-in-weight feeders on a twin-screw extruder.

feeders, and the extruder becomes a "slave" to the feeders. This method of feed is typical for twin-screw extruders as shown in Figure 6.2. The primary functions of the feeder are to regulate the mass-transfer properties of the process, ensure constant material throughput, maintain formulation consistency, introduce the ingredients in the proper order, and provide collection and acquisition data to enable process validation and lot traceability.

Alternatively, single-screw extruders can be flood-fed, where the hopper sits over the feed throat opening and the extruder screw rpm determines the throughput. In order to properly choose the right feeder technology for the process, it is critical to evaluate the material characteristics that affect the flowability of the material as well as the required measured accuracy.

6.2   EVALUATION OF MATERIAL CHARACTERISTICS TO ASSESS FEEDER CHOSEN

A number of material characteristics can affect the performance of the feeder. The characteristics of the material to be handled will often narrow the feeder technology selection. A typical list of these characteristics is shown in Table 6.1.

The properties of these characteristics aid in the classification of most materials into one of four categories: floodable, free flowing, difficult to flow, and cohesive/sticky. With a simple manual test, one can make a preliminary determination about how to classify a material. Take a fistful of material in hand and squeeze it into a ball. If the material squirts out and doesn't form that ball, it is likely to be floodable. If the material does not escape the hand when squeezed, nor does it form a ball when compacted, it can be considered free flowing. If the material is string-like (like fibrous

TABLE 6.1

Characteristics That Affect Flowability

Material Characteristics

Bulk density—loose and packed-consolidated
Particle size, shape, and aspect ratio, size consistency
Moisture and temperature sensitivity
Angle of repose
Internal angle of friction
Kinematic angle of surface friction
Gas permeability
Particle friability
Compressibility and springback

---

materials), it is considered difficult to flow. Finally, if the material makes a ball when squeezed and retains its shape when released, the material can be categorized as cohesive/sticky.

As shown in Table 6.2, these characteristics and flowability categories all have a variety of effects on the feeder type and configuration chosen.

6.2.1 DEFINITION OF ACCURACY IN EVALUATING FEEDER PERFORMANCE

To fully define feeder accuracy and resultant performance for a batching or continuous operation, it is necessary to address three separate and distinct areas of feeder performance: repeatability, linearity, and stability. Repeatability reports how consistent the feeder's discharge rate is at a given operating point, linearity assesses how accurately the feeder discharges at the requested average rate over its full operating range, and stability gauges performance drift over time. Repeatability is the performance statistic most familiar to feeder users. It quantifies the short-term level of consistency of discharge rate. Repeatability is of importance to quality assurance because it measures the expected variability of the discharge stream, and hence of the product itself. The repeatability measurement is made by taking a series of carefully timed consecutive catch samples from the discharge stream, weighing them, and then calculating the ± standard deviation of sample weights expressed as a percentage of the mean value of the samples taken.

It is important to note that the repeatability statistic reveals nothing at all about whether the feeder is delivering, on average, the targeted rate. Repeatability only measures the *variability* of flow rate. It is the linearity statistic that reports how well the feeder delivers the desired average rate throughout the feeder's operating range. Perfect linearity is represented by a straight-line correspondence between the setpoint and the actual average feed rate throughout the feeder's specified turndown range from its design full-scale operating point. To perform a linearity measurement, typically ten consecutive catch samples are obtained and weighed at each of the following flow rates: 5%, 25%, 50%, 75%, and 100% of full scale. (The smallest tested flow rate should be at the feeder's maximum turndown.)

TABLE 6.2
Material Characteristics and Effects on Feeder

Material Characteristics	Definition	Effect on Flowability and Feeder Selection
Bulk density—loose	Material weight per unit volume (e.g., kg/L)	Affects feeder hopper volume chosen based on capacity as well as flow rate for volumetric feeding.
Bulk density—packed	Same as above after applying pressure to product	Affects feeder hopper volume chosen, as well as option for refill design in continuous feeding. Bulk density can change with applied pressure. If pressure changes affect the bulk density, a potential for flow problems may exist.
Particle size	Actual size of individual particles (e.g., mesh or micron)	Consistency of both size and shape of particles will affect material flow. Larger particles often flow better than finer sized ones.
Particle morphology	Shape of particles—i.e., needle versus round	Needle shapes flow less easily. Round shapes "roll" off each other to make material more free flowing.
Aspect ratio (AR)	Ratio of particle length to width	Needle shapes (high AR) are less free flowing.
Moisture content	Percent of moisture (in food applications this can also be fat content) in bulk solids	Materials with higher moisture or fat content have a tendency to pack and be more cohesive. Some materials that flow from a 1-ft-diameter bin opening with low moisture may need an opening > 9 ft when at 12% moisture.
Temperature sensitivity	Sensitivity of product to temperature increase	If heat-sensitive material is exposed to an increase in temperature before the feed process, flowability may be compromised.
Angle of repose	Angle to the horizontal that a bulk solid makes as it flows, unconstrained onto a flat, level surface	The higher the angle of repose, the more cohesive the product. It is also an indication of the friction exerted between material particles.
Kinematic angle of surface friction	Angle of surface friction between the bin wall and bulk solids	Will determine the angle of hopper design for the feeder as well as indicate the ability to get material to the feed device.
Gas permeability	Ability of product to be aerated	Pellets have high gas permeability and therefore do not easily "flood." Alternatively, materials like fine fumed silica have poor gas permeability and will thus "flood" easily.
Compressibility	Sensitivity of product to pressure	Helps to determine how material will pack or bridge in a feeder hopper.

A perfectly performing feeder is worth little if it can't maintain its performance over the long haul. Many factors can potentially contribute to performance drift, including feeder type, control and weigh system stability, the handling characteristics and variability of the material, the feeder's mechanical systems, maintenance, and the operating environment itself. Drift is detected by calibration checks and is typically remedied by a simple weight span adjustment. The user will ultimately determine the appropriate frequency of calibration checks based on operational experience.

6.2.2 PREPARATION OF THE DRY INGREDIENTS FED TO THE EXTRUDER

Once the material characteristics are evaluated, there are still a number of options in the evaluation of the method of feed to the extruder. When feeding the ingredients to the extruder, they are fed in accordance with a correct ratio as defined by the recipe of the formulation. As stated above, in some cases a premix of these ingredients is done utilizing feeders in a batch dispensing system. After the mix is complete, these premixes can be fed via starve feeding or gravity, depending on the type of extruder being used. When batch dispensing, feeding devices are also used to accurately dispense the individual ingredients into a blender or intermediate bulk container (IBC) for batch tumble blending. This dispensing can be done either by gain-in-weight (GIW) or loss-in-weight (LIW) batching. An example of LIW batching is shown in Figure 6.3.

6.2.3 BATCH DISPENSING OF DRY INGREDIENTS

In order to understand the principles of both batch LIW and GIW dispensing, it is important to first understand the technologies of volumetric versus gravimetric feeding.

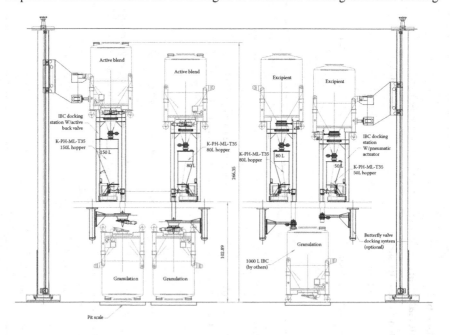

FIGURE 6.3 Pharmaceutical dispensary layout.

6.2.3.1 Volumetric Feeding

A volumetric feeder, as shown in Figure 6.4, feeds a certain material volume per unit time (such as cubic feet or liters per hour) to a process. The bulk material is discharged from a hopper with a constant volume per unit of time by regulating the speed of the feeding device. The actual volume of material fed is determined through calibration. In general, the feeding accuracy of any volumetric feed device is dependent upon the uniformity of the material flow characteristics and the bulk density.

In the case of volumetric screw feeders, the feed system consists of a hopper, material discharge device or feed screws, and controller. This is the most common volumetric feed device, and its material discharge device is a screw (or screws) that rotate at a constant speed to meter material at a predetermined volume-per-revolution discharge rate from the hopper to the process. The controller monitors and controls the feeder's screw speed, which determines the material's discharge rate. Typically, volumetric feeders are open-loop devices that cannot detect or adjust to variations in the material's density. Due to the open loop concept, headload variations and material buildup on the feed device change the volume-per-revolution relationship, throwing off calibration without any outward sign.

Three factors affect volumetric screw feeder accuracy: the consistency of delivered volume per screw revolution, the accuracy of screw speed control, and material density variability. For example, in cases of screw feeding of cohesive materials, it is possible in volumetric mode to have relatively no material discharging while the screws are running, caused by bridge building or packing in the hopper. Similarly, flooding can also remain undetected since the feeder has no way of "knowing" the out-of-control condition. Since the feed rate in a volumetric feeder is purely a

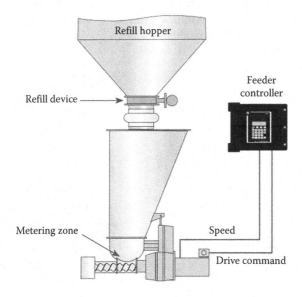

FIGURE 6.4 Volumetric screw feeder.

function of speed, the feeder and the process below have no way of detecting this upset condition. Often times, even the use of level sensors in the feed hopper may not alert the process about this upset in a timely fashion, thus affecting the accuracy of the feeder and the performance of the process below.

Understandably, the highest accuracy in volumetric screw feeders, such as the one shown in Figure 6.5, can be attained on free-flowing materials that fill the screw consistently and whose density is reasonably constant regardless of hopper level. It should also be noted that volumetric screw feeders represent an economical solution to many process feeding applications, as opposed to the higher costs of equivalent gravimetric or loss-in-weight designs.

6.2.3.2 Gravimetric or Loss-in-Weight Feeders

Unlike the volumetric screw feeder, a loss-in-weight (LIW) feeder is a gravimetric feeder that directly measures the material's weight to achieve and maintain a predetermined feed rate that's measured in units of weight per time. The bulk material or liquid is discharged from a hopper by weighing the material being fed and regulating the speed of the feeding device. The weighing system with control compensates for nonuniform flow characteristics and variations in bulk density, and therefore it provides for a high degree of feeding accuracy.

By definition, gravimetric feeders measure the flow's weight in one fashion or another and then adjust feeder output to achieve and maintain the desired setpoint. As a comparison, volumetric feeders do not weigh the flow; they operate by delivering a certain *volume* of material per unit time from which a weight-based flow rate is inferred by the process of calibration. The LIW feeder, as shown in Figure 6.6, consists of a hopper, refill device, weight-sensing device (typically either a digital or analog load cell), feeder (typically a volumetric screw feeder powered by a variable-speed motor), and controller. Before operation, an operator programs the controller to discharge material at a predetermined feed rate (or setpoint) measured in units of weight per time (such as pounds per hour).

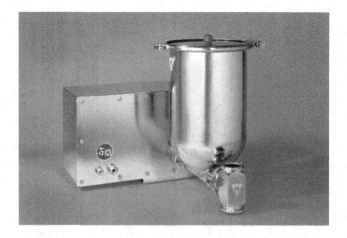

FIGURE 6.5   Volumetric screw feeder.

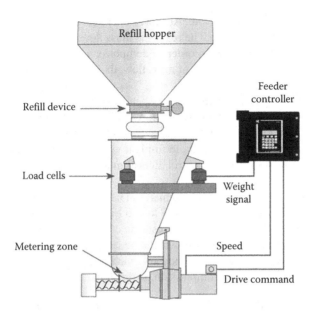

FIGURE 6.6 Loss-in-weight feeder.

As the feeder discharges material, system weight declines. The speed of the metering device is controlled to result in a per-unit-time loss of system weight equal to the desired feed rate. A typical loss-in-weight feeder controller adjusts feeder speed to produce a rate of weight loss equal to the desired feed rate setpoint.

The most common type of gravimetric feeder device used in the pharmaceutical industry is the loss-in-weight screw feeder, such as that shown in Figure 6.7. A LIW feeder calculates the mass flow rate (quantity per time) by dividing the

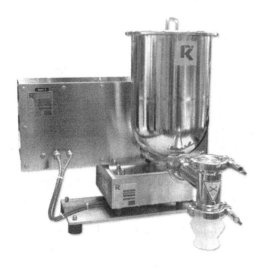

FIGURE 6.7 Pharmaceutical loss-in-weight feeder.

weight reduction by the time interval. At short time intervals, the weight is measured and transmitted to the controller. The real time mass flow rate is calculated from the weight reduction per unit time. In order to compensate for the difference between the setpoint and the measured value of mass flow, the screw motor speed is continuously modified.

Loss-in-weight feeder performance is dependent on three areas that are closely linked: (1) the mechanical configuration of the feeding device and any material flow-aid used in the feeder hopper, (2) the accuracy and speed of weight measurement and the immunity of the weighing system to in-plant vibration and temperature fluctuations, and (3) the response of the control algorithm and the available features of the control algorithm.

Loss-in-weight feeding affords broad material handling capability and thus excels in feeding a wide range of materials from low to high rates. With this technology, a constant mass flow is ensured, thus also ensuring consistent product output from the process below. For this reason, loss-in-weight feeders are typically used for continuous processes in the pharmaceutical industry, such as hot melt extrusion, extrusion granulation, continuous direct compression, and coating.

6.2.3.3   Types of Batch Weighing Feed Devices for Dry Ingredients

After transfer from the material source, the ingredients are usually delivered to the batching station. This station can include volumetric metering devices, such as screw feeders or valves, which deliver the product to a hopper on load cells. This method is called gain-in-weight (GIW) batching. Alternatively, the station can include gravimetric feeding devices, such as screw or vibratory feeders, mounted on load cells or scales, which deliver the product to the process by means of LIW batching. As outlined below, in some cases where small amounts of microingredients or APIs are required for a total overall batch, both methods are employed: LIW feeders for the micros and minors, and GIW batchers for the major ingredients.

6.2.3.4   Gain-in-Weight Batching

In GIW batching, volumetric metering devices sequentially feed multiple ingredients into a collection hopper mounted on load cells, as illustrated in Figure 6.8. Each feeder delivers approximately 90% of the ingredient weight at high speed, slowing down toward the end of the cycle to deliver the last 10% at a reduced rate to ensure higher accuracy. The GIW controller monitors the weight of each ingredient and signals each volumetric feeder to start, increase or reduce speed, or stop accordingly. Once all the ingredients have been delivered, the batch is complete and the mixture is discharged into the process below. It should be noted that this type of batching method is sequential for each ingredient, and therefore results in a longer overall batching time than with LIW batching (outlined below) if the number of ingredients is high.

Gain-in-weight type arrangements can be utilized with the receiving hopper on load cells or a weigh scale if the percentage accuracy requirement of the material received is within 0.5% of the total batch weight, depending upon the resolution of

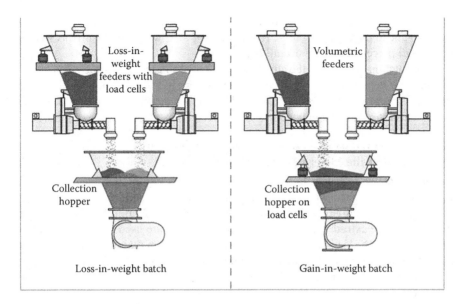

FIGURE 6.8   LIW vs. GIW batch principles.

the scale or analog load cell below (e.g., most floor scales may have a total resolution of 0.02% of the full scale range). If the material weighed in is within the resolution range, the receiving vessel may be fed by means of a volumetric device, such as a twin-screw feeder. The volumetric twin-screw feeder is used not only to accurately meter the flow of the weighed material to the receiving vessel, but also to eliminate any possibility of segregation of the mix when delivering it to the vessel below. It should be noted, however, that in most cases where accuracies of 0.1%–0.5% are required, and the required metered components' amounts are much less than the scale resolution requirements, the LIW feeder design is recommended.

6.2.3.5   Loss-in-Weight Batching

LIW batching is used when the accuracy of individual ingredient weights in the completed batch is critical or when the batch cycle times need to be very short. Also, shown in Figure 6.5, gravimetric feeders operating in batch mode simultaneously feed multiple ingredients into a collection hopper. Similar to GIW batching, a batch cycle is comprised of two phases. During the first phase, 90% of the batch weight (as determined by the preprogrammed recipe) is delivered as quickly as possible. In the second phase, the last 10% is fed in a slower "dribble" mode to ensure an accurate batch weight equal to ±0.1% of the desired setpoint. Adjustment of the delivery speed (on/off, fast/slow), as well as the ability to quickly change batch setpoints, is set using the LIW batcher controls.

Once all of the ingredients have been delivered, the batch is complete and the mixture is delivered to the process below. Since all ingredients are being delivered at the same time, the overall batch time and further processing times downstream are greatly reduced. This method of batching is often used for microingredients (such as APIs) due to the highly accurate requirement of their weight in the mix as well as their small percentage of the overall batch.

LIW batching also offers the advantage of a much shorter batch time when batching multiple ingredients. Since each LIW feeder has its own weighing system, several gravimetric feeders operating in batch mode can simultaneously feed multiple ingredients into a collection hopper.

6.2.3.6 Continuous Dispensing of Dry Ingredients to Either the Mixer or Directly to the Extruder

As an alternative to batch dispensing and batch blending the premix prior to the extruder, today's pharmaceutical manufacturers are using continuous loss-in-weight feeding of each individual ingredient directly into the continuous mixer and/or directly into the extruder. In this case, multiple feeders are used to proportion multiple ingredients based upon weight. Running materials simultaneously in the proper ratio essentially promotes homogenous mixing with the extrusion device.

Continuous pharmaceutical feeders can be supplied in both volumetric and gravimetric configurations. However, it should be noted that volumetric feeders are generally not used for metering dry ingredients into extruders for pharmaceutical applications because of the high fluctuations in the mass flow rate and difficult flow characteristics of many micronized excipients and APIs.

In a continuous loss-in-weight feeding operation, a feeding device with a hopper containing material to be fed is placed upon a platform scale or suspended via a suspension scale weighing system. The weight of the feeding device and the hopper is electronically tared. The bulk material is discharged from the hopper by the feeding device and the resultant weight loss per unit of time is determined by the weighing and control system. This actual weight loss per unit of time is compared to a desired weight loss per unit of time based upon a desired continuous feed rate setpoint. Any difference between the actual and desired weight loss per unit of time results in a correction to the speed of the feeding device. For example, if an overfeed condition occurs due to an abrupt increase in material density, sensed weight falls below desired (setpoint) weight, triggering a reduction in feeder device speed to return to the setpoint value. Additionally, since the integrated error associated with the overfeed is known, this speed may be further reduced to immediately and precisely compensate for the overfeed condition. The opposite occurs with an underfeed condition.

When the hopper reaches a predetermined minimum weight level, the LIW control is briefly interrupted and the hopper is refilled as illustrated in Figure 6.9. With some manufacturers, during the refill period, the controller regulates the speed of the feeding device based upon the historic weight and speed information that was accumulated during the previous weight loss cycle. This prevents overfeeding of material during the refill cycle due to changes in headload of material and filling of material into the screws. This is also critical for maintaining feed rate performance within specification on a second to second basis. The loss in weight feeder principle is most accurate when using a high resolution, fast responding, vibration-immune weighing system combined with self-tuning controls.

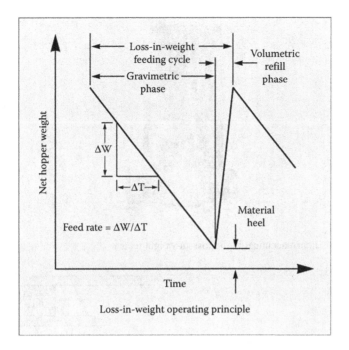

FIGURE 6.9   Continuous loss-in-weight operating principle.

6.2.3.7   Continuous Dispensing of Liquid Additives to the Extruder

Liquids can be fed through a variety of pumps (such as gear, piston, and peristaltic pumps), all equipped with a variable speed drive. The mass flow rate can be measured either via a mass flow meter with a PID (proportional–integral–derivative) controller or load cells. A PID controller is a control loop feedback mechanism commonly used in industrial control systems. A PID controller continuously calculates an error value as the difference between a measured process variable and a desired setpoint.

As an alternative, the mass flow rate can be measured and controlled by a liquid tank (Figure 6.10) placed on load cells with the same loss in weight control described above. Instead of changing the screw speed, the same signals are used to control the pump speed.

The benefits of a mass flow meter versus a load cell arrangement are that there are no special refill devices required and the controls are fairly simple. The benefits of the loss-in-weight arrangement include easier calibration, lack of a pressure drop experienced by the measuring device, suitability for liquids in excess of 150°C, and most importantly, higher accuracy in feed and control.

6.2.4   FEEDER TYPES USED IN PHARMACEUTICAL EXTRUSION OPERATIONS

6.2.4.1   Vibratory Feeders

In the case of a vibratory feeder, the material is metered by means of vibration. As shown in Figure 6.11, by adjusting the amplitude of the vibration, a set amount of material can

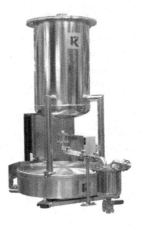

FIGURE 6.10   Pharmaceutical liquid loss-in-weight feeder.

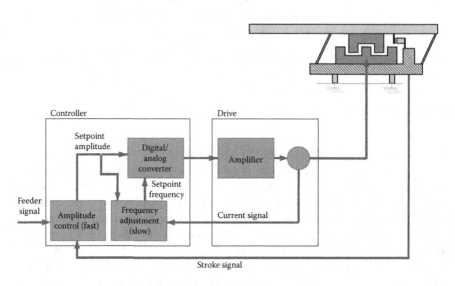

FIGURE 6.11   Vibratory feeding principle.

be delivered. These devices can be provided in both gravimetric and volumetric options, and they are often well suited not only for free-flowing materials, but also materials with high aspect ratios. A loss-in-weight vibratory feeder is shown in Figure 6.12.

In vibratory loss-in-weight feeding, the system controls the motion of the tray. The amplitude of vibration is adjusted in accordance with the weight setpoint. This motion includes tray displacement and rate of oscillation. In general, these feeders are usually not well suited for the metered feed of cohesive materials, since the vibration effect may cause the material to clump in the delivery tray, thus delivering the product inconsistently to the process below. However, it should be noted that they have been successful for very low rate feeding, in cases where extremely cohesive materials may bind to screw feeders. In these cases, the vibration is so minimal that

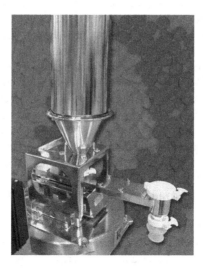

FIGURE 6.12   Pharmaceutical vibratory LIW feeder.

it does not cause excessive clumping of material, but rather exerts just enough force to feed the material evenly to the process below.

6.2.4.2 Single- or Twin-Screw Feeders

Screw feeders represent the most versatile feed technology for most bulk solids. Given the material characteristics, a variety of screw configurations varying in both screw pitch and diameter are available to cover a wide variety of feed ranges. In addition, screw feeders can have a single- or twin-screw design, as shown in Figure 6.13.

Of special note is the basic distinction between the material handling capabilities of twin-screw versus single-screw design. Where two screws intermesh and corotate, the result is the formation of relatively sealed, forward moving pockets of material. Thus, the twin-screw feeder acts similar to a positive displacement pump to first capture floodable or poor-flowing materials and then forcibly moving them to discharge.

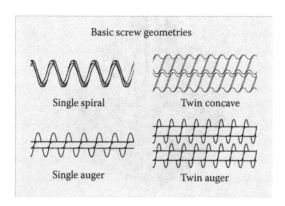

FIGURE 6.13   Screw configurations available for twin-screw and single-screw feeders.

In addition, an added advantage, similar to that of the twin-screw extruder, is the self-wiping action of the screws that helps to keep the screw surfaces clean and free of buildup. Single screws, whether in a spiral or auger type design, do not possess this type of pumping action, and thus are not recommended or appropriate for floodable or cohesive, poor-flowing materials. Due to the high turndown ratio and flexibility of design, screw feeders can also be provided to feed extremely accurately at rates as low as 20 gm/hr, with screws as small as 12 mm in diameter, as shown in Figure 6.14.

Twin-screw feeders are often the technology of choice for pharmaceutical operations because of their sanitary design, inclusion of stainless steel, easy disassembly, and adherence to cGMP and FDA design guidelines for pharmaceutical equipment. Additional options are also available that include designs for completely contained feeding of potent compounds, ATEX and explosion proof electricals, and integration of wash-in-place retractable spray balls.

It is important to note that any screw feeder accuracy is largely dependent upon consistent screw fill. To ensure this consistent screw fill, there are a number of flow-aid devices that may be required in the feeder's hopper to ensure that the process material flows into the feeding device as uniformly as possible. Again, the more stable or uniform the material flow is, the easier it is for the weighing and control system to provide optimal second to second performance. Several types of material flow aids are available, such as:

Mechanical hopper agitators: These stir the material and break down any bridging or rat-holing of the material. These agitators can include horizontal type configurations mounted by the screws to facilitate flow into the screw area and possibly vertical agitators that provide additional agitation in the hopper above. Vertical agitators often include a separate motor and require additional headroom for the feeder. In addition, they can become a cleaning concern.

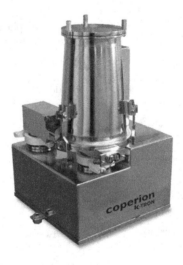

FIGURE 6.14 Twin-screw microfeeder.

Vibration on the feeder hopper: In the case of loss-in-weight feeders, this vibration can cause interference with the loss-in-weight signal if the control system cannot filter out this vibration. In addition, constant uncontrolled external vibration can cause excessive packing of the material within the hopper. Alternatively, some new control technologies are available that utilize vibration applied to the hopper and use an external drive tied directly into the weight system controls. This drive operates at a variable frequency and amplitude based on the weighing and control system detecting nonuniform material flow by weight. This real-time device activates the external vibration when there is an upset in the loss in weight signal. By detecting changes in the signal, it can detect conditions prior to bridging or rat holes, and prevent these from happening at all. This technique provides added benefits in that it eliminates headroom and cleaning concerns and avoids compaction of the process material because only the necessary amount of vibration is applied to the material to assure uniform material flow.

Flexible side walled feeders: These feeders gently agitate materials. It should be noted, however, that they do not have stainless steel surfaces and may wear or create contamination concerns.

6.2.5 THE IMPORTANCE OF REFILL ON A CONTINUOUS LIW SYSTEM

The design of the refill system for a LIW feeder that is feeding a continuous extrusion process can be almost as critical as choosing the right feeder technology. When refilling a loss-in-weight feeder, it is imperative that the refill devices be reliable to maintain a constant flow of either the API or excipient to the process within a specific refill time limit. This time limit must be relatively short, in order to allow the feeder to return to a true gravimetric operation, and ensure constant mass flow of the product to the process. The method of refill, reaction time of the refill device, and also the size of the refill hopper are all critical variables in ensuring an accurate and consistent flow of material to the LIW feeder.

6.2.6 LIW REFILL DEFINED

Two basic ways exist to refill the feeder hopper: the manual method and the automatic method. The manual method implies that a quantity of bulk solids is tossed into the feeder hopper by the plant operator and the process continues. The automatic method implies that dosing machinery under control of the feed system will add material to the feeder hopper from an upstream supply as shown in Figure 6.15.

In the past, the traditional method of maintaining feed was simply to utilize a constant metering speed throughout the refill phase—a speed corresponding to the metering speed associated with gravimetric control just prior to entering the refill phase. If, for example, the metering speed averaged 60 rpm just prior to the system sensing the need to refill the supply hopper, the screw speed would be maintained at that 60 rpm for the duration of the refill operation. After refill is completed, the material has settled, and the feeder senses an appropriately declining system weight, the feeder is returned to gravimetric operation in which metering speed once again becomes the parameter of control.

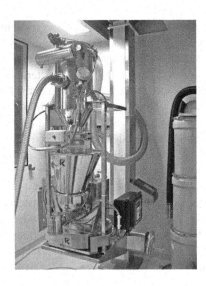

FIGURE 6.15   LIW feeder with butterfly valve and pneumatic refill.

6.2.7   REFILL CONTROL ALGORITHMS

The older method of simply utilizing a constant refill speed mitigates two significant problems in accurate feed to the process below. First, the feeder is only acting as a volumetric device, without any sensitivity to material density changes within the hopper. Second, upon reentry to true loss-in-weight control, abrupt changes in feeder speed can occur, resulting in a sometimes extended period of off-spec flow until the feeder settles at the new proper speed. These abrupt speed changes occur due to the fact that screw fill efficiency changes during refill, and material density at the bottom of the hopper can be somewhat higher than it was prior to refill.

To remedy these problems, it is sometimes necessary to utilize control measures during refill to compensate for the increasing density or headload of material about to be discharged. This can be achieved by gradually altering feeder speed in such a manner as to precisely mirror the effects of increasing density and headload. To determine the appropriate speed at any given material level in the refill process, the relationship between flow rate and feeder control output (termed feed factors) is memorized during the entirety of the preceding gravimetric phase of operation. Then, during refill, reference is made to this array of feed factors, called refill array. The appropriate motor speed can then be applied based on the sensed system weight as the hopper is filled. This correlation among mass flow, net hopper weight, and motor speed during the refill cycle is shown in Figure 6.16.

By taking this more sophisticated approach, it is possible to smoothly exit the refill phase and return to true gravimetric operation. Additionally, by controlling feeder speed during refill based on the most recent performance history, reverting to volumetric performance is avoided and gravimetric accuracy is essentially preserved.

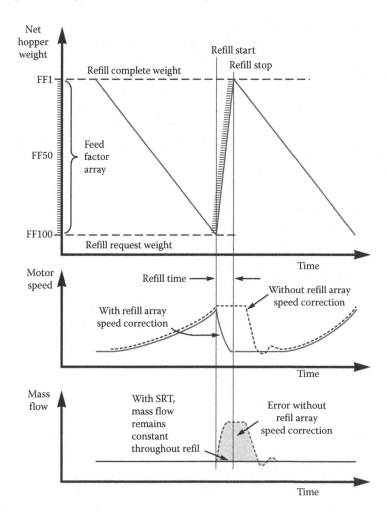

FIGURE 6.16   Refill array and loss-in-weight feeder performance.

6.2.7.1   Refill Times and Material Effects on Refill

As a rule, the refill period should be about 6–10 seconds. This duration ensures positive control over the incoming material but is so short that minor flow variations should not perturb the downstream processes. However, the material characteristics described in Section II of this chapter should also be evaluated. Each of these material characteristics will greatly affect not only the flow out of the hopper but also how quickly the hopper is refilled. For example, if the bulk material has a high gas permeability (i.e., if gas can escape rapidly from the solid), the refill can occur as rapidly as is feasible. On the other hand, if the bulk material has a very low permeability rate (i.e., the gas expands the bulk material and doesn't quickly escape to return the solid to its resting condition), care must be taken during refill, because these materials often become floodable in this condition or at least suffer significant bulk density changes.

If flooding of the bulk solid begins during refill, the product could easily flush out of the loss-in-weight feeder. Air entrainment effects resulting in underfeed conditions during and immediately after refill can significantly alter bulk density, since the control system is using control data from earlier in the run, when the product density was much higher. Air entrainment comes from rapidly refilling the feed hopper, such that air, being unable to quickly escape, passes through the incoming material to the region of lower pressure above in the refill hopper. Venting of the weighed hopper can minimize the problem, but now dust collection and, in the case of active materials, filtration must be arranged. Adequate venting will assist in material settling and aid in a quicker return to true gravimetric operation.

6.2.7.2 Refill Hopper Sizing

Another issue that often arises with refill systems is determining how often the feeder should refill to get the best performance. This is also dependent on the properties of the material, behavior of the bulk solid during transfer from the refill bin to the weighed hopper, and responsiveness of the weight measurement system to rapidly changing weight values that occur when frequent refills occur. If the system is refilled more frequently, the feeder is spending more time in volumetric control. However, if headroom and space are not an issue, the weighed hopper size can be made larger, thus having the feeder in volumetric control for less time. The longer a feeder remains in volumetric control, the more likely it is to drift away from delivering the desired setpoint. Table 6.3 outlines some of the benefits and pitfalls of refill hopper sizing.

6.2.8 REFILL DEVICES

The flow rate from the refill device must be sufficient to avoid exceeding the refill time limit. Additionally, the flow cutoff action of the selected device must be quick and sure. A slow tapering off of the refill flow needlessly lengthens refill time, and any leakage of the refill device may cause an unavoidable measurable weight disturbance, but will always result in a flow error in the positive direction.

There are several choices on the type of refill device utilized above the feeder hopper. Options include knife gates, modulating butterfly valves, or in the case where extreme control and accuracy is required (low rate feeding), the use of alternate metered devices such as volumetric screw feeders. This is illustrated in Figure 6.17. In addition, the use of pneumatic loaders above the butterfly valve or rotary airlock is often employed to transfer the material to a receiver above the feeder hopper.

A knife gate or a slide gate might be acceptable if the feeder hopper is large and consumes most of the vertical space between the weighed hopper and the refill hopper, and if modulation of the gate valve is feasible for the given bulk material flow characteristics. Problems arise when the refill system does not take into consideration the capacity of the feeder hopper, the flow properties of the bulk solid, and the distance and potential storage volume of bulk solids that can occur between them.

For example, in refilling a feeder hopper from an IBC, supersack, or large hopper, the volume of the product in these vessels will often times exceed the volume of the

TABLE 6.3

Benefits and Issues for Refill Systems Discharging into Both Large and Small Feeder Hoppers

Hopper	Benefits	Problems
Small	• Uses more sensitive scale for potentially higher accuracy • Requires less vertical space • May spend less time in volumetric control during filling • Quick to clean, less surface area	• Refill system is more stressed by a higher cycle rate • If refill system fails, less time is available to correct problem before emptying • Powder may not de-aerate in a timely manner • For difficult flowing powders, a special refill system may be required to extract product from the refill bin
Large	• Fewer refills, easier on the refill system • Bulk material flow may be better in a larger hopper • More time is available to correct a refill failure • More settling time is available for the powders • Refill may be easier with difficult powders since a larger hopper inlet opening is possible	• Potentially less accurate weighing at setpoint because of the large weight of material being weighed • Takes up more vertical space • Larger hopper, more surface area, more cleaning time required • Feeder supports must be more robust • Long emptying times may permit consolidation and packing of bulk materials, making withdrawal difficult

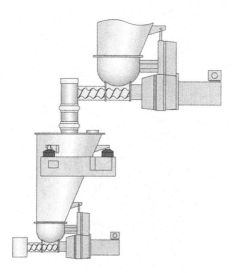

FIGURE 6.17   Refill of LIW feeder using volumetric feeder.

feeder hopper. Clearly, it is impossible to control the refill without overfilling the feeder hopper, unless a time window is established for the opening and closing cycle of the refill valve. This time window can be calculated based on bulk density of the material, the angle of repose that dictates the settling leveling the feeder hopper, and the flow rate through the refill device. It should also be noted that when discharging from bins or IBCs that may be equipped with flow aid devices (e.g., vibrators or live bottom bins), special care must be taken to isolate the vibration of these devices from the feeder hopper, in order to prevent interference with the loss-in-weight feeder weight measuring device.

Pneumatic receivers that operate under a dilute or dense phase vacuum transfer principle are often used as refill devices, particularly for continuous operations, as illustrated in Figure 6.18. The pneumatic system utilizes negative pressure to suck the material required to refill into a separate mounted and supported vacuum receiver. The receiver is filled to a determined level and then holds this material charge until the feeder below requests a refill. The level of fill in the receiver is determined by level sensors. At the point of refill request by the feeder below, the discharge valve opens and the receiver contents are discharged into the feeder hopper. At the same time as this release, a gas pulse is sent through the filter housed in the vacuum receiver, in order to release any entrained particulate or material that may have settled on the filter. The filter material can vary, with options including laminated membrane type materials, for quick release and easy clean properties.

After the material is dumped into the feeder hopper below, the valve is shut again and then the receiver vacuum cycle immediately begins, in order for the pneumatic

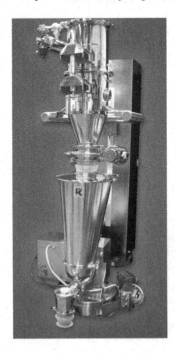

FIGURE 6.18 Loss-in-weight feeder with butterfly valve and pneumatic receiver.

receiver to be instantly ready for the next refill request. The use of pneumatic receivers as refill devices allows for an uninterrupted source of refill from bags, drums, IBCs, or supersacks.

6.2.9   WEIGHING TECHNOLOGIES USED IN LIW FEEDING

Any loss-in-weight process controller requires accurate high speed measurement of material weight changes in order to provide optimal feeder control and performance, especially on a second to second basis. The weighing system must also be able to filter out erroneous measurements due to in-plant vibrations or disturbances and be stable over changes in process room or process material temperatures. Two types of weighing technologies are typically used in loss-in-weight feeders. They are (1) analog strain gauge technology and (2) digital vibrating wire technology. The higher the resolution of weight measurement and the faster those weight measurements are taken, the better the information that will be provided to the control algorithm to work and the better any vibration filtering algorithm will work. In addition, almost all weighing systems provide temperature compensation. The exact temperature range should be verified, as this can affect the long-term stability of feeder performance.

6.2.10   LOAD CELL RESOLUTION

In order to be sensitive to low mass flow rates, load cells must have an extremely high resolution. For example, a typical scale with an analog load cell for feeding bulk solids at low mass flow rates can have a weighing range of 32 kg and a resolution of 1:65,000. This scale can detect approximately 500-mg weight changes. Typically weight changes per second should be approximately five times higher than the minimum resolution, which is equivalent to 2.5 g/sec (9 kg/hr). When feeding at this rate it takes the controller 20 sec to detect whether the setpoint is reached within a deviation of ±1%. If the mass flow rate is below 9 kg/hr, it becomes even more difficult to detect improvements of gravimetric control versus volumetric control. Therefore, any mass flow rate below 9 kg/hr may not even see a significant improvement with gravimetric control.

Conversely, a typical platform scale with a digital load cell with a weighing range of 24 kg and a resolution of 1:4,000,000 can actually detect 6 mg. The limit value can therefore be reduced from 9 kg/hr to approximately 108 gm/hr. This is significant for low mass flow rates, such as those that may be for low formulation percentage APIs and also for high required second to second accuracy. In addition, higher resolution also results in improved feeder accuracy for high mass flow rates as well.

6.2.11   INFLUENCES ON WEIGHING TECHNOLOGIES

Due to the high accuracies required in the pharmaceutical industry, a number of additional influences on the weighing system must be taken into consideration when designing and setting up the loss-in-weight feeder and refill system. These process considerations include isolation and balancing of the feed weigh assembly, minimizing external vibrations, and isolating external pressure or vacuum influences on the weigh scale. These external influences can be even more influential at even lower feed rates.

6.2.12 Weight Balancing

It is important to position the feeder so that no external forces or friction can influence the weighing. Flexible connections to any other part of the system, such as at the product or refill inlet and product discharge, help to isolate the feeding system, as shown in Figure 6.19. In addition, any electrical cabling or flexible tube connections for the pneumatic drives or cleaning nozzles must be isolated from the weigh scale. These connections should not be stretched to avoid external forces on the scale.

6.2.13 Influences of Vibration

In-plant shock and vibration can also corrupt the weight measurement, destroying the basis for feed rate control. Since LIW feeder operation depends on accurate weight measurements of the material in the hopper, the feeder and weight-sensing device must be isolated from any external vibration created by other equipment in the process. Vibration can impose artificial forces on the feeder that cause weighing errors. This requires installing the feeder so that the weight-sensing device is shielded from vibration effects. It is important to ensure that the feeder has a stable mounting, flexible connections, and shock mounts, and that no strong air currents occur near the feeder. In addition, modern load cells and control algorithms are able to discriminate between the load to be measured and the transient forces imposed by vibration. In order to distinguish between these two, a sophisticated digital filtering algorithm can be applied to identify and extract frequency components characteristic of in-plant vibration.

6.2.14 Pressure

A feeder's refill cycle increases air pressure in the hopper due to the sudden inflow of material. Any positive air pressure acts equally toward all sides and pushes up on the hopper lid and the refill valve. Because the force in the inlet area is not applied

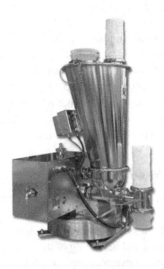

FIGURE 6.19 LIW feeder with flexible connections on inlet and discharge.

to the hopper lid but to the refill valve above, pressure forces inside the hopper are not balanced. Due to the inlet opening, forces acting up on the lid are lower than those acting down oppositely on the floor of the hopper. The higher forces acting down result in an increase in the weight signal. The loss-in-weight controller would interpret the increased weight signal to mean that mass flow is slowing and react by erroneously increasing the feeder output, creating a mass flow error.

Hopper pressure issues can also have other causes such as a clogged vent filter, a dust collection system connected to the hopper vent, or a nitrogen blanket applied to the hopper. Sometimes, the dust collection systems or nitrogen blankets are connected across many feeders and when any of the feeders refill, the others see pressure disturbances.

A pressure fluctuation at the feeder discharge also distorts the feeder's weight signal if the outlet is sealed with a cap. Pressure increases in the discharge tube push up on the cap, which, if it is connected to the feeder, pushes up on the feeder and reduces the measured weight. To mitigate pressure fluctuations on the outlet, the cap may be isolated from the feeder by a flexible bellows rigidly mounted to an outside structure. In addition, discharge pressure problems may be caused by extruder back pressure or extruder screw pulsations.

Traditionally, these troublesome pressure fluctuations have been compensated for by mechanical means (Figure 6.20). However, factors such as mechanical tolerances,

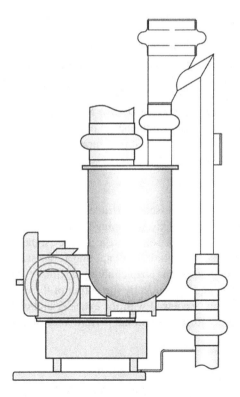

FIGURE 6.20   Mechanical design for pressure compensation.

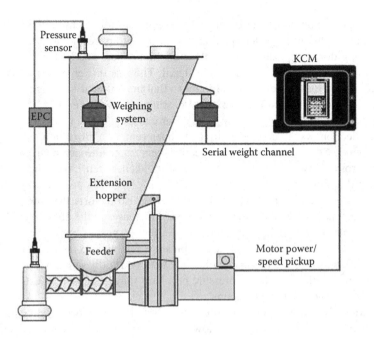

FIGURE 6.21 Electronic pressure compensation.

the alignment, number, age of the flexible bellows, etc., can impact the mechanical pressure compensation and prevent it from fully compensating for the forces generated by changing pressures, making this costly solution deficient. In addition, flexes provide additional side and vertical forces, thus affecting the hysteresis of the scale.

Alternatively, instrumentation and control algorithms to electronically monitor and compensate for this pressure influence can be supplied. An example of a loss-in-weight feeder with this type of pressure compensation is shown in Figure 6.21.

6.3   SUMMARY

As outlined above, the use of twin-screw extruders coupled with highly accurate LIW feeding and refill systems is quickly becoming the manufacturing process of choice when developing pharmaceutical solid dosage forms. Higher accuracy feeders and integrated refill systems are essential to maintaining a consistent output in all continuous operations. As illustrated in the chapter above, a number of key factors will affect the feeder performance and subsequently the output of the extruder. It is imperative that all of these factors be reviewed with the extruder and/or feed and refill system supplier in detail in order to ensure optimal performance of the extrusion system.

BIBLIOGRAPHY

1. United States Food and Drug Administration. Current Good Manufacturing Practices, 21 CFR, Parts 210 and 211.

2. K-Tron Process Group, Smart refill technology in loss-in-weight feeding, Processing Magazine, Grand View Media Group, Birmingham, AL, March 2004.

3. Boilard, TG, Feeder selection for pharmaceutical extruder applications, *Medical Pharmaceutical Extrusion Conference*, Technical Paper delivered December 2001.

4. Ghebre-Sellassie, I, Martin, C, Pharmaceutical Extrusion Technology, Marcel Decker, New York, 2003.

5. Billings, JP, Bradley, RO, Damon, RH Jr, Hejzlar, S, Nielson, HA, Paelian, O, Platt, FL, Quinn, D, Shapiro, BH, Terms and definitions for the weighing industry, Scale Manufacturers Association, Inc, Washington DC, 1975.

6. Martin, C, Continuous mixing of solid dosage forms via hot-melt extrusion, *Pharmaceutical Technology*, Vol. 32, Issue 10, October 2008.

7. Crowley, MM, Zhang, F, Repka, MA, Thumma, S, Upadhye, SB, Kumar, S, McGinty, JW, Martin C, Review article: Pharmaceutical applications of hot melt extrusion: Part I, *Drug Development and Industrial Pharmacy*, 2007.

8. Nowak, S, Feeder accuracy and design: Critical parameters in continuous pharmaceutical operations, Pharmaceutical Online, May 2007.

9. Nowak, S, Choosing the right refill design for pharmaceutical loss-in-weight feeders, Pharmaceutical Online, March 2008.

10. Wilson, DH, Smart refill technology in loss-in-weight feeding, Processing Magazine, March 2004, Feeding Technologies for Plastic Processing, Hanser Publishing, Cincinnati, Ohio.

11. Doetsch, W, Material handling and feeder technology, *Pharmaceutical Extrusion Technology*, Marcel Decker Inc, New York, 2003.

7 Rheology, Torque, and Oscillatory Rheometers

*Scott T. Martin, Fengyuan Yang,
and Thomas Durig*

CONTENTS

The rheological characterization of molten materials for pharmaceutical extrusion processes is an important facet in many stages of product development. This characterization can be in the form of specific (absolute) rheological determination of an expected phenomenon (flow, temperature, time, relative humidity dependence, etc.) or a general (relative) "rating" of the system in comparative terms (expected degradation, product inspection, resistance to process and storage, etc.). Recently, both torque and oscillatory rheometers have been applied to the research and development of pharmaceutical hot melt extrusion (HME) for preparing API-polymer amorphous solid dispersions, melt granulation, and profile extrudate. In this chapter, we summarize a review of the fundamentals of both torque and oscillatory rheology by covering their basic principles, setups, and methods. In addition, we highlight several applications by utilizing viscoelastic properties of the polymer and API-polymer system gathered from a small sample size to assess, guide, and optimize the formulation development via HME.

7.1   TORQUE RHEOLOGY

A torque rheometer system is an extremely effective tool that has found application in characterizing rheological properties. Although traditionally used for plastic and food processes, this device has been embraced by the pharmaceutical industry to develop and produce wide-ranging formulations for solid dosage forms.

A torque rheometer is an instrument that is widely used in studying formulations, developing pharmaceutical dosage forms, and characterizing polymer (for example) flow behavior by measuring viscosity-related torque caused by the resistance of the material to the shearing action of the melting process. Its fundamental usefulness relates to the versatility of the instrument to simulate development or manufacturing processes within a small-scale "laboratory environment."

Before describing the system itself, it is important to define the primary characterization parameter obtained through the use of the instrument—torque. Torque can be described as the effectiveness of a force to produce rotation, and its mathematical function would equal the product of the force applied and the perpendicular distance from the line of action to the instantaneous center of rotation. By definition, torque can be described as

$$M = F \times r$$

where M is the torque, F is the force applied, and r is the radial arm (distance from the center of rotation to the force applied). Units of torque are typically given in m g, N m, or ft-lb (see Figure 7.1). The usefulness of this measurement in the characterization of a material and/or process lies in the comparative analysis of the torque registered by the system. This gives the user a "measure" of the resistance of the material to the process (and conditions) at hand. Through methodical variation of these parameters—materials and processes—a thorough comparison of materials and a potential for optimization of the process can be achieved. This can lead to useful functionality for the user in many areas of testing, ranging from standard quality control to pilot-scale investigations and production processing.

Torque rheometers have been in existence for nearly a century, originally finding application within the baking industry (flour dough quality control). Although the configurations have experienced several evolutions—purely mechanical, electronic, and microprocessor controlled—the basic goal of materials/process characterization

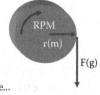

$M = F \times r$, where...
M = Torque
F = Force applied
r = Radial arm (distance from center of rotation to force applied)

FIGURE 7.1   Definition of torque.

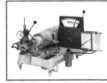

Mechanical torque rheometer
The mechanical torque rheometer system was truly that–it relied upon a lever arm, weight, and dashpot configuration (dynamometer) to physically sense deflection due to motor resistance. The system proved quite useful for testing purposes, however due to its mechanical nature calibration was difficult and frequently required. In addition, numerous external 'modules' were necessary for the control/monitoring of parameters such as temperature and pressure.

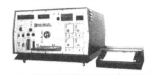

Electronic torque rheometer
The next generation of torque rheometers were built primarily to address the inconveniences of the mechanical. The system was semi-automatic, relatively compact with most 'modules' and features (calibration, analysis) built in, and featured a unique measuring system that introduced a transducer to monitor axial movement of a lever arm/idler gear configuration.

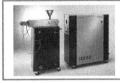

Microprocessor-controlled torque rheometer
This most recent evolution of the torque rheometer provides a complete incorporation of all facets of testing within one versatile, compact system. It allows for the user to not only control but also monitor, collect, and analyze information from a variety of signal sources. In addition, the system offers a variety of range-specific strain gauges, positioned directly in-line to the output shaft which thus produces a true torque signal with excellent resolution.

FIGURE 7.2 The evolution of the torque rheometer.

has been well preserved (see Figure 7.2). What has been learned is currently being applied to develop GMP products.

The torque rheometer system has been developed primarily in a "building-block" fashion that allows the combination of different types of instruments to be mated to the torque rheometer, which is utilized as the instrument's main-drive motor. These instrument additions are in actuality "simulators" of the varying processes and include miniaturized mixers (batch compounders), twin-screw extruders (continuous compounders), single-screw extruders (product processing instruments), and a host of auxiliary equipment to complete the "simulation" (see Figure 7.3).

It is important to note that although the torque rheometer is used as the main drive, this is not its primary function. An accurate and application-specific drive is important for the system; however, the torque rheometer's true utility is derived from its ability to process not only all of the signals from the sensors (temperature, pressure, feeding, ancillary conditions, etc.) but also primarily to maintain precise monitoring of the torque on the system. This is accomplished with a torque transducer (or load cell) positioned in line with the attached sensor. An added feature of modern torque rheometer systems is an easily removable load cell (see Figure 7.4), which allows for application-specific matching of the load cell to the required testing range (to obtain better resolution in the torque signal).

A walk-through procedure applicable to generalized torque rheometry testing would be as follows:

1. A system (or sensor) is defined, based upon the objective of the process simulation.
2. Process conditions for initial testing are defined (materials, temperatures, instrument speed, etc.). It is noted as "initial" because the modification of these to review the response/outcome is commonly the objective of the testing.

3. Testing is performed and optimized (if necessary).
4. Information through testing is collected. This information can include not only the testing parameters and variables (torque, set temperatures, resultant materials temperatures, resultant materials pressures, etc.) but also the material in its final form.
5. The analysis is performed based upon the results.

The typical output objective for testing is material and/or process characterization. This can be broken down into four areas of particular torque rheometry interest. These would be as follows:

Viscosity—the internal resistance of a fluid to flow under a defined shear rate and resultant shear stress

Elasticity—a property of a material by virtue of which it tends to recover its original size and shape following deformation

Shear sensitivity—the nature of a material to break down structurally when exposed to shear stresses (during processing)

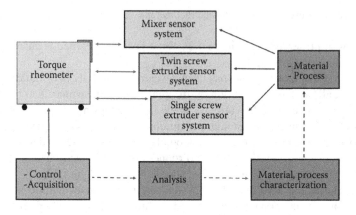

FIGURE 7.3 Block diagram of torque rheometer process.

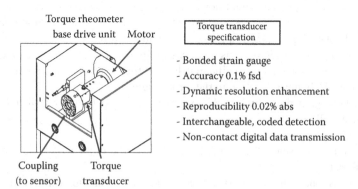

FIGURE 7.4 Removable load cell.

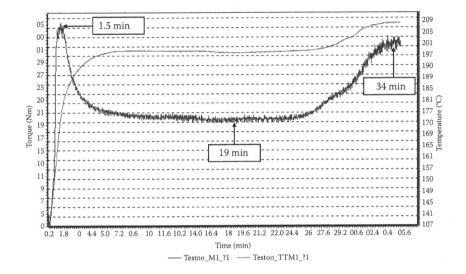

FIGURE 7.5 Batch mixer rheograph example.

Temperature sensitivity—the response of a material to its thermal history (during processing)

As an example of a common torque rheometer experiment and the results obtained, please refer to Figure 7.5. The graph, also known as a rheograph (torque vs. time curve), shows the response of a material to a process simulated by a torque rheometer/batch-mixer system. Torque and melt temperature are critical parameters to provide insight into the viability of the formulation being evaluated.

An evaluation technique quite common to rheograph data includes the observation of a torque signal at significant points (or times) during the testing. These data can be used to compare against a standard material, to indicate physical or chemical state changes, or to determine the work required for processing the material.

7.2 TORQUE RHEOMETER WITH BATCH-MIXING SENSOR

Now that some general definitions for the system have been defined, more detail as to the specific sensors and their applications will be given. Although not an extrusion device, it is important to understand the miniature batch-mixing sensor, which often serves as the starting point for formulation development. Many materials that are utilized for pharmaceutical products are essentially a combination of different material types, chosen to impart the benefits of the individual properties. However, theoretical compounds often do not perform as predicted because of material incompatibility, unforeseen chemical reactions between components, or the unexpected impartation of detrimental properties from individual components of the blend. A torque rheometer with a batch-mixing sensor provides a means by which the user can simulate compounding on a small, tightly controlled system to offer a useful prediction of these combinations. In addition, the system provides a means by which the compounding conditions for known formulations can be optimized.

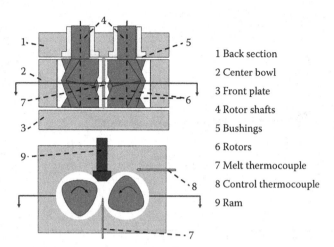

1 Back section
2 Center bowl
3 Front plate
4 Rotor shafts
5 Bushings
6 Rotors
7 Melt thermocouple
8 Control thermocouple
9 Ram

FIGURE 7.6   Batch mixing system.

The standard mixer system consists primarily of a central bowl section hollowed out to resemble a "figure eight." Within each lobe of the "eight" a rotor blade is housed, the type of which is chosen depending on the level of shear the user wishes to impart to the sample. These blades are rotated in opposing directions and at varying speeds in order to promote good flow/mixing and optimum shearing action between the two lobes. The mixer chamber is completed through the incorporation of a front and back plate, which essentially close off and seal the bowl at both ends. A loading device and ram are utilized to introduce the sample into the chamber and define the final volume within the system (the lower portion of the ram actually forms the top wall of the mixing chamber) (see Figure 7.6).

As has been described, the mixing system consists of three separate sections (back plate, center bowl, and front plate). In addition to allowing for ease of disassembly (useful in cleaning), this also allows for individual temperature control in each of the three sections (a specific number of cartridge heaters are typically embedded within each section, along with a respective control thermocouple). This is important within miniaturized mixing systems as even slight temperature variations of a few degrees can cause dramatic changes in the results. This is important, as a significant degree of the heat energy resultant within the system is a result of the shear energy imparted from the motor and rotating screws (shear heating). For this reason, cooling is also available to attempt to maintain a proper temperature level (air cooling channels are typically routed through the central bowl; air flow is automatically controlled via programmed solenoid actuation). And finally, as there will exist definite differences between the set temperature and the actual temperature of the material (mainly because of shear heating), a melt thermocouple is typically incorporated in the center bowl and protrudes within the chamber itself (refer to Figure 7.6). This signal provides an additional parameter that is utilized for material/process characterization.

There are a number of variables incorporated within the mixing system that allow for the manipulation of the resultant mixing mechanism. As noted, one that is extremely important would be the shear (or shear rate) induced upon the sample. This variable can be manipulated through the use of different rotor blades, the programming of different rotor speeds, and through bowl temperature modifications (as the viscosity of many materials is temperature dependent as well as shear dependent). Other variables that can affect the outcome (or efficiency) would include sample size or percentage loading, set temperature, and residence time during each stage of the experiment (the user may wish to incorporate a number of staged condition sets to expand the information obtained).

A number of testing procedures have become standardized in the usage of a torque rheometer/batch-mixing system combination. A few examples, along with the results obtained, are described below.

7.2.1 Batch Differentiation

Pharmaceutical formulations can often be differentiated through the associated torque (relative viscosity) levels under varying degrees of shear. Typical usage for this type of test would be to predict the success/failure of a modification made to a "good" formulation (or standard). For example, Material A with a certain level of "additive" has been processed within a torque rheometer/batch-mixer system and gives a respective rheograph (see Figure 7.7). In the interest of improving the compound's efficacy, the users are investigating the processing response of Material A with different additive levels.

It is evident that specific changes can be noted between the torque curves for the two different formulations. The levels of torque for the two systems react differently within the first four min of testing, although after that point both compounds seem to stabilize at a certain similar value (approximately 23 N m). Beyond approximately 13 min, however, it is important to note that a significant increase in the formulation with limited stabilizer can be seen. On the other hand, the material with increased

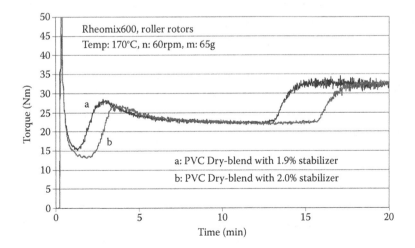

FIGURE 7.7 Batch differentiation rheograph.

stabilizer continues on with a stable torque signal until almost 16 min. As a synopsis, it could be concluded that by reducing the amount of additive within the formulation, the users have reduced the amount of time before degradation will take place within the system by approximately three min. However, this does not mean that the experiment was a failure—it could be the case that the residence time for the actual manufacturing (extrusion) process can accept this reduction in "stable time."

7.2.2 SAMPLE COMPOUNDING FOR EXTERNAL EVALUATION

One important feature of a torque rheometer/batch-mixer system is the ability to compound small quantities of materials for external evaluation. A typical mixing system can operate with as little as 50 g of material, which is often sufficient for standard torque rheometry evaluation as well as sample collection during varying stages of the compounding process (see Figure 7.8). Specialized systems are also available that operate with as little as 6 g of material.

Within this test, the standard procedure was modified to incorporate a collection of the material at specified time intervals for visual inspection.

7.2.3 SPECIALIZED ADAPTATIONS FOR SPECIFIC TESTING

As has been mentioned, the torque rheometer system provides the user with great flexibility in testing protocol. This can prove exceptionally beneficial for very specific testing requirements in that the system can be readily adapted to meet these needs. One case in which a system has been modified that is used in the rubber industry is to determine the conductivity of rubber compounds as a measure of the dispersion of carbon black.

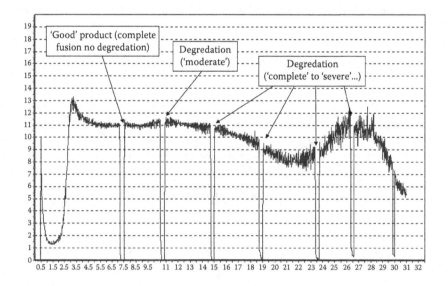

FIGURE 7.8 Sample evaluation with data collection.

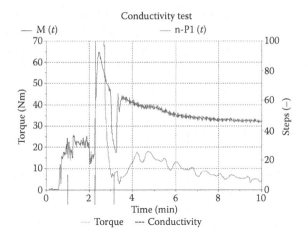

FIGURE 7.9 Conductivity measurement.

A common testing procedure within the rubber industry involves the blending of rubber with carbon black within a torque rheometer system. Based on varying levels of shear, a relative measure of the degree of an additive's incorporation can be made directly through the observation of the torque signal. This information gives a good indication of the dispersion of carbon black within the base material. Within this experiment, however, the batch mixer has been modified to incorporate a conductivity sensor in place of the common melt thermocouple (in the central bowl). The chamber wall then would act as a secondary electrode and, depending on the dispersion of carbon black within the base resin, a specific value of conductivity will be measured. This method provides an additional manner in which the degree of dispersion of carbon black can be evaluated (see Figure 7.9).

7.3   TORQUE RHEOMETER WITH TWIN-SCREW EXTRUDER SENSOR

A torque rheometer with twin-screw extruder sensor is in many ways similar to the batch mixer combination. The system allows the user to blend various types of materials and additives for the production of a compound; however, an important difference is that this system allows simulation for a continuous production. In addition, more complex configurations and operations are available with the continuous system, which is not feasible for batch processes.

In general, twin-screw systems are utilized for continuous compounding (mixing) applications. This process may result in a final product being formed or may act as an intermediary step in its development. Whatever the case, the addition of a torque rheometer system to the twin-screw extruder allows the user to simulate this task while maintaining a very tight level of control over the various parameters involved (screw speed, zone temperatures, feeding systems, post extrusion devices, etc.). In addition, experimental signals such as melt temperatures, pressures, and output rates are monitored to assist in an analysis of the development. Just as a batch mixer allows the user to investigate a material and simulated process, the twin-screw extruder allows for an actual small-scale compounding process to be performed and optimized in real time under processing conditions and constraints.

The following detail a few examples of common applications for twin-screw extrusion/torque rheometer systems.

7.3.1 SAMPLE PRODUCTION WITHIN A COUNTERROTATING, CONICAL TWIN-SCREW SYSTEM

The importance of torque rheometer systems is evident, as they have been applied for many years to the PVC plastics used in medical devices, such as tubing. A good complement to this test would be the utilization of a laboratory conical twin-screw system for the creation of a sample based on these PVC materials. Figure 7.10 shows how a correlation can be made between the residence time or process time for the material within the extruder, as a complement to degradation information obtained from a batch-mixing system.

7.3.2 CLINICAL TRIALS WITHIN A COROTATING, PARALLEL TWIN-SCREW SYSTEM

One of the most beneficial facets of the torque rheometer system is that it provides the user with a great degree of control over not only the processing parameters but also the environment within which the system is run. The units are often referred to as "lab scale," clearly describing the fact that these devices are smaller than their production-sized counterparts. This reduction in size also means that in general all operations performed on these systems can be accomplished with a greater degree of flexibility and ease—startup, maintenance of the run, sample collection, shutdown, and cleaning. This can be of great interest for small-scale clinical studies, as commonly performed within the pharmaceutical industry.

In order to further facilitate this ability, many systems have been designed to exaggerate this ease of usage. An example might be a corotating twin-screw extruder with a 15- to 30-mm screw diameter and a clamshell design barrel, which allows users to fully disassemble and investigate all portions of the device. This provides

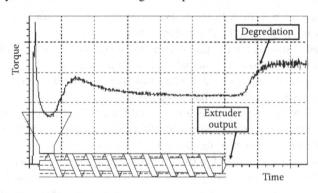

FIGURE 7.10 Residence time and degradation correlation for PVC compound from batch mixer applied to the extrusion process.

great utility not only for the shutdown and cleaning of the unit, but also in simple shear investigations—during a trial the system can be stopped (drive unit) and temperatures within the extruder lowered to solidify the materials within. The top portion of the barrel can then be removed and a visual examination of the sample's progression (and shear history) down the extruder screws can be made. Further morphology studies could then also be made through the collection and comparison of samples at varying positions within the extruder.

7.3.3 MICROCOMPOUNDING

A large portion of applications for torque rheometer systems stems from the research and development of new materials. One reason for this lies in the cost of these materials, which can be thousands of dollars per kilogram. An additional cause could be a lack of availability of large sample sizes, often the situation with new and experimental materials. Whatever the case, taking advantage of a system that utilizes samples in gram sizes as opposed to kilogram quantities is certainly beneficial. A microscale compounder does exactly this.

A microscale compounder is essentially a system that allows for the user to compound very small quantities of material in a style as close to traditional extrusion as possible (see Figure 7.11). Predominant systems currently on the market offer a conical extrusion design. Some provide a "backflow" channel, which enables the user to maintain the testing material within the system as long as desired, thus defining the residence time. The unit itself is typically instrumented to control and measure a number of different testing parameters (torque, temperature, and pressure), and visualization software is also available to assist with data handling and analysis. Studies are possible with as little as 6 g with this type of device.

An experiment performed using a microcompounder can be seen in Figure 7.12, which demonstrates a reactive extrusion process utilizing a bypass valve. The use of

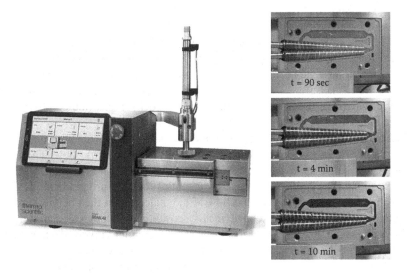

FIGURE 7.11   Twin-screw microcompounder with clamshell barrel and bypass valve.

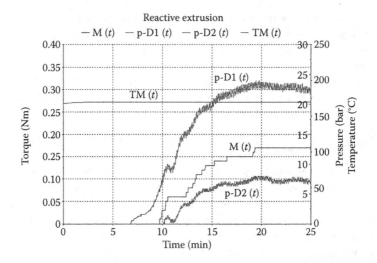

FIGURE 7.12 Reactive extrusion analysis of microcompounder.

a bypass valve allows the material to recirculate in the system and demonstrates that the time to reaction begins at approximately seven min and stabilizes after approximately 18 min. This information can assist in assessing processing parameters for this material within production.

7.4 TORQUE RHEOMETER WITH SINGLE-SCREW EXTRUDER SENSOR

The flow mechanisms for single-screw systems promote a constant, positive displacement of material, which enables a stable, surge-free pressurization to the exit (die) of the system and the creation of a "good," unvarying product.

In addition to production simulation and quality control, a torque rheometer and single-screw extruder can also be utilized for an absolute measurement of a sample's properties. In essence, absolute viscosity information can be obtained by assembling a system that simulates traditional piston-type capillary flow within an extrusion process. Both measurements utilize the same measuring principles; however, the mode in which the process melt is prepared and delivered to the capillary varies between the two.

In terms of the base measuring principle, a test sample is forced through a capillary (rod or slit) of known geometry with a constant volumetric flow. The sample creates, depending upon its viscosity, a flow resistance that results in a pressure gradient along the capillary. This measurement of the pressure gradient provides a calculated shear stress. The volume flow of the material can then be measured and used to calculate the shear rate. The melt viscosity can then be calculated through the division of the shear stress by shear rate. The calculations involved depend on the geometries of the capillaries in question (different for slit and rod types). In addition, several corrections are necessary to account for error-inducing effects within the capillary (entrance pressurization) and to correlate for non-Newtonian flow.

Extruder-type capillary rheometers use a laboratory extruder to prepare the process melt stream and feed the capillary die. The variation of screw speed of the extruder sets different shearing rates. The flow rate of the test material is either measured using one of several balance methods (manual, semiautomatic, or automatic) or controlled through the use of a melt pump system. The advantages associated with using an extruder to simulate an extrusion process are inherently obvious.

7.5 OSCILLATORY RHEOLOGY

Other experiments often used to characterize the rheological properties of a molten polymeric system are oscillatory shear. Oscillatory rheometers have been the most popular instrument for measuring rheological properties of polymeric melt in the plastic industry because oscillatory shear experiments enable easier measurement of the storage and loss moduli than the relaxation experiments that required generating a step stress or strain. In a typical oscillatory experiment, a sinusoidal wave of stress or strain is applied to the subject and the corresponding strain or stress is measured and fitted to a sinusoidal function. In fact, this fitting process works as a filter that can significantly reduce the noise that is nonsinusoidal or others rather than an imposed function. In addition, the noise rejection is enhanced with the increase of repeating test cycles. In comparison, a step stress or strain measurement depends on the time, and the noise rejection is achieved by repeating the entire experiment and averaging multiple runs together. In contrast, oscillatory shear, whose time scale is determined by the frequency of oscillation, is an easier and more accurate way to study the relaxation behavior of polymeric melts.

Before introducing the detailed fundamental terminologies in oscillatory rheology measurement, it is important to define some primary characteristics of materials, including elasticity, plasticity, viscoelasticity, and phase angle. Key differences between materials can be easily identified when measuring the time dependence of stress (strain) response to an applied strain (stress) at a single frequency. As shown schematically in Figure 7.13, if a material is ideally elastic, then the resultant stress (strain) is proportional to the applied strain (stress), and the proportionality constant is the shear modulus of the material. Moreover, the resultant stress (strain) is always exactly in phase with the applied sinusoidal strain (stress), where $\delta = 0$. Conversely, if a material is purely plastic, then the resultant stress (strain) in the sample is proportional to the rate of applied strain (stress), where the proportionality constant is the viscosity of the material. In addition, the applied strain (stress) and the measured stress (strain) are out of phase, with a phase angle $\delta = \pi/2$. The mechanical behaviors of polymers are complicated by the fact that many polymers are essentially viscoelastic, so their rheological properties lie between those of a purely elastic solid and those of a plastic liquid. The viscoelastic material shows a response that contains both in-phase and out-of-phase contributions and these contributions reveal the extents of elastic-like and plastic-like behavior. As a consequence, the total stress (strain) response shows a phase shift δ with respect to the applied strain (stress) that lies between that of an elastic solid and plastic liquid, $0 < \delta < \pi/2$.

As mentioned above, the basic concept of an oscillatory shear experiment is to introduce a sinusoidal shear deformation (strain) or stress to the sample and measure the resultant stress or strain response. For most currently commercially available

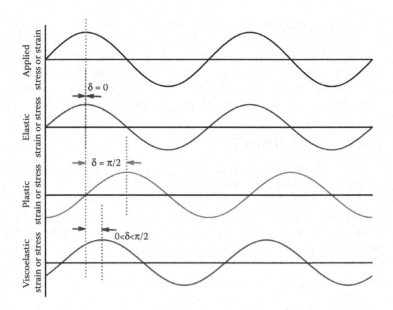

FIGURE 7.13 Schematic strain (stress) response to applied stress (strain) for an ideal elastic material, a purely plastic material, and a viscoelastic material.

oscillatory rheometers, they are either operated in a strain-controlled mode or in a stress-controlled mode. For a typical strain-controlled rheometer, the sample is subjected to a homogeneous deformation (strain) given by a motor, and a transducer is used to monitor the responding stress response from the material. Specifically, the motor generates a strain that is as close as possible to a sine wave:

$$\gamma = \gamma_0 \sin(\omega t)$$

When the applied strain amplitude is sufficiently small, the resultant stress response is within the linear region and can be fitted with a sinusoidal function. Specifically, the resulting stress can be measured by a transducer and written in terms of the stress amplitude (σ_0) and the loss angle (δ), which is a function of frequency, as below:

$$\sigma(t) = \sigma_0 \sin(\omega t + \delta)$$

Here, a new term of amplitude ratio, $G_d = \sigma_0/\gamma_0$ is defined and introduced, so the results of an oscillatory shear stress can be written in terms of the storage (G') and loss (G'') moduli as functions of frequency:

$$\sigma(t) = \gamma_0 [G'(\omega)\sin(\omega t) + G''(\omega)\cos(\omega t)]$$

where G' and G'' are calculated from G_d and δ as follows:

$$G' = G_d \cos(\delta)$$

$$G'' = G_d \sin(\delta)$$

Sometimes, it is useful to consider the storage and loss moduli to be the imaginary and real components of the complex viscosity, η^*. Thus, an alternative representation of oscillatory shear data in terms of complex viscosity can be defined as

$$\eta^* = \eta' - i\eta''$$

where the real and imaginary components are functions of frequency and related to the storage and loss moduli as follows:

$$\eta' = G'' / \omega$$

$$\eta'' = G' / \omega$$

Normally, the absolute value of the complex viscosity is of interest because it can be correlated with the steady-shear viscosity by the Cox-Merz rule.

In practice, the experimental data of oscillatory shear are converted into a set of discrete $G(t)$ according to a generalized Maxwell model. The discrete relaxation expressions of G' and G'' can be written as follows:

$$G'(\omega) = \sum_{i=1}^{N} \frac{G_i(\omega\tau_i)^2}{[1+(\omega\tau_i)^2]}$$

$$G''(\omega) = \sum_{i=1}^{N} \frac{G_i(\omega\tau_i)}{[1+(\omega\tau_i)^2]}$$

Because the generalized Maxwell model is widely used in the interpretation of the linear viscoelastic behavior of polymer melts, the appropriate models for polymers can be easily obtained by presenting the storage and loss moduli by taking just one term of the above summations. If both storage and loss moduli are plotted on a double logarithmic plot, we note that at low frequency, the storage modulus approaches a line with a slope of two, while the loss modulus approaches a line with a slope of one. At high frequency, the storage modulus goes to a constant, while the loss modulus approaches zero.

Another key term obtained from the oscillatory shear test is the loss factor, tan (δ), or damping factor, with a unit of 1 and definition as follows:

$$\tan\delta = \frac{G''}{G'}$$

The loss factor is calculated as the quotient of the loss and storage modulus. Therefore, it represents the ratio of the plastic and the elastic portion within a viscoelastic material. In general, $0 \leq \tan(\delta) \leq \infty$ is always holding because δ is a function of frequency and follows $0 \leq \delta \leq \pi/2$. Ideal elastic behavior is specified in terms of tan $(\delta) = 0$ and $\delta = 0$ because G' completely dominates G''. In contrast, the ideal plastic behavior is expressed as tan $(\delta) = \infty$ and $\delta = \pi/2$, since here G'' completely dominates G'. If elastic and plastic behavior exactly balance each other, then tan $(\delta) = 1$ and $\delta = \pi/4$. Polymers are viscoelastic materials, which behave as plastic or elastic, depending on how fast (at what frequency) they flow or are deformed in the process.

7.6 OSCILLATORY GEOMETRY AND EXPERIMENT

The fundamentals of oscillatory rheology and measurement discussed above are applied to both strain-controlled and stress-controlled rheometers. A walkthrough procedure applicable to a generalized oscillatory rheological test would be as follows:

1. A system (oscillatory geometry) is selected, mainly based on the intrinsic properties of the subject.
2. An oscillatory experiment (amplitude, frequency, time, or temperature sweep) is defined, based on the objective of the system studied or process simulated.
3. A sample (preprepared specimen) is properly loaded into the rheometer and the test is performed and optimized (if necessary).
4. Information is collected through testing. This information can include not only the testing parameters and variables (modulus, viscosity, loss factor, strain, frequency, time, and temperatures), but also the specimen in its final state.
5. The analysis is performed based on the results.

The typical objective of oscillatory rheology testing is material and/or process characterization. To achieve this goal, both the selection of a suitable geometry and the design of an appropriate oscillatory experiment for a given system are very critical. In this section, we will focus on the details of the initial two steps of the procedure, including both introduction and selection of oscillatory geometry and introduction and design of the oscillatory experiment. Figure 7.14 displays several conventionally used geometries for an oscillatory rheometer, including concentric cylinders, cone and plate, parallel plates, and torsion rectangular. Before discussing the design of appropriate oscillatory experiments for a specific objective, it is worth introducing the fundamentals of individual geometry options and discussing how to select a suitable geometry for a given system.

1. The typical concentric-cylinder geometries include an outer cylinder (cup) and an inner cylinder (rotor). Both cylindrical components show the same symmetry axis if they are mounted in the working position. An oscillatory test has two operating modes: either the Searle method or the Couette method. Specifically, the Searle method sets the rotor in motion and the cup is stationary. In contrast, the Couette method operates the cup in motion and the rotor is stationary. In industrial laboratories, most rheometers work using the Searle mode and only a few are designed for the Couette method. Therefore, the following discussion and calculation are based on concentric

geometry operated according to the Searle principle. The definition of the rheological properties (strain and strain rate, stress, and viscosity) discussed above can also be applied here despite the rounded areas of the cylinder walls, as long as a relatively narrow gap is used. For a typical concentric-cylinder measuring system, the shear stress, shear rate, and viscosity are all related to the rotor surface. Then

$$\tau_i = \frac{M}{(2\pi \cdot L \cdot R_i^2)}$$

$$\dot{\gamma}_i = \frac{(2 \cdot R_e^2)}{(R_e^2 - R_i^2)} \cdot \omega$$

$$\eta = \frac{\tau_i}{\dot{\gamma}_i} = \frac{(R_e^2 - R_i^2)}{4\pi \cdot L \cdot R_e^2 \cdot R_i^2} \cdot \frac{M}{\omega}$$

where M is the torque, L is the length of the cylinder part of the rotor, R_i is the radius of the rotor, R_e is the radius of the cup, and ω is the angular frequency.

In addition, other specialty geometries, including various vanes, helical, and starch pasting impeller rotors, as well as large diameter and grooved cups, are available for the concentric cylinders. These special concentric-cylinder geometries are very valuable for characterizing dispersions with limited stability and bulk materials with larger particulates. Moreover, a solvent trap is available, which includes a base reservoir and a two-piece cover that is mounted to the shaft of the rotor. The solvent trap provides a vapor barrier for sealing the environment inside the cup and prevents solvent evaporation. As indicated in Figure 7.14, concentric cylinder geometries are commonly used for testing low viscosity fluids and dispersions, especially the pourable liquids. Examples of materials that are suitable for concentric-cylinder

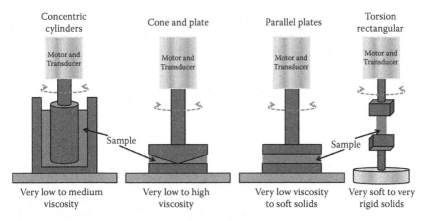

FIGURE 7.14 Schematic illustration of oscillatory geometry options.

geometry include low-concentration polymer solutions, paint, and pharmaceutical suspensions such as cough medicine and baby formula. One disadvantage associated with the geometry is the requirement of a large amount of sample material.

2. The cone-and-plate geometry consists of a lower plate and an upper cone that has a conical profile with a truncated tip. The gap between the cone and plate in the working position is determined by the imaginary tip of the cone, which should touch the lower plate. When an oscillatory test is being conducted, the cone is set in motion and produces a uniform shear rate profile through the gap, while the plate is stationary. In a typical cone-and-plate measuring system, the shear stress, shear rate, and viscosity can be written as follows:

$$\tau = 3M / (2\pi \cdot r^3)$$

$$\dot{\gamma} = \omega / \theta_0$$

$$\eta = \frac{\tau}{\dot{\gamma}} = 3M\theta_0 / (2\pi \cdot \omega \cdot r^3)$$

where M is the torque, r is the radius of the plate, ω is the angular frequency, and θ_0 is the angle between the cone and the plate. If a small-angle oscillatory shear mode is applied by a cone-and-plate geometry, then the rheological properties (storage, loss modulus, and complex viscosity) mentioned above can be written as follows:

$$G' = \frac{3M_0\theta_0\cos\delta}{2\pi r^4 \phi_0}$$

$$G'' = \frac{3M_0\theta_0\sin\delta}{2\pi r^4 \phi_0}$$

where M_0 is the torque amplitude, ϕ_0 is the angular amplitude of the oscillation, and δ is the phase angle. From the storage and loss modulus and the angular frequency (ω), the complex viscosity can be calculated as

$$|\eta^*| = \sqrt{\left(\frac{G'}{\omega}\right)^2 + \left(\frac{G''}{\omega}\right)^2}$$

Upper cone geometries are available with cone angles of 0.02, 0.04, and 0.1 radians. By changing the diameter and cone angle, the measurement range of stress and strain or shear rate can be varied to capture the widest range of test conditions. Moreover, a solvent trap is available with a two-piece cover that is mounted to provide a vapor barrier to seal the gap environment between the cone and plate.

The cone and plate geometry is suitable for testing liquids with low to high viscosity. In addition, the geometry only requires a very small amount of sample and can provide high shear rate measurements. Major limitations associated with this geometry are as follows: (1) Samples with a larger particle size or three-dimensional structures are not suitable for the geometry. (2) A long relaxation time is required for highly viscous samples. (3) Isothermal experiments are preferred over temperature sweeps, because of the strong influence of the equipment-dependent thermal expansion on the narrow gap dimension.

3. The parallel-plates geometry possesses a similar setup as the cone-and-plate system but replaces the upper cone with a plate. Both upper and lower plates have a flat surface and the dimensions of the plates are defined by the plate radius r. The gap between the plates is set to be h, which is much smaller than r, and normally the ratio $(2r/h)$ is between 10 and 50. During measurement, the parallel-plates geometry produces an uneven shear rate field across the plate radius (highest on the rim and zero in the center of the plate) because of the rotation kinematics. To overcome the error caused by the nonconstant shear rate profile, a correction procedure must be considered for a rotational measuring mode. However, when a small-angle oscillatory shear is carried out, no correction is needed because of the minimal strain amplitude. For a typical parallel-plates measuring system operated in a small-angle oscillatory mode, the shear stress, shear rate, and viscosity at the rim can be written as follows:

$$\tau = 3M / (2\pi \cdot r^3)$$

$$\dot{\gamma} = r\omega / h$$

$$\eta = \frac{\tau}{\dot{\gamma}} = 3Mh / (2\pi \cdot \omega \cdot r^3)$$

where M is the torque, r is the radius of the plate, ω is the angular frequency, and h is the gap between the plates. In addition, other rheological properties, including storage, loss modulus, and complex viscosity, can be written as follows:

$$G' = \frac{2hM_0 \cos\delta}{\pi r^4 \phi_0}$$

$$G'' = \frac{2hM_0 \sin\delta}{\pi r^4 \phi_0}$$

where M_0 is the torque amplitude, ϕ_0 is the angular amplitude of the oscillation, and δ is the phase angle. From the storage and loss modulus and the angular frequency (ω), the complex viscosity can be calculated using the same equation as the cone-and-plate system.

Different plate geometries are available with diameters of 8, 25, 40, and 50 mm. By changing the diameter, the measurement range of stress and strain or shear rate can be varied to capture the widest range of test conditions. Moreover, a range of materials of construction and plate surface treatments are available to guarantee reliable results by avoiding the risks of wall slip or wall depletion. Also, a solvent trap is available to provide a vapor barrier to seal the gap environment between the plates.

Parallel-plates geometry is very powerful for testing liquids with low to high viscosity, soft solids, gels, polymer melts, and materials with a large particle size and long relaxation time. In addition, the geometry requires a very small amount of sample material and is very effective at preventing sample slip. In comparison with cone-and-plate geometry, parallel-plates geometry is preferred for temperature sweeps. But parallel plates are not good for nonlinear studies due to the uniform shear rate profile.

4. Typically, torsion rectangular geometry is used to characterize solid or rubbery materials. It is a very powerful tool for measuring the glass transition and subglass transitions of polymers. As shown in Figure 7.14, a stiffer sample is clamped with its long axis coaxial with the rheometer's rotational axis. Rectangular samples can vary between 0.3 and 6 mm in thickness, up to 12 mm in width, and 40 mm in length. The torsional test consists of twisting a specimen under the oscillatory rotation of torque applied at one end and keeping the other end fixed. In order to correlate the material parameters, such as strain (γ) and stress (τ), with the rheometer responses, such as rotation angle (θ) and torque (M), two geometry constants, the strain constant K_γ and stress constant K_τ, are introduced:

$$K_\gamma = \frac{\gamma}{\theta}$$

$$K_\tau = \frac{\tau}{M}$$

When a rectangular specimen is used to measure torque and rotation angle, the following equations are applied to calculate the strain and stress constants:

$$K_\gamma = \frac{\gamma}{\theta} = \frac{t}{l}\left[1 - 0.378 \cdot \left(\frac{t}{w}\right)^2\right]$$

$$K_\tau = \frac{\tau}{M} = \frac{3 + 1.8 \cdot \left(\dfrac{t}{w}\right)}{wt^2} \cdot 1000 \cdot g$$

where t is the thickness of the specimen, l is the actual specimen length between the clamps, w is the width of the specimen, and g is the gravity

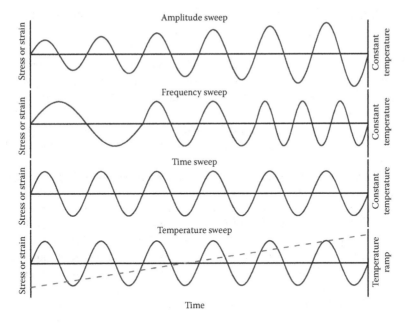

FIGURE 7.15 Schematic illustration of oscillatory experiment modes.

constant. From the strain and stress constants, the shear modulus, the ratio of stress and strain, can be calculated as

$$G = \frac{\tau}{\gamma} = \frac{K_\tau M}{K_\gamma \theta}$$

Torsion rectangular geometry allows solid samples, both soft and very rigid, to be characterized with reliable results because it minimizes the risk of sample slip. Moreover, it also enables the measurements in a temperature- and/or humidity-controlled environment. In general, the specimen for torsion rectangular geometry is simple to prepare, but occasionally it is limited by its stiffness.

Once a suitable geometry is identified for a given system, designing an appropriate oscillatory experiment becomes crucial to meet the objectives of the study, which could be material characterization and/or processing simulation. So far, an oscillation shear test is the most powerful way to characterize the viscoelastic properties of materials. Both elastic and plastic characteristics of the material can be studied by imposing a sinusoidal strain (or stress) and measuring the resultant sinusoidal stress (or strain) along with the phase difference between the two sinusoidal waves (input and output). Moreover, many key processing parameters, such as deformation, stress, processing speed, time, and temperature, can be simulated by an appropriately designed oscillatory experiment, because viscoelastic properties of the system can be monitored as a function of deformation amplitude, frequency, time, and temperature. Figure 7.15 illustrates different oscillatory experiment modes that are very useful for both material characterization and processing simulation.

1. In a typical amplitude sweep mode, the frequency and temperature are held constant and the viscoelastic properties are monitored as the strain is varied. Strain sweep tests are normally used to identify the linear viscoelastic region. Tests within the linear viscoelastic region provide a useful structure-property relationship because a material's molecular arrangements are never far from equilibrium and the response is a reflection of internal dynamic processes.

2. In a frequency sweep mode, the temperature and strain are held constant and the viscoelastic properties are monitored as a function of frequency. Because frequency is the inverse of time, the frequency sweep curve shows the time dependence of the mechanical response, with short times (high frequency) corresponding to solid-like behavior and long times (low frequency) corresponding to liquid-like behavior. The magnitude and shape of the frequency sweep curves depend on the molecular structure. Frequency sweeps are typically run over a limited range of 0.1–100 rad/s. Time-temperature superposition (TTS) is often used to extend the frequency range by running a series of frequency sweeps at different temperatures.

3. In a time sweep mode, the temperature, strain, and frequency are all held constant, while the viscoelastic properties of a system are measured as the time is running. Oscillation time sweeps are important for tracking how the material structure changes with time, especially under the processing conditions of interest. This mode is widely used for kinetically monitoring a curing reaction, fatigue studies, structure rebuild, and other time-dependent investigations.

4. Measuring the viscoelastic properties over a range of temperatures is an extremely sensitive technique for measuring glass transition temperature and any subglass transition movements of a system. In a temperature sweep experiment, a linear heating or cooling rate is applied. Typical heating or cooling rates are on the order of 1–5°C/min. The material response is monitored at one or more frequencies with constant amplitude. Data can be recorded at user-defined time intervals.

Based on a carefully selected geometry and well-designed rheological experiments, the rheological properties of a given polymer system can be studied as functions of several key parameters, such as stress, strain, strain rate, frequency, temperature, and time. Because the rheological response of the polymer melt is very sensitive to small changes in the molecular structure, rheology is the most convenient method to characterize polymers. In practice, the rheology-polymer structure relation makes rheology the ideal tool to design polymeric structure with optimal processability and desired performance. Due to the sensitivity of the process to the polymer structure, the material structure needs to be controlled within tight tolerances to guarantee a good processability. The viscoelastic nature of the melt may cause wanted and unwanted anisotropy flow during the process, which may eventually affect the performance of the final product. Besides providing direct information on processability, the rheology of the solid and melt phase can also be related to the performance of the end product.

Although rheology has shown strong capabilities in the characterization of polymer structure, optimization of processability, and evaluation of performance, it is worth mentioning that the rheological behavior is not a direct representation of the polymer structure. Key information including physical, chemical, and thermal properties of the system is still lacking based solely on rheological study. For a complex system like an API-polymer system (multicomponent and phase system), the structure-rheology relationship is still ambiguous. Therefore, additional characterizing methods, such as microscopy, nuclear magnetic resonance (NMR) spectroscopy, x-ray diffraction spectroscopy (XRD), and differential scanning calorimetry (DSC), have to be used in conjunction with the rheological measurement to isolate the contributions of different structural elements and provide comprehensive information of the system of interest.

7.7   OSCILLATORY RHEOLOGY APPLICATIONS

To begin with, this section introduces a few commonly used pharmaceutical polymers for the HME process. Polymer systems have played indispensable roles in many industries, including food, pharmaceutical, and cosmetic, due to their unique structures and performances. Over the past few decades, polymers have been extensively applied to the pharmaceutical industry, ranging widely from material packaging to manufacture of the most sophisticated drug delivery systems. For instance, the use of polymers has evolved from a simple gelatin capsule shell into materials that provide great benefits and clinical promises for the final dosage forms, including enhanced bioavailability and stability, controlled release, and targeted therapy of the active pharmaceutical ingredient (API). In a conventional solid dosage form, the polymers can act as diluents, binders, disintegrants, and/or coating films. Recently, polymers have also been used as a carrier for poorly water-soluble API to enhance solubility, stability, and bioavailability. API-polymer amorphous solid dispersions can significantly enhance the bioavailability of poorly soluble API. Compared to the crystalline form, amorphous API often exhibits higher solubility due to the absence of lattice energy. Moreover, polymers in a solid dispersion can act as crystallization inhibitors to prevent recrystallization of the amorphous API, giving the API good physical stability. Different processing techniques, such as HME and spray drying, have been employed to prepare API-polymer amorphous solid dispersions. In particular, HME is a continuous, versatile, and solvent-free process that enables dispersing an API into a polymer excipient more efficiently than other processing methods. Therefore, HME processing has gained a great deal of attention from the pharmaceutical industry and groups of polymers suitable for HME processing have been developed. Table 7.1 summarizes a number of commercially available polymers (pharmaceutical grade) for HME processes, including polyvinylpyrrolidone and its copolymer, cellulose derivatives, polymethacrylates, polymethacrylic acid, and poly(ethylene) oxide. Among them, povidone and cellulose derivatives are two major categories of polymers that have been widely applied in HME processes to prepare an API-polymer amorphous solid dispersion. Here, we focus on these polymers, and the details are as follows:

TABLE 7.1
Commercially Available Polymers (Pharmaceutical Grade) for Hot Melt Extrusion

Polymer Category	Brand Name	Chemical Structure	Manufacture
Polyvinylpyrrolidone and Copolymer	Polyvinylpyrrolidone (PVP)*: Plasdone™ K, Kollidon®		Ashland Inc., BASF Corporation
	Vinyl pyrrolidone-vinyl acetate (6:4) copolymer (copovidone): Plasdone™ S-630, Kollidon® VA 64	n:m=1.2	
Cellulose Derivatives Polymers	Hydroxypropyl cellulose (HPC): Klucel™	R=H or CH$_2$CH(OH)CH$_3$	Ashland Inc., Dow Chemical Company, Shin-Etsu Chemical Co., Ltd.
	Hydroxypropyl methyl cellulose (HPMC): Benecel™, AFFINISOL™	R=H or CH$_3$ or CH$_2$CH(OH)CH$_3$	
	Hypromellose acetate succinate (HPMCAS)**: AquaSolve™, AFFINISOL™, Shin-Etsu AQOAT®	R=H or CH$_3$ or CH$_2$CH(OH)CH$_3$ or COCH$_3$ or COCH$_2$CH$_3$	
Others	Polymethacrylates and polymethacrylic acid: Eudragit® ***	****	Evonik Industries, Dow Chemical Company
	Poly(ethylene) oxide: POLYOX™		

Note: * Available in several molecular weight grades. ** Available in three grades varying in the extent of substitution of acetyl and succinyl groups (L, M, and H), and in two particle sizes (F and G). *** Available in several grades varying in modular weight and/or structure. **** Modular structure changes depending on polymerization.

1. Polyvinylpyrrolidones, or povidones, are water-soluble polymers obtained by radical polymerization of N-vinylpyrrolidone. Povidones are available in different grades that are structurally similar but have different molecular weights. Povidone, shown in Table 7.1, is a linear polymer with different degrees of polymerization, which results in polymers of different molecular weights. Povidone is widely used in solid dosage forms. In tablet formulations, povidone solution is used as a wet granulation binder. Povidone can also be incorporated into powder blends in the dry form and granulated *in situ* by the addition of other solvents. Recently, povidone has been applied as a dissolution-enhancing agent in oral formulations for poorly soluble drugs involving processes such as HME. Depending on the grades, the glass transition temperatures vary from 130°C to 176°C for low molecular weight grade and high molecular weight grade, respectively. Theoretically, selecting the HME processing temperature about 40°C higher than the glass transition temperature is required. In practice, however, adding API to the povidone system decreases the processing temperature due to the plasticizer effect of API.

2. The copolymer of polyvinylpyrrolidones and polyvinyl acetate, or copovidone, is 6:4 linear random copolymer of N-vinylpyrrolidone and vinyl acetate. It is produced in the same way as soluble polyvinylpyrrolidone, by the free-radical polymerization reaction. Because vinyl acetate is not soluble in water, the synthesis is normally conducted in an organic solvent. The applications of copovidone rely mainly on its good binding and film-forming properties, and the relatively low hygroscopicity. Because of these properties, copovidone is used as a binder in the production of granules and tablets by wet granulation, as a dry binder in direct compression, and as a film former in coatings on tablets. In addition, copovidone is used as a carrier and dissolution-enhancing agent in oral formulations for poorly soluble drugs in the HME process, because it acts as solubilizing agent, dispersant, and crystallization inhibitor. The optimal HME processing temperature window for copovidone ($T_g = 107°C$) is in the range from 140°C to 180°C. However, in certain API-copovidone systems, the processing temperature can be reduced to a lower temperature because of the plasticizer effect of API.

3. Cellulose is a polymer consisting of linearly linked units of D-glucose. Because of the presence of a large number of hydroxyl and ether groups in the glucose units of polymer chains, celluloses have high intra- and intermolecular hydrogen bonding, which results in crystallinity in native cellulose and also imparts water-insoluble properties to cellulose. Typically, celluloses are converted to cellulose derivatives by partially or fully reacting the hydroxyl groups of glucose units with different reagents. Most cellulose derivatives are predominantly amorphous and water soluble because the substituents cause a breakup of the hydrogen bonds. Depending on the type of reagent used during derivatization, the physicochemical properties of these cellulose derivatives vary and therefore may have different applications in pharmaceutical formulations and HME processes. Three typical cellulose derivatives that have been applied in HME processes are listed in Table 7.1 and their properties are as follows:

3.1. Hydroxypropyl cellulose (HPC) is a cellulose derivative in which some of the hydroxyl groups on the cellulose backbone have been hydroxypropyl acted. Because each of the added hydroxypropyl groups introduces a secondary hydroxyl group to the polymer and the new hydroxyl group can be further hydroxypropyl acted during the reaction, the obtained HPC typically has an additional chain extension. HPC is a nonionic water-soluble cellulose derivative with a remarkable combination of different properties. It combines organic solvent solubility, thermoplasticity, surface activity, and stabilizing properties of other water-soluble cellulose polymers. HPC is widely used in solid oral dosage forms as a binder, a coating film, and a controlled-release matrix former. Typically, in an HME process, HPC is recommended as an HME aid and is coprocessed with other cellulose derivatives to bring down the processing temperatures of the polymers. HPC is commercially available in different grades corresponding to different average molecular weights.

3.2. Hydroxypropyl methylcellulose (HPMC) is a partly methylated and hydroxypropyl-acted cellulose derivative. It is commercially available in several types with different degrees of substituent and molar substituent and different molecular weights. Similar to the preparation of HPC, the added hydroxypropyl group introduces a secondary hydroxyl group that can also be further hydroxypropyl acted during the preparation of HPMC, giving rise to an additional chain extension. Variations in the ratios of methoxy and hydroxypropyl substitutions and molecular weight affect HPMC's resultant properties such as organic solubility, thermal gelation temperature in aqueous solution, swelling, diffusion, and drug-release rate. In practice, HPMC is used in solid oral dosage forms as a binder, a coating film, and a controlled-release matrix. It is the polymer of choice in the preparation of hydrophilic matrix tablets because it rapidly forms a uniform, strong, and viscous gel layer, which protects the matrix from disintegration and controls the rate of drug release. HPMC also has been tailored to possess a relatively lower glass transition temperature and improved melt rheological properties, which enable it to be extruded through HME at lower processing temperatures. In addition to improved processability, the modified HPMC also maintains advantages as the precipitation inhibitor during dissolution.

3.3. HPMCAS is synthesized by the esterification of HPMC with acetic anhydride and succinic anhydride. In a typical reaction, a carboxylic acid, such as acetic acid, is used as a medium and an alkali carboxylate, such as sodium acetate, is used as a catalyst. HPMCAS maintains the structural diversity of the starting HPMC, such that the added hydroxypropyl group introduces a secondary reaction site that can also be hydroxypropyl acted, giving rise to a chain extension. HPMCAS is available in several grades with varying fractions of substitutions, mainly of acetyl (2.0%–16.0%) and succinyl (4.0%–28.0%) groups.

HPMCAS is insoluble in gastric fluid but starts to swell and dissolve at a pH above 5, and its dissolution pH increases as the ratio of acetyl over succinyl substitution increases. Traditionally, HPMCAS is used for enteric film coating of tablets. However, today HPMCAS is also utilized as an amorphous solid dispersion polymer for drug solubility enhancement. HPMCAS has been successfully used to prepare solid dispersions via the HME process and has shown a superior anticrystallization effect when compared to other cellulosic and vinylpyrrolidone polymers. Because the amount of side chain substitution or the ratio of different substituents in HPMCAS is tunable, it affects the relative hydrophilic-hydrophobic balance of the API-polymer system. When using HPMCAS as carriers for amorphous solid dispersion of poorly soluble APIs, different grades have the potential to form distinct API-polymer interactions, such as hydrogen bonding and hydrophobic interaction with API molecules. But, one limitation associated with HPMCAS is the potential degradation occurring at the elevated processing temperatures necessary for the HME process. Dissociation of the side chains and the formation of volatile materials (free acetic acid and succinic acid) under extreme processing conditions could react with the drug or other excipients. Also, the crosslinking of HPMCAS at a higher temperature could result in a decrease in the drug dissolution rate. For these reasons, it is better not to extrude an API-HPMCAS system at a temperature greater than 180°C.

Because the polymer is a major component of the final drug products prepared by HME, the melt rheology of polymers and/or API-polymer mixtures that determine the system's processability should be considered key factors in selecting suitable candidates and parameters for an HME process. It is necessary to understand their rheological behavior when subjected to mechanical stress, heat, and time that are analogous to real HME processing conditions. Moreover, macroscopic rheological behavior reflects the structural properties of a given system, which often affect the usability of the system for a given application. In the following text, we highlight several case studies of oscillatory rheology applications for characterizing polymers, evaluating API-polymer dispersion, and optimizing HME processing parameters.

7.7.1 CASE STUDY 1: CHARACTERIZATION OF POLYMER

As mentioned above, it is important that a small angle oscillatory experiment be conducted within the linear viscoelastic region, where the applied strain deformation is sufficiently small so that the subject's molecular arrangements are never far from equilibrium. In this manner, the linear viscoelastic response is a reflection of the internal dynamic processes. In order to determine the strain limit of the linear viscoelasticity, a sweep with increasing strain amplitude at a constant frequency needs to be performed. As long as the rheological responses remain constant, the deformation is within the linear viscoelastic range. Figure 7.16 shows a strain sweep

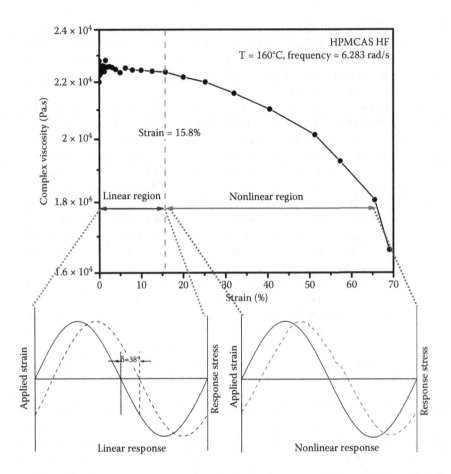

FIGURE 7.16 Oscillatory strain sweep of HPMCAS-HF at 160°C and 6.283 rad/s and higher harmonic strain-stress response.

on HPMCAS HF grade melt in a parallel-plates geometry at 160°C and 6.283 rad/s. At low strains, the complex viscosity is independent of the strain amplitude up to a critical strain of 15.8%. Beyond the critical strain, the behavior is nonlinear and the complex viscosity begins to decrease significantly in magnitude. In addition to the viscoelastic properties, the rheometer can collect higher harmonic information as shown in the figure. As long as the test is conducted within the linear region, the measured response stress can be fitted into a sinusoidal function similar to the applied strain wave but showing a delayed phase angle, which is 38° for this particular system. In contrast, once the applied strain is beyond the critical limit of the linear region, the response stress cannot be fitted into a sinusoidal function anymore and obvious deviation of the response stress from a sinusoidal function can be observed. In practice, the strain limit for a linear viscoelastic region is highly material dependent and should always be checked for an individual system. If the oscillatory measurements are to be performed over a wide range of temperatures, conducting strain sweeps at different temperatures is highly recommended, because the linear viscoelastic region becomes narrow at low temperature. In addition, the strain limit is also dependent on the frequency at which it is tested. In general, the linear viscoelastic region determined by using a low frequency may not be applicable at a significantly higher frequency. It is also worth mentioning that some polymers may show a strikingly nonlinear stress response as the strain deformation is increased, which suggests a fundamental change of the material properties under shear from the equilibrium properties at rest. However, such nonlinear data are often disregarded because the physical origins of this behavior remain poorly understood.

7.7.2 CASE STUDY 2: EVALUATION OF MODEL SOLID DISPERSIONS

Linear viscoelasticity has been used to characterize polymer melts and is sensitively dependent on the subject's structures. This study aims to assess several model solid dispersions by using oscillatory rheology and to correlate their viscoelastic responses with structures. As shown in Figure 7.17, a model API, clotrimazole, is compounded with copovidone to form solid dispersions (50:50 wt) via various techniques with different mixing capabilities. As illustrated in the figure, simple physical mixing leads to a poorly mixed blend manifested by the existence of large API crystalline content and heterogeneous distribution. Cryogenic milling significantly improves mixing of the two components as a result of reduced particle size and increased contact surface area. In contrast, HME processing results in a homogenous amorphous solid dispersion because of its inherent mixing efficiency. Figure 7.17 also displays frequency sweeps of copovidone and different model solid dispersions measured at 130°C. Under this circumstance, most of the API crystals are preserved and embedded in the polymer melt. As shown in the figure, copovidone exhibits a typical entangled polymeric melt behavior manifested by a significant drop of storage modulus in the high-frequency range and an approximate rubbery plateau in the intermediate frequency range. Because of the low temperature used, however, the lowest frequency applied here reflects an insufficient time scale to permit the unraveling of entanglements, displaying a slope of 0.81. API crystalline particles and molecules significantly decrease the storage modulus in this system. Within the low-frequency region, a drop in modulus becomes more rapid as the dispersion of API is improved, reflected by the gradually increasing slope. In particular, the extrudate exhibits a slope of 1.86 at 0.4 rad/s and eventually reaches an unmeasurable level, approximating closely the theoretical value of 2 from the linear viscoelastic Maxwell model at the terminal zone. The storage modulus versus frequency of different solid dispersions indicates that the incorporation of API results in a plasticizing effect on the polymer matrix. Moreover, the crystalline/aggregated forms of API exhibit more elastic response than their amorphous/dispersed counterparts.

7.7.3 CASE STUDY 3: OPTIMIZATION OF HME PROCESSING TEMPERATURE

The production of amorphous solid dispersions via HME relies on elevated temperature and prolonged residence time, which can result in potential degradation and

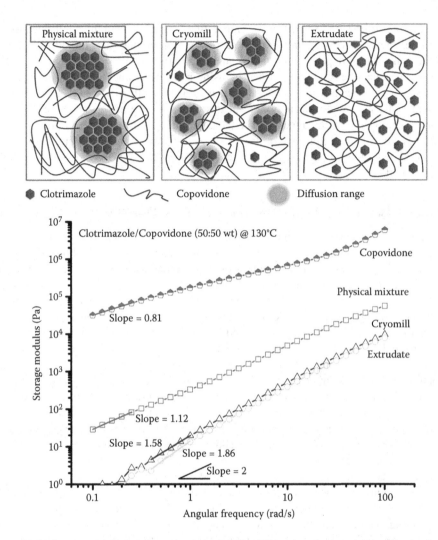

FIGURE 7.17 Model solid dispersions prepared by different methods and an oscillatory frequency sweep of copovidone and clotrimazole/copovidone (50:50 wt) model solid dispersions at 130°C.

decomposition of thermally sensitive components. In this case study, the rheological properties of an API-polymer physical mixture are utilized to guide the selection of appropriate HME processing temperature. Complex viscosity and damping factor of a nifedipine-copovidone system as a function of temperature are depicted in Figure 7.18. For the pure copovidone, the complex viscosity is over 105 Pa.s at the starting temperature of 130°C and gradually decreases at higher temperatures. With the incorporation of 50 wt% of nifedipine, a decrease in complex viscosity is observed across the entire temperature range. Initially, the plot for the physical mixture appears to run parallel to that of pure copovidone; however, as the temperature rises above 145°C, the complex viscosity of the physical mixture dramatically

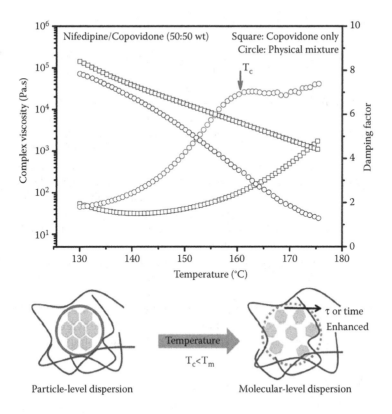

FIGURE 7.18 Oscillatory temperature sweep of copovidone and nifedipine/copovidone (50:50 wt) physical mixture and schematic depiction of the critical temperature.

drops, signifying the plasticizing effect of the dissolved nifedipine molecules on copovidone. However, there is no peak or bump observed for the physical mixture in complex viscosity that can be attributed to the dissolution of nifedipine or melting point of the crystalline nifedipine (173°C). Practically, the smooth transition of complex viscosity leads to difficulty in locating the exact critical temperature at which the nifedipine becomes completely dispersed at the molecular level into copovidone. In contrast, the damping factor, a ratio of loss modulus to storage modulus, displays a relatively high sensitivity to structural changes and holds potential for identifying an appropriate HME processing temperature. In particular, the curve for copovidone exhibits a parabolic shape with a minimum around 140°C, implying that the molecular chain mobility increases when the temperature exceeds T_g. Physically, the material may still remain very stiff due to chain entanglements and therefore not be extrudate by HME. Scientifically, this is the rationale for the practice of selecting the optimal extrusion temperature to be ~40°C higher than T_g. The damping factor of the physical mixture as a function of temperature successfully captures a transition bump at 160°C, which can be correlated with a critical transition temperature (T_c), at which the crystalline API starts dissolving into the polymeric matrix to achieve molecular-level mixing. Practically, in the preparation of amorphous solid dispersion by HME processing, the processing temperature is often raised above the melting point of the API to convert crystalline materials into amorphous ones. However, the most significant aspects of this study are the rational determination of the critical temperature, which may be below the melting point of the API, and optimization of the HME processing temperature based on a rheological study of polymer/API physical mixtures. It is observed that when the copovidone/nifedipine (50 wt%) mixture was extruded at the identified critical temperature of 160°C, which is approximately 13°C below the melting point of nifedipine, a smooth and transparent extrudate with the majority of crystalline API converted into amorphous form could be obtained. In addition, as the temperature reaches or surpasses the critical point, further increasing the temperature has limited contribution to API dispersion. The molecular-level dissolution of the API molecule into the polymer melt is highly dependent on contact surface area and residence time. Therefore, both distributive and dispersive mixing and prolonged residence time may significantly enhance the dissolution of API as depicted in Figure 7.18. In other words, adding kneading elements with high shear force in screw design, generating API-polymer contact surface, or prolonging the residence time may be helpful to guarantee the formation of amorphous solid dispersion via HME, even at a relatively low processing temperature that can be substantially below the melting point of the crystalline API. Most importantly, in this manner, one probably could avoid potential risks of thermal degradation and decomposition of thermal-sensitive components due to overheating.

7.8 SUMMARY

The adaptability of the torque rheometer to adhere to changing needs of markets, materials, processes, and the ever-demanding user is remarkable. Torque rheometer systems have, through the years, proven themselves over and over again in meeting these requirements for change and diversity, and they are now being applied to pharmaceutical extrusion applications. Moreover, the most important feature of torque rheometer is versatility. The ability to measure common characteristics of materials and processes is certainly essential.

On the other hand, oscillatory rheology is another very powerful tool for characterizing viscoelastic properties of the polymer and API-polymer system. Comprehensive rheological studies of the polymer and API-polymer system could provide insightful information for the structure and processability of materials. Many key findings associated with the underlying mechanisms of formation of amorphous solid dispersion via HME could be accomplished by rationally designed oscillatory experiments. Eventually, all these findings could facilitate the development of novel formulations and products via HME.

8 Foam Extrusion

Graciela Terife and Niloufar Faridi

CONTENTS

8.1 INTRODUCTION

The terms "foams" and "cellular structures" refer to porous solids with either closed or open cells. Closed-cell foams, Figure 8.1a, can be visualized as a honeycomb structure, and open-cell foams, Figure 8.1b, as a rigid sponge.

Application of foams is widespread in both the food and plastic industries. Some examples of foams in the food industry include bread, cakes, puffed cereals, and snacks. Some of the typical applications of foamed products in the plastic industry include insulation (thermal, acoustic, and electrical); floating devices; shock mitigation; packaging; and cushioning, among others. The end use, as well as the performance and properties of polymeric foams, strongly depends on their physical characteristics. For example, open-cell foams, where all the cells are interconnected, are used for applications that require high permeability to gases and higher capacity to absorb fluids and moisture [1–3]. On the other hand, closed-cell foams—where each cell is isolated from the rest—are preferred for thermal, noise, and electrical insulation over open-cell foams [3].

Foaming has proven to provide clear benefits to manufacturing and performance of drug products as listed below:

(a)　　　　　　　　　　　　　　　　　　(b)

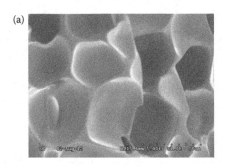 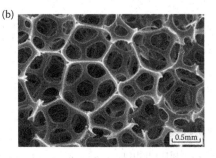

FIGURE 8.1 SEM images of (a) a closed-cell foam, and (b) an open-cell foam (Reprinted from *International Journal of Solids and Structures*, 42, Gong, L., S. Kyriakides, and W.Y. Jang, Compressive response of open-cell foams. Part I: Morphology and elastic properties, 1355–1379, Copyright (2004), with permission from Elsevier).

Enhanced efficiency of the extrusion process

- Plasticization of the polymers by gas enables lower processing temperatures, avoiding degradation of the active pharmaceutical ingredient (API) and/or excipient
- The Joule-Thomson effect enables cooling of the extrudate without the requirement for forced cooling via chilled rollers or air
- Porous structure facilitates milling of the extrudate resulting in higher yield and higher efficiency

Improved compaction robustness

- Increased tablet compactibility and decreased lubrication sensitivity during compression

Improved product performance

- Enhanced dissolution

8.2 FOAMING MECHANISMS

Cellular structures can be commercially manufactured through continuous processes, such as foam extrusion, or through batch or semicontinuous processes, such as injection molding. From a general perspective, the foaming process can be described through the following elementary steps: (1) dissolution of a gas in a polymer-based formulation, (2) cell nucleation, (3) bubble growth, and (4) stabilization of the cellular structure. These elementary steps are shown schematically in Figure 8.2.

Gas dissolution in the polymer is often carried out under pressure. The manufacturing process dictates the method of introducing the gas and the solubilization mechanism. Once the gas is completely dissolved, forming a single phase with the polymer, a thermodynamic instability is induced by a rapid increase in temperature or drop in pressure. As the system seeks a lower free-energy state, gas molecules will

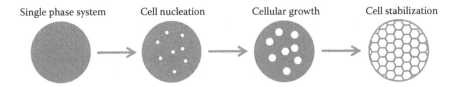

Single phase system   Cell nucleation   Cellular growth   Cell stabilization

FIGURE 8.2 Elementary steps of the foaming process.

cluster, promoting nucleation and bubble formation. Once nuclei are formed there are two possible paths forward. The nuclei will either grow or die. Growth happens by diffusion of gas from the bulk (polymer + API + gas melt) into the nuclei. Nuclei disappear or die in two ways: 1) if pressure is too high, the bubbles collapse, or 2) the nuclei merges or coalesces with other nuclei or bubbles. Cell growth is limited by the diffusion rate and stiffness of polymer/gas solution. The last step of a foaming process is stabilization of the bubbles, which is controlled by variations in foam processing conditions. If the cell membranes surrounding a bubble remain intact, the foam has closed cells. If the membranes rupture, some or all of the cells will be open.

8.2.1 Cell Nucleation

There are two major types of nucleation in polymer foaming, homogeneous and heterogeneous. When nucleation occurs without the presence of any impurities, it is called homogeneous nucleation. Heterogeneous nucleation typically occurs due to impurities in the polymer itself or in the presence of added nucleating agents. The nucleation step at high energy regions governs cell morphology of the foam for both homogeneous and heterogeneous nucleation.

The change in free energy of the system during nucleation is described by Equation 8.1; here the first term on the right side of the equation corresponds to a reduction in free energy as the gas molecules are incorporated into the bubble. The second term on the right side of the equation corresponds to an increase in free energy due to the formation of a new surface, and it is associated interfacial energy [4].

$$\Delta G = -V_b \Delta P + A\gamma \tag{8.1}$$

where ΔG is the change of free energy during nucleation, V_b is the nucleus volume, $\Delta P = P_{sat} - P_{atm}$ is the difference between saturation pressure (P_{sat}) and atmospheric pressure (P_{atm}), A is the surface area of the nucleus, and γ is the surface energy of the polymer-bubble interface [4,5].

Based on molecular kinetics, the nucleation rate (J) can be expressed as [4,6,7]

$$J = Be^{(-\Delta G/\kappa T)} \tag{8.2}$$

where ΔG is the free energy barrier that needs to be overcome for cell nucleation to occur; κ is the Boltzmann's constant; T is the system temperature; and B is the product of a frequency function and the concentration of either gas or nucleating agent, for homogeneous and heterogeneous nucleation, respectively. The free energy barrier, ΔG, is lower if a bubble is nucleated on the surface of a second phase (heterogeneous nucleation), such as solid additives, impurities, and the equipment wall surface, compared to the case where the bubble is nucleated in the bulk phase of the polymer-gas solution (homogeneous nucleation).

In conclusion, the above expressions show that concentration of the gas molecules and the number of the heterogeneous nucleation sites impose positive influence on the nucleation process, while the interfacial tension plays a negative role.

8.2.2 BUBBLE GROWTH

Once critical size nuclei are formed, gas dissolved in the polymer diffuses into the gas bubbles, and as a result, the pressure inside the bubbles increases, subjecting the polymer to biaxial tension and deformation. The rate of cell growth depends on the gas diffusion rate, external pressure on the foam, current cell size, heat transfer affecting melt temperature, and polymer strength (i.e., polymer-gas viscoelastic properties) [8–11].

From Equation 8.1 it can be inferred that the system is more stable with fewer and larger cells. Therefore, cell combination or coalescence is thermodynamically favored during bubble growth.

Another important relationship is given by the Young-Laplace equation (see Equation 8.3). This indicates that the internal pressure of the bubble keeps increasing as gas diffuses into the cell, until it is balanced by the surface tension of the polymer-bubble interface and the viscoelastic properties of the melt.

$$\Delta P_b = \frac{2\gamma}{r} \tag{8.3}$$

where ΔP_b is the bubble's internal pressure change, γ is the surface tension of the polymer-bubble interface, and r is the radius of the bubble.

In addition, the gas pressure in a small bubble is greater than in a large bubble, with the difference given in Equation 8.4.

$$\Delta P_{1,2} = 2\gamma_{bp}\left(\frac{1}{r_1} - \frac{1}{r_2}\right) \tag{8.4}$$

where $\Delta P_{1,2}$ is the difference in pressure between cells with radii of r_1 and r_2. Thus, gas tends to diffuse from the smaller bubble into the larger one.

8.2.3 STABILIZATION OF THE CELLULAR STRUCTURE

Cell stabilization can occur by use of cell stabilizers and surface tension depressants. In addition, an increase in viscosity of the polymer phase by cooling or further polymerization can influence foam stability significantly [12].

Shrinkage is another issue that influences stabilization of foams after production. Shrinkage usually occurs in closed-cell foams when a partial vacuum develops inside the cell at a time when the cell structure is not strong enough to resist the excess pressure of the atmosphere over that within the cells.

Successful closed-cell foams are produced when the cell membranes are sufficiently strong enough to withstand rupture at the maximum foam rise. The modulus of the polymer is increased rapidly to a high level so that the cells are dimensionally stable in spite of the development of a partial vacuum within the cells. On the other hand, a critical element in producing open-cell foams is the adjustment of the foaming rate and the rate of stabilization so that at the peak of the foam rise many cell membranes are thin and rupture, but the ribs of the cells are strong enough to stop the rupture [12].

8.3 MATERIALS FOR FOAMING

The blowing agent or foaming agent is added to a formulation as the source of the gas used to produce a foamed structure. Two major types of blowing agents can be used for foaming: chemical blowing agents (CBAs) or physical blowing agents (PBAs). When CBAs are used, a gas is produced via a chemical reaction, while PBAs are introduced as a liquid or as supercritical fluid. This chapter focuses on the use of PBAs for foaming operations since these are of greater interest in pharmaceutical applications.

In addition to the type of blowing agent, the solubility and diffusivity of the gas in the melt as well as the viscoelastic properties of the molten polymer are among the material parameters playing an important role during the various stages of foaming.

8.3.1 PHYSICAL BLOWING AGENTS

In the case of PBAs, these can either be permanent gases or volatile compounds [13]. Within the pharmaceutical space, nitrogen (N_2) and carbon dioxide (CO_2) are examples of permanent gases while water (H_2O) is a volatile compound; key properties of these are listed in Table 8.1. Examples of their use in the plastic and pharmaceutical industries can be found in the literature [14–17]. However, the use of water to manufacture drug products may be limited due to chemical and physical stability risks. In the food industry, CO_2 and H_2O are commonly used to produce puffed snacks and cereals via a foam extrusion cooking process [18,19].

The solubility of physical blowing agents in a polymer is of great importance during foaming operations. Gas solubility also has a direct impact on the rheological properties of the material and, as a result, on the foam morphology and its final properties. Various in-line and off-line methods have been used to measure the solubility of PBA in polymers. In-line gas solubility determination techniques are generally based on viscosity measurements [20–22] and optical methods [23,24]. Pressure decay and gravimetric

TABLE 8.1
Properties of Commonly Used Physical Blowing Agents

PBA	Density at 23°C [g/cm³]	Boiling Point [°C]	Critical Temperature [°C]	Critical Pressure [MPa]
N_2	1.146	–	−147	3.40
CO_2	1.811	−78.5	31	7.39
H_2O	1.000	100	374.1	22.10

Source: Throne, J.L., *Thermoplastic Foam Extrusion. An Introduction.* 2004, Hanser: Munich. Germany.

methods are the most commonly used off-line measurement techniques [24–26]. These methods provide between 5 and 7% accuracy in the solubility determination [26].

Gas solubility in polymers increases as the pressure is increased, but decreases as the temperature is increased. The latter is due to increased mobility of both the gas and solid phases, making it more difficult for the gas to remain within the melt.

The solubility of gases in polymers as a function of pressure is known to follow Henry's law [21,23,24,27] through the following expression:

$$S = k_p P_{CO_2} \tag{8.5}$$

where S is the volume of gas dissolved at standard temperature and pressure (STP), 273 K and 1 atm, conditions per unit weight of the polymer [cm^3(STP)/g]; k_p is the Henry's Law constant; and P_{CO_2} is the saturation pressure.

Furthermore, the temperature dependence of k_p follows the following Arrhenius expression:

$$k_p = k_{po} \exp\left(\frac{-E_s}{RT}\right) \tag{8.6}$$

where T is the absolute temperature, R is the universal gas constant, k_{po} is the temperature-independent Henry's law constant, and E_s is the heat of the solution. Table 8.2 shows the values of the latter two constants determined for copovidone and hydroxypropyl methylcellulose acetate succinate (HPMCAS).

8.3.2 POLYMER PROPERTIES

Polymer properties that influence the foaming process include melt shear and elongational viscosity, melt strength, and for semicrystalline polymers, the rate of crystallization.

In general, melts with high viscosity, particularly with high extensional viscosity, are needed for foaming. This is very important since a dissolved gas may act as a plasticizer, reducing the overall viscosity. In addition, melts with high elasticity and

---

TABLE 8.2
Henry's Law Constant and Heat Solution for Copovidone and HPMCAS

Polymer	Gas	k_{po} [cm^3 (STP)/g atm]	E_s [L atm/mol K]
Copovidone	CO_2	1.72×10^{-3}	0.511
	N_2	1.97×10^{-4}	0.684
HPMCAS	CO_2	1.09×10^{-3}	0.547
	N_2	1.35×10^{-5}	0.899

Source: Brown, C.D. et al., in *ANTEC 2011*. 2011, Society of Plastic Engineers: Boston, MA. USA. pp. 1224–1228.

high normal stress differences are needed during the extensional portion of the bubble inflation to create high resistance to stretching for stabilization of the growing bubbles. At the end of the bubble growth process during the final biaxial stretching, high melt elasticity to resist blowout, moderately high elongational viscosity (as long as it does not interfere with processability of the material), and rapid crystallization are needed.

Shear viscosity of a polymer without gas is commonly determined using a capillary rheometer by measuring the force required to push the molten polymer at a constant temperature and at various rates through a capillary tube. Measuring shear viscosity of a polymer containing dissolved gases is far more difficult due to the difficulty in maintaining enough pressure to prevent degassing. Various in-line methods (in-line rheometers, helical barrel rheometers [20,28]) are used to measure the shear viscosities of polymer-blowing agent solutions.

The polymer resistance to stretching is proportional to the rate of stretching. This proportionality is commonly called "extensional" or "elongational viscosity." Elongational viscosity of a material is directly related to its melt strength and therefore its ability to foam and create a cellular structure. Elongational viscosity measurements can be performed on a SER Universal Testing Platform Xpansion Instruments LLCd (SER-HV-R01) [29].

Melt strength (or melt elasticity, or melt extensibility) is the ultimate force at which a polymer melt can be greatly stretched without fracture or melt separation. Elasticity inhibits explosive initial bubble formation and allows rapid cell inflation and membrane stretching in low density foaming. Extensional rheometers, such as Rheotens from Gottfert's, are devices that measure both melt strength and extensibility simultaneously by combining the capillary rheometer with a device that pulls the melt away from the die at increasing rates and draw ratios. Crosslinking, branching, copolymerization, and blending are examples of methods for enhancing the melt strength of a polymer.

8.4 FOAM EXTRUSION PROCESS WITH PHYSICAL BLOWING AGENTS

During gas-assisted hot melt extrusion (HME) or foam extrusion (fHME), a gas is dissolved in the molten polymer-API system inside an extruder. Figure 8.3 shows schematically the elementary steps during the fHME process. Prior to gas injection,

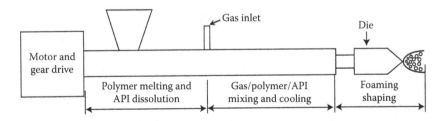

FIGURE 8.3 Schematic representation of the foam extrusion process. (Adapted from Lee, S.T. and D. Scholz, in *Polymeric Foams Series*, ed. S.T. Lee. 2009, CRC Press: Boca Raton, FL [31].)

the foam extrusion process is equivalent to the conventional HME process. Following gas injection, the gas must be dissolved in the melt and the "solution" has to be cooled to increase the melt viscosity and melt elasticity to provide the necessary melt strength to sustain the cellular structure without collapsing. Finally, foaming occurs along the die as the pressure is rapidly dropped to atmospheric conditions [23,30].

8.4.1 GAS INJECTION AND DISSOLUTION IN THE MELT STREAM

During a foam extrusion operation, a gas has to be introduced and dissolved in the molten polymer. If PBA is used, the gas is injected into the barrel during HME. The process must be designed to prevent the gas from escaping through the feed throat or along the die. This is accomplished through "melt seals" or fully filled screw sections. The melt seal upstream from the gas injection site is primarily achieved though screw design by utilizing flow restricting screw elements. In descending order of efficacy, the following elements enable formation of the melt seal: reversing conveying elements, reversing kneading blocks, and neutral (90°) kneading blocks. Furthermore, the injection pressure of the physical blowing agent must be lower than the maximum pressure along the melt seal to assure the gas remains inside the twin-screw extruder (TSE) and available for dissolution.

Dissolution of the gas in the melt is achieved through a combination of dispersive and distributive mixing.

8.4.2 CELL NUCLEATION

Depressurization along the die is the driving force for cell nucleation during a foam extrusion process. Figure 8.4 shows a schematic representation of the cell nucleation mechanism along a capillary die during the foam extrusion process. To assure a stable and robust process, the gas must be fully dissolved in the melt as it enters the die, forming a single phase with the molten polymer. Bubble nucleation is then triggered at a critical pressure (P_c). At this critical pressure, the system becomes oversaturated, favoring phase separation, i.e., nucleation [15,32].

As depicted in Figure 8.4, the pressure along a strand or capillary die drops linearly along its length. Equation 8.7 shows this relationship for non-Newtonian fluids [34].

$$\Delta P_d = K' \left(\frac{4Q}{\pi R^3} \right)^n L \tag{8.7}$$

where ΔP_d is the die's pressure drop (the pressure difference between a capillary's entrance and exit, points A and B in Figure 8.4); Q is the volumetric flow rate; R is the capillary radius; L is the length of the capillary; and K' and n are the consistency and flow indexes of the melt.

The four key variables controlling cell nucleation are gas concentration, concentration of the nucleating agent (if one is added to the formulation), depressurization rate, and pressure drop. In general, an increase in any of these four variables will result in foams with smaller cells and higher cell density (i.e., number of cells per

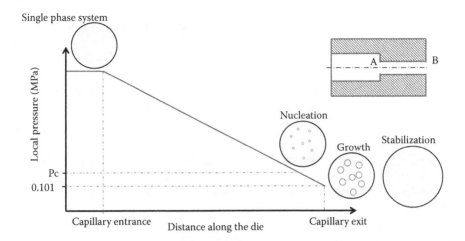

FIGURE 8.4 Schematic representation of the foaming mechanism during fHME. (Adapted from Terife, G., *Foaming of Amorphous Drug Delivery Systems Prepared by Hot Melt Mixing and Extrusion*. 2013, New Jersey Institute of Technology: Newark, NJ [33].)

unit volume) [15,32]. In order to avoid flow instabilities along the die, ideally the process should be designed to maximize both pressure drop and depressurization rate. From Equation 8.7 it can be concluded that an increase in pressure drop and/or depressurization rate can be achieved by die design or process throughput. Another strategy for controlling pressure would be by controlling process stream temperature, thus affecting polymer viscosity.

8.4.3 Cellular Growth and Stabilization

For a given formulation, with specific composition and set gas concentration, temperatures of the process stream and die are the key variables in controlling the kinetics of cellular growth and stabilization. As mentioned before, cell coalescence is thermodynamically favored; therefore, it is essential to control the viscoelastic properties of the product to mitigate extensive breakage of cell walls and/or shrinkage. Therefore, careful balance between die temperature and process stream temperature is the key for controlling cell coalescence, which is shown schematically in Figure 8.5.

The main function of die temperature is freezing the skin of the extrudate. This prevents gas loss via diffusion through the outer portion of the extrudate. It should be noted that if this temperature is too low, the skin fractures as the core expands continuously. On the other hand, product temperature is important in controlling the viscoelastic properties of the material. As a general rule, material needs to be cooled to increase its viscosity so it can undergo biaxial deformation, as bubbles form and grow, without breaking or collapsing. Although cooling of the melt can be done within the length of the twin-screw extruder, in some cases, additional cooling is needed. Methods for additional cooling include use of a tandem extruder (ideally a single-screw extruder) or static mixers [35].

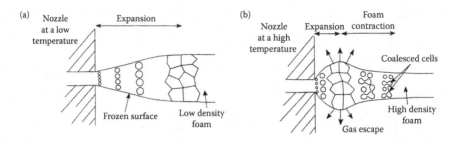

FIGURE 8.5 Schematics of cell growth and stabilization through die temperature: (a) optimum die/melt temperature and (b) high die/melt temperature. (From Park, C.B., A.H. Behravesh, and R.D. Venter, *Polymer Engineering & Science*, 1998. 38(11): pp. 1812–1823.)

8.5 APPLICATION OF FOAMING EXTRUSION OF PHARMACEUTICS

Research on fHME has focused on the following areas: (1) PBAs as fugitive plasticizers, (2) foams to facilitate milling operations, and (3) enhancing API release rate from solid dispersions.

8.5.1 Physical Blowing Agents as Fugitive Plasticizers

Addition of plasticizers to HME formulations is often necessary. Some APIs are susceptible to thermal degradation under HME processing conditions and potentially become inactive or lose functionality [36]. Similarly, many polymeric excipients in the market have a very narrow processing window and/or high viscosities, making processing without plasticizers very difficult. However, adding permanent plasticizers may be unfavorable to the formulation for several reasons:

- Plasticizers added to a formulation with the sole purpose of enabling processability of the intermediate constitute "dead weight" in the final dosage form. This may have a negative impact on patient adherence if the dosage form becomes too large.
- Plasticizers are in general low-molecular-weight compounds that may be lost via volatilization or migration during storage, resulting in unexpected changes in product performance during the shelf life of the drug product.
- The mechanism of action in plasticizers results in an increase in the overall mobility of the system; thus, it may be detrimental to the stability of the system, reducing the shelf life of the product.

The reasons outlined above make the use of a transient plasticizer very attractive during the HME process. This approach would allow reduction of the processing temperatures without negative effects on the long-term stability and performance of the drug product with a permanent plasticizer.

It is well known that once a PBA is dissolved in a polymer it can act as a plasticizer, making it a great candidate as a "fugitive" plasticizer. Carbon dioxide can decrease the viscosity for poly(methyl methacrylate) and polystyrene up to 80 and 70%, respectively [37].

The plasticization effect of PBA can be studied by varying the processing conditions (such as melt temperature, polymer flow rate, and gas content) and observing their effect on the melt viscosity while monitoring phase separation under supercritical and non-supercritical conditions [38,39]. Phase separation of the blowing agent during the extrusion process can be assessed using an optical cell along with a microscope by monitoring if any gas bubbles are observed in the glass window. Viscosity of the system can be determined in-line as a function of shear rate, temperature, and gas content for one-phase homogenous systems and indirectly through changes in the extruder torque, die, and melt pressures, which can be used as an indication of changes in the viscosity of the formulation.

A schematic of the gas-assisted extrusion process along with the monitoring system described above is shown in Figure 8.6. When the gas is injected at a specific

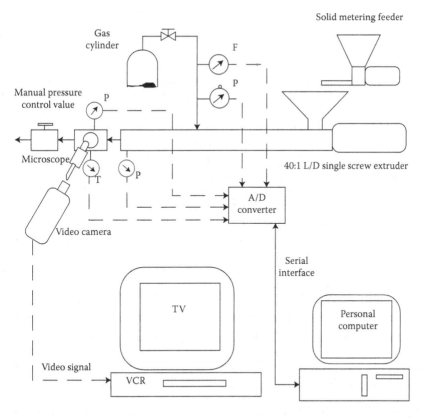

FIGURE 8.6 Schematic of the gas assisted extrusion process for viscosity measurements (Polymer Processing Institute, Newark, NJ). (From Faridi, N. In-Line Measurement of Solubility of Physical Blowing Agents in Polymer Melt. [cited 2017]; Available from: http://www.polymers-ppi.com/old/foam/solub.html.)

flow rate, if the die pressure is high enough, the gas would remain dissolved in the melt and a homogenous melt phase is observed. However, at higher gas pressures and lower die pressures, gas bubbles appear in the melt. The onset of the appearance of gas bubbles is an indication of a two-phase system, i.e., a phase separation where the gas amount is above its solubility in the polymer melt, and thus processing parameters such as die pressure cannot be used for viscosity calculation of the polymer-gas system.

The melt viscosity can be determined from the measured pressure drop (ΔP) and volumetric flow rate of the polymer in a capillary tube (Q), by using the following rheological equations [34]:

$$\eta_{app} = \frac{\tau_w}{\gamma_{app}} \tag{8.8}$$

$$\tau_w = \frac{\Delta P}{L} \frac{R}{2} \tag{8.9}$$

$$\gamma_{app} = \frac{4Q}{\pi R^3} \tag{8.10}$$

where η_{app} is the apparent viscosity, γ_{app} is the apparent shear rate, τ_w denotes the shear stress at the capillary wall, L is the length of the capillary tube, and R is the radius of the capillary.

The setup shown in Figure 8.6 was used to study the viscosity variations of a HPMCAS-API formulation containing different concentrations of CO_2. Figure 8.7 shows the viscosity as a function of temperature for this system measured at an apparent shear rate of 570 s^{-1}. The viscosity data show that CO_2 is an efficient plasticizer for HPMCAS-API formulation, lowering the viscosity of the melt by 20%–50% depending on the operating conditions. This plot helps in choosing the processing conditions such as percent of plasticizer and temperature to process a certain melt viscosity. It should be noted that a shear rate of 570 s^{-1} is a calculated shear rate at the die wall surface under the specific flow rate; the average shear rate in the extruder should be lower than this number and the plasticization effect is expected to be more significant at lower shear rates.

Several researchers have evaluated the plasticizing effect of CO_2 on pharmaceutical relevant systems by monitoring extruder torque during manufacture.

Verreck et al. [36,40,41] evaluated the effect of CO_2 as a plasticizer during the HME process in an 18-mm twin-screw extruder by determining the minimal temperature at which the maximum torque of the extruder was reached with and without injecting CO_2. In the absence of API, they reported a decrease in minimum temperature for copovidone, Eudragit® E100 (EPO), and ethyl cellulose (EC) of 30°, 15°, and 65°C, respectively [40]. The same study was performed using two binary systems: itraconazole/EC [36] and itraconazole/copovidone [41]. In the former case, the minimum processing temperature was decreased by 30°C and 65°C and in the latter case by 5°C and 10°C, depending on API loading.

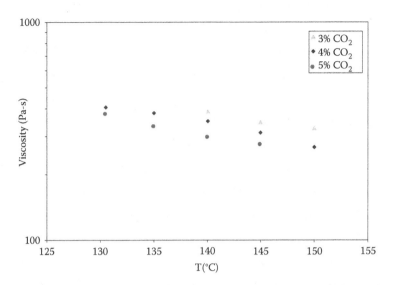

FIGURE 8.7 Viscosity of HPMCAS-API with various CO_2 concentrations as a function of temperature (measurements performed at shear rate of 570 s^{-1}).

Nikitine et al. [42] observed a 27%–43% reduction in torque by injecting CO_2 when extruding EPO in a 30-mm single-screw extruder. Nagy et al. [43] also observed a decrease in torque of 7 to 20% by using CO_2 as a PBA during compounding of the binary system of Carvedilol and EPO in a 30-mm single-screw extruder. Lyons et al. [44] also observed a decrease in torque and die pressure upon CO_2 injection in a 16-mm corotating twin-screw extruder.

Verreck et al. [45] used CO_2 as a fugitive plasticizer during compounding of p-amino salicylic acid—which is highly sensitive to thermal degradation—with EC in an 18-mm twin-screw extruder. The authors observed that through a conventional HME process, 17% of the API decomposed during compounding, but by using CO_2 as a fugitive plasticizer, the processing temperatures were reduced and the amount of decomposed API was reduced to 5%.

8.5.2 FOAMS TO FACILITATE MILLING

HME intermediates need to be milled to produce the final dosage form. Milled HME intermediates are further processed to produce tablets, dry powder-filled capsules or in suspensions for liquid formulations. However, extrudates tend to be very difficult to mill into suitable particle sizes with a narrow distribution. Furthermore, high energy milling is needed due to the inherent toughness of the extruded material, which results in localized heating, which further results in softening of the material and mesh blinding.

Weng et al. [14] demonstrated a significant increase in milling yields for HPMCAS upon foaming at the lab scale utilizing a Fitz mill. The milling yields for foamed

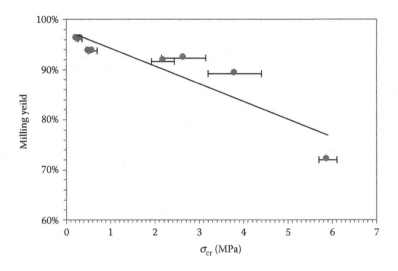

FIGURE 8.8 Milling yield as a function of critical compressive stress (σ_{cr}) form HPMCAS foamed extrudates produced using PBAs. (Adapted from Weng, J. et al., in *ANTEC 2015*. 2015, SPE: Orlando, FL.)

extrudates ranged from 72 to 96%, while the yield for unfoamed extrudate was 59%. Among the foamed samples, the yield was a function of the mechanical properties of the foamed material, specifically the critical compressive stress (see Figure 8.8). It should be noted that mechanical properties of the foam are a function of cell sizes, wall thicknesses, and foam density.

Verreck et al. [36,40,41] evaluated at small scale the impact of foam extrusion on milling efficiency for HME products. The studies were carried out using pure polymer excipients [40] and two polymer-API pairs [36,41]. Compounding and foaming was carried out in an 18-mm corotating TSE, employing CO_2 as the PBA. In all cases, the particles produced by grinding foamed extrudates had smaller measured average particle size, higher porosity, and bigger specific surface area than the particles produced from unfoamed extrudates, thus improving the milling efficiency of drug products.

In summary, it has been shown in the literature that the milling process of foamed extrudates is more efficient than that of unfoamed extrudates, and as expected, it yields smaller particles with higher surface area and porosity.

8.5.3 FOAMS TO INCREASE API RELEASE RATE

Solid dispersions manufactured via HME result in particles that have very low porosity. This may slow down penetration of body fluids into the sample and, thus, hinder API release [46]. Therefore, foaming could be used to increase surface area of the particles and reduce particle size to facilitate dissolution. Several researchers have observed an enhancement in dissolution rate when intermediates were produced via fHME.

Verreck et al. [36] observed an increase in release rate for the itraconazole/EC system upon foaming. By the end of the dissolution test, the amount of API released from the foamed samples was approximately 11-fold higher than that from unfoamed samples.

Lyons et al. [44] also observed an increase in API release rate by using foamed samples. HME and foam extrusion of a ternary system comprising carvedilol, polyethylene oxide (PEO), and EPO was carried out in a 16-mm corotating twin-screw extruder, with CO_2 as the PBA.

Nagy et al. [43] observed only a slightly faster API release for ground foams compared to the particles produced by milling unfoamed extrudates. Compounding and foaming of the carvedilol/EPO formulation was carried out in a 30-mm single-screw extruder, and CO_2 was used as the PBA.

In all cases, the increase in release rates of API was attributed to higher surface area of the milled fHME compared to milled HME samples. In the case of itraconazole/EC formulation, foaming yielded smaller particles.

REFERENCES

1. Gong, L., S. Kyriakides, and W.Y. Jang, Compressive response of open-cell foams. part i: morphology and elastic properties. *International Journal of Solids and Structures*, 2005. 42(5): pp. 1355–1379.
2. Shutov, F.A., Cellular strucuture and properties of foamed polymers, in *Handbook of Polymeric Foams and Foam Technology*, D. Klempner and K.C. Frisch, Editors. 1991, Hanser: New York, NY. USA. pp. 16–46.
3. Mills, N., *Polymer Foams Handbook. Engineering and Biomechanics Applications and Design Guide*. First ed. 2007, Elsevier: Burlington, MA. USA. 535.
4. Colton, J.S. and N.P. Suh, The nucleation of microcellular thermoplastic foam with additives: part i: theoretical considerations. *Polymer Engineering & Science*, 1987. 27(7): pp. 485–492.
5. Kumar, V. and N.P. Suh, A process for making microcellular thermoplastic parts. *Polymer Engineering & Science*, 1990. 30(20): pp. 1323–1329.
6. Saunders, J.H., The formation of urethan foams. *Rubber Chemistry and Technology*, 1960. 33(5): pp. 1293–1322.
7. Saunders, J.H. and R.H. Hansen, The mechanism of foam formation, in *Plastic Foams - Part I*; 1972, Marcel Dekker: New York. pp. 23–108.
8. Barlow, E.J. and W.E. Langlois, Diffusion of gas from a liquid into an expanding bubble. *IBM Journal of Research and Development*, 1962. 6(3): pp. 329–337.
9. Amon, M. and C.D. Denson, A study of the dynamics of foam growth: analysis of the growth of closely spaced spherical bubbles. *Polymer Engineering & Science*, 1984. 24(13): pp. 1026–1034.
10. Holl, M.R. et al., Cell nucleation in solid-state polymeric foams: evidence of a triaxial tensile failure mechanism. *Journal of Materials Science*, 1999. 34(3): pp. 637–644.
11. Tadmor, Z. and C.G. Gogos, *Principles of Polymer Processing*. 2 ed. 2006, Wiley-Interscience: Hoboken, NJ. USA.
12. Saunders, J.H. and D. Klempner, Fundamentals of foam formation, in *Polymeric Foams and Foam Technology*, D. Klempner and K.C. Frisch, Editors. 2004, Hanser: Ohio, 5–14.
13. Throne, J.L., *Thermoplastic Foam Extrusion. An Introduction*. 2004, Hanser: Munich. Germany.

14. Weng, J. et al., Correlation between foam extrusion process parameters, mechanical properties and pharmaceutical downstream processing, in *ANTEC 2015 Proceedings*. 2015, SPE: Orlando, FL.
15. Han, X. et al., Continuous microcellular polystyrene foam extrusion with supercritical CO_2. *Polymer Engineering & Science*, 2002. 42(11): pp. 2094–2106.
16. Sahmoune, A., Foaming of thermoplastic elastomers with water. *Journal of Cellular Plastics*, 2001. 37(2): pp. 149–159.
17. Nakamichi, K. et al., Evaluation of a floating dosage form of nicardipine hydrochloride and hydroxypropylmethylcellulose acetate succinate prepared using a twin-screw extruder. *International Journal of Pharmaceutics*, 2001. 218(1–2): pp. 103–112.
18. Moraru, C.I. and J.L. Kokini, Nucleation and expansion during extrusion and microwave heating of cereal foods. *Comprehensive Reviews in Food Science and Food Safety*, 2003. 2(4): pp. 147–165.
19. Cho, K.Y. and S.S.H. Rizvi, New generation of healthy snack food by supercritical fluid extrusion. *Journal of Food Processing and Preservation*, 2010. 34(2): pp. 192–218.
20. Todd, D.B., C.G. Gogos, and D. Champarampopoulos, *Helical Barrel Rheometer*, P.P. Institute, Editor. 1998. United States. pp. 1–7, US patent US005708197A.
21. Lee, M., C.B. Park, and C. Tzoganakis, Measurements and modeling of PS/supercritical co_2 solution viscosities. *Polymer Engineering & Science*, 1999. 39(1): pp. 99–109.
22. Choudhary, M. et al., Measurement of shear viscosity and solubility of polystyrene melts containing various blowing agents. *Journal of Cellular Plastics*, 2005. 41(6): pp. 589–599.
23. Zhang, Q. and M. Xanthos, Material properties affecting extrusion foaming, in *Polymeric Foams. Mechanisms and Materials*, S.T. Lee and N.S. Ramesh, Editors. 2004, CRC Press: Washington, D.C. USA, pp. 11–138.
24. Faridi, N. and D.B. Todd, Solubility measurements of blowing agents in polyethylene terephthalate. *Journal of Cellular Plastics*, 2007. 43(4–5): pp. 345–356.
25. Sato, Y. et al., Solubilities and diffusion coefficients of carbon dioxide in poly(vinyl acetate) and polystyrene. *Journal of Supercritical Fluids*, 2001. 19(2): pp. 187–198.
26. Tomasko, D.L. et al., A review of CO_2 applications in the processing of polymers. *Industrial & Engineering Chemistry Research*, 2003. 42(25): pp. 6431–6456.
27. Brown, C.D. et al., Evaluation of foaming of pharmaceutical polymers by CO_2 and N_2 to enable drug products, in *ANTEC 2011 Proceedings*. 2011, Society of Plastic Engineers: Boston, MA. USA. pp. 1224–1228.
28. Pabedinskas, A., W.R. Cluett, and S.T. Balke, Development of an in-line rheometer suitable for reactive extrusion processes. *Polymer Engineering & Science*, 1991. 31(5): pp. 365–375.
29. Sentmanat, M., B.N. Wang, and G.H. McKinley, Measuring the transient extensional rheology of polyethylene melts using the ser universal testing platform. *Journal of Rheology*, 2005. 49(3): pp. 585–606.
30. Lee, S.T., *Foam Extrusion. Principles and Practice*. 2000, Technomic Publishing Company, Inc.: Lancaster, PA. USA. 344.
31. Lee, S.T. and D. Scholz, Polymeric foams, technology and developments in regulation, process, and products. In *Polymeric Foams Series*, ed. S.T. Lee. 2009, CRC Press: Boca Raton, FL, 338pp.
32. Han, X. et al., Effect of die temperature on the morphology of microcellular foams. *Polymer Engineering & Science*, 2003. 43(6): pp. 1206–1220.
33. Terife, G., *Foaming of Amorphous Drug Delivery Systems Prepared by Hot Melt Mixing and Extrusion*. 2013, New Jersey Institute of Technology: Newark, NJ.
34. Brydson, J.A., *Flow Properties of Polymer Melts*. 2nd ed. 1981, Butler and Tanner Limited: Great Britain. 226.

35. Park, C.B., A.H. Behravesh, and R.D. Venter, Low density microcellular foam processing in extrusion using CO_2. *Polymer Engineering & Science*, 1998. 38(11): pp. 1812–1823.

36. Verreck, G. et al., The effect of supercritical CO_2 as a reversible plasticizer and foaming agent on the hot stage extrusion of itraconazole with EC 20 cps. *Journal of Supercritical Fluids*, 2007. 40(1): pp. 153–162.

37. Elkovitch, M.D. and D.L. Tomasko, Effect of supercritical carbon dioxide on morphology development during polymer blending. *Polymer Engineering & Science*, 2000. 40(8): pp. 1850–1861.

38. Lee, S.M. et al., High-pressure rheology of polymer melts containing supercritical carbon dioxide. *Korea-Australia Rheology Journal*, 2006. 18(2): pp. 83–90.

39. Faridi, N. *In-Line Measurement of Solubility of Physical Blowing Agents in Polymer Melt.* [cited 2017; Available from: http://www.polymers-ppi.com/old/foam/solub.html]

40. Verreck, G. et al., The effect of pressurized carbon dioxide as a plasticizer and foaming agent on the hot melt extrusion process and extrudate properties of pharmaceutical polymers. *Journal of Supercritical Fluids*, 2006. 38(3): pp. 383–391.

41. Verreck, G. et al., The effect of pressurized carbon dioxide as a temporary plasticizer and foaming agent on the hot stage extrusion process and extrudate properties of solid dispersions of itraconazole with PVP-VA 64. *European Journal of Pharmaceutical Sciences*, 2005. 26(3–4): pp. 349–358.

42. Nikitine, C. et al., Controlling the structure of a porous polymer by coupling supercritical CO_2 and single screw extrusion process. *Journal of Applied Polymer Science*, 2010. 115(2): pp. 981–990.

43. Nagy, Z.K. et al., Use of supercritical CO_2-aided and conventional melt extrusion for enhancing the dissolution rate of an active pharmaceutical ingredient. *Polymers for Advanced Technologies*, 2012. 23(5): pp. 909–918.

44. Lyons, J.G. et al., Preparation of monolithic matrices for oral drug delivery using a supercritical fluid assisted hot melt extrusion process. *International Journal of Pharmaceutics*, 2007. 329(1–2): pp. 62–71.

45. Verreck, G. et al., Hot stage extrusion of p-amino salicylic acid with ec using co_2 as a temporary plasticizer. *International Journal of Pharmaceutics*, 2006. 327(1–2): pp. 45–50.

46. Andrews, G.P. et al., Physicochemical characterization and drug-release properties of celecoxib hot-melt extruded glass solutions. *Journal of Pharmacy and Pharmacology*, 2010. 62(11): pp. 1580–1590.

9 Melt Pelletization and Size Reduction

Powder to Pellets and Powder to Powder

Christopher C. Case, Albrecht Huber, and Kathrin Nickel

CONTENTS

9.1 INTRODUCTION

Pelletization is a downstream operation for a melt extrusion process where materials are taken from a device such as an extruder or melt pump, pumped through a die, cooled, and cut into a "pellet." Many products enter their first solid or densified state in a "pellet" form. This pellet, typically 3 mm in size or less, is then processed in another extruder and milled for tableting or for capsule filling. The main goal of pelletization is to facilitate the consistent feeding, transport, and packaging of the pellets. Generally, the pellet itself is made up of multiple components that have been compounded in a device, such as a twin-screw extruder, so that the material has the desired properties. Sometimes, chill rolls with pin breakers are used to accomplish the same goal.

Primarily used in the plastic industry, pelletization came into being due to a few simple facts. Many products needed to be transported from one place to another in a uniform particle size. Also, the pellet may need to be subsequently fed into another piece of

183

equipment for further processing. Finally, the particle size often needs to be very similar to achieve an accurate and continuous feed rate. All factors that make a pellet desirable for a plastic pellet also apply to a pharmaceutical process. Nearly every machine built for the pelletizing process for pharmaceutical applications is constructed of stainless steel product contact areas. Out of necessity, however, some components such as pneumatic cylinders, bearings, and seals might still be manufactured from oxidizing materials.

Downstream systems come in several designs and are selected based upon the material characteristics, throughput rate, and lot size. The following is a simple description of commercially available pelletizers and chill rolls with pin breakers that are used to make small/compounded particles in preparation for subsequent downstream process operations.

9.2 STRAND PELLETIZERS

The strand pelletizer was developed in the 1950s to cut strands into a canister-like final product. This is accomplished by forcing the product through a strand die that produces spaghetti-like strand(s). The strand is then pulled through some type of a cooling medium by the feedrolls of the pelletizer and cut to length. The diameter of the final pellet is controlled by the diameter of the orifice and the speed at which the feedrolls are pulling the strand. Almost all products will be "drawn down" in diameter upon exiting the die. As seen in Figure 9.1, the feedroll speed is usually set in a ratio to the rotor or cutting head based on the number of cutting edges and the desired pellet length.

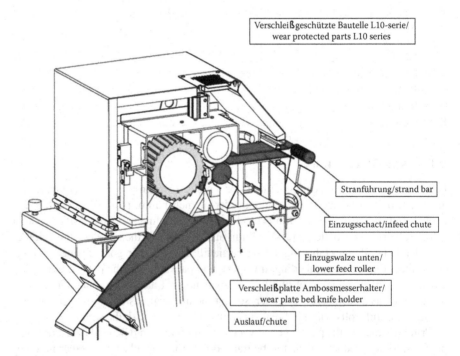

FIGURE 9.1 Close-up strand pelletizer.

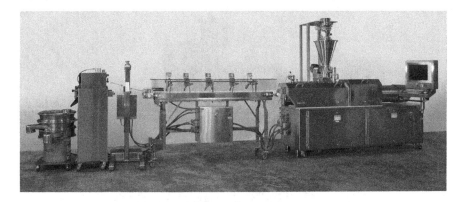

FIGURE 9.2   Twin-screw extruder with in-line gauging and downstream pelletizing system.

Prior to the pelletizer, the strands must be cooled. For the plastics industry, the strands are typically drawn through a water bath by the pelletizer feedrolls. Upon exit of the water bath and before the pelletizer, an air stripper device removes moisture from the surface of the strands by means of compressed air, an air blower, or by vacuum.

As many pharmaceutical products cannot contact water, the cooling bath is often replaced with a cooling belt or static cooling table. Cooling belts can be stainless steel with liquid "spray" cooling underneath the belt to facilitate additional heat exchange. Belts can also be constructed of a covering or plastic mesh compliant with Food and Drug Administration (FDA) guidelines. Auxiliary blowers utilizing ambient or refrigerated air streams can be specified to assist the cooling process as shown in Figure 9.2.

If the strands exhibit enough elasticity, another alternative is to utilize a series of grooved stainless steel rolls that are cored for liquid cooling. The "grooving" of the rolls will increase the surface contact for better heat transfer capabilities, as well as assist in sizing the shape of the strands.

9.3   DIE FACE PELLETIZERS

An alternative to strand pelletization is a process referred to as "die face" pelletizing. With this method, the strand is cut at the die face in a molten form and cooled via air or liquid. The advantage of this system, if workable, is that the problem of strand breakage during the cooling phase is eliminated. Die face pelletizing is not a wide spectrum with regard to the range of materials that can be processed, and start-up procedures need to be defined more carefully. However, if the process is amenable, die face pelletizing is often preferred over the strand systems defined above.

9.4   AIR QUENCH DIE FACE PELLETIZERS

A die face pelletizing method that is often preferred for pharmaceutical applications is where the melt stream exits horizontally through a streamlined die and is cut by a flywheel or spring loaded cutter at the die face. After the "cut," pellets can be conveyed to either a vibratory cooler/separator or fluidized vibratory unit, where the cooling process is finished.

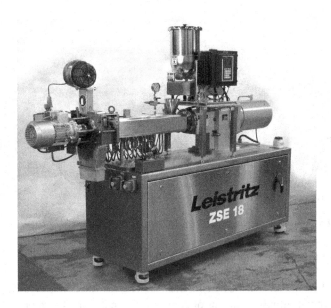

FIGURE 9.3   Twin-screw extruder with hot face pelletizer attachment.

Additional product drying is possible if a heated air supply is supplied for convey-ing. Air quench pelletizing is ideal for formulations that have a high level of inert materials, such as desiccant compounds. Air quench pelletizing should be tested for specific products because many formulations cannot be processed this way, as some products tend to smear at the die face. An example of this type of system, which works well for higher viscosity and highly filled process melts, is shown in Figure 9.3.

For materials that have a tendency to smear, the use of Vortex tubes to direct chilled air at the die face facilitates die face cutting. Another alternative is to utilize atomizers to mist the die area for borderline formulations. Pellets produced via the air quench method are often slightly deformed in cooling and are generally deemed less aesthetically appealing than other methods described.

9.5   UNDERWATER AND WATER RING PELLETIZERS

Underwater pelletizing describes a method where molten product is fed through a die with a series of holes in a circular pattern. When the product emerges from the die, it is cut into pellets by the rotating blades, with the pellet immediately solidifying in the water. The water/pellet slurry is then pumped to a spin dryer for dewatering and surface drying, returning the process water to the central system. As seen in Figure 9.4 below, the underwater pelletizer is recommended for lower-viscosity materials that can withstand water contact and retain temperature but cannot be cut in air.

Another die face design is a water ring pelletizer, where the pellets are cut at the die face in air and "flung" into a slurry discharge, which is pumped into a centrifugal dryer where the pellets are separated from the water. Most commercial water ring pelletizers discharge vertically downward, which is generally not suited for pharma-ceutical applications, as the increased residence time and the flow stagnation often

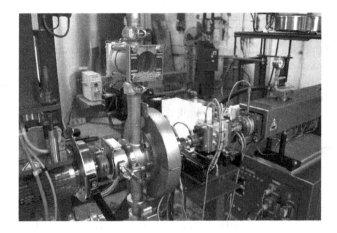

FIGURE 9.4 Close-up underwater pelletizing assembly.

adversely affect the product properties and make cleanout more difficult. However, commercial units that integrate a horizontal die design similar to the underwater pelletizing method described above can eliminate this problem.

9.6 VIBRATING RING DROPPO PELLETIZERS

A unique pelletizing method that handles the low-viscosity materials in an innovative way is the Vibrating Ring Droppo Pelletizer. By pumping the material through a small vibrating head, an array of pellet sizes can be produced. The pellet size depends on the frequency of the head. The typical viscosity range is 100–300 cP. The Droppo method is capable of the production of uniform spherical droplets and offers an alternative for pelletizing low-viscosity melts and liquids that do not form strands. Pellet formation is achieved by the harmonic vibration applied to the melt in a die head. Surface tension causes the flow to break into small droplets. The droplets produced become spherical pellets with an extremely narrow pellet size distribution. There is no mechanical cutting involved. Depending on the viscosity and the surface tension

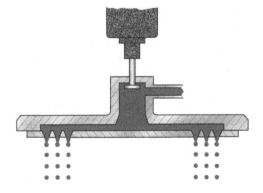

FIGURE 9.5 Vibrating Ring Droppo Pelletizer schematic.

of the melt, drops with diameters from 0.3 to 4.0 mm are generated by varying the frequency and the size of the die holes (as demonstrated in Figure 9.5).

After exiting the die, the droplets fall through a cooling tower that uses air, nitrogen, water, or water spray to solidify the product. The height of the tower is dictated by the materials, the throughput rate, and the method of cooling. The resulting spherical pellet can offer the ideal pellet shape for exact dosing and homogenous mixtures, where equal material flow and high-bulk density are required.

9.7 MICROPELLETIZING

Micropellets are small, free-flowing, spherical or semispherical units, made up of fine powders or granules of bulk drugs and excipients. They can be coated and are very often used in controlled-release dosage forms. As an intermediate product, they are filled in capsules or sachets or directly pressed into tablets. There are various reasons to produce micropellets, such as

- Improvement of free-flowing properties
- Defined shape and weight to improve the appearance of the product
- Prevention of dust formation (process safety)
- Increased bulk density by decreasing bulk volume
- Controlled-release application (low surface area versus volume)
- Film coating possibilities to support multiple unit pellet systems (MUPS)

The "standard" pellet size produced is approximately 3 mm. Larger pellets, up to 20 mm, are possible but uncommon. More typically, the goal is to extrude pellets of 1 mm or smaller, which is preferred for feeding in small single-screw extruders and micromolding machines. All of the pelletizing methods described above may be used to make micropellets, with varying degrees of modifications and probability of success.

For strand micropelletizing, the speed of the pull rolls requires a drive that is independent and can be synchronized with the cutter rpm. The speed of the pull rolls determines the linear speed of the strands; the faster the cutter rpm, the shorter the pellet. Due to geometrical limitations associated with the pull roll/bed knife/ cutter assembly, this method has only been successful in producing pellets approximately 0.8 mm in length and larger. Another alternative is to use a flywheel cutter, as described in the "Shape Extrusion" chapter of this book.

For any of the die face pelletizers, the number and the diameter of the holes in the die are dramatically increased. As the pellets are very small (in the 400-Am range), die blockage, material handling, and classification can become challenging. Often times, dies for micropelletization operate at higher pressures than for standard pellets, which may necessitate the use of the gear pump front end attachment to build pressure to the die, particularly for a pelletizing system that is mated to a starve-fed twin-screw extruder.

For low-viscosity carriers, the Vibrating Ring Droppo Pelletizer, as described above, might be the ideal choice for micropellets. Figure 9.6 shows an actual Leistritz micropelletizer (LMP 18 2.0). The pelletizer can be operated with one or two knives up to 3000 rpm. Cooling and transport of the pellets is performed by vacuum conveying, and blade pretension is adjustable through the control panel.

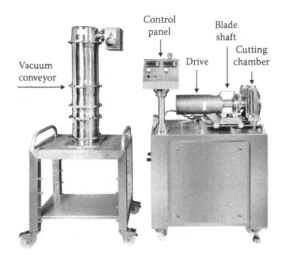

FIGURE 9.6 Leistritz micropelletizer (LMP).

Typical pellet sizes range between 0.8 and 1.2 mm and trials with smaller die holes of 0.3 mm have been performed. Figure 9.7, for example, shows a scanning electron microscope (SEM) of Eudragit® RS pellets made with a 1-mm die. Micropelletizers for pharmaceutical applications work when the extruder pushes the material over a cone through the die holes. Rotating knives then cut the melt directly when it exits the die head. Figures 9.8 and 9.9 illustrate the pelletizer die and the cutting device.

9.8 PROCESS TECHNOLOGY

Due to the relatively small diameters of the die holes, pressure can easily go up to 200 bars, resulting in an increased melt temperature. As a rule of thumb, a 40-bar

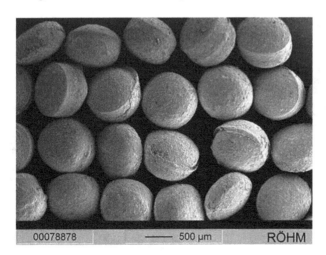

FIGURE 9.7 SEM picture of Eudragit® RS pellets (Source: Evonik).

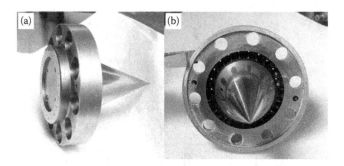

FIGURE 9.8 Die with mounted cone side view (a) and back view (b).

pressure increase results in a 20°C temperature rise. To diminish this effect of increasing temperature due to high pressure, gear pumps are often used because they are able to build up the pressure more efficiently than an extruder. Additionally, the shear in the extruder can be reduced while using a gear pump, lowering the melt temperature. This, in turn, will result in a wider operating window. On one hand, higher throughputs can be obtained; on the other hand, lower shear for sensitive active pharmaceutical ingredients (APIs) will enhance the quality of the end product. The differences of working with or without a gear pump are depicted in Figure 9.10. Another advantage of hot die face pelletizing is a narrower particle size distribution as compared to other existing cutting methods. This can be seen in Figure 9.11, which shows a comparison of the particle size distribution of pellets made with the LMP compared to milled strand granules. Besides the die diameter and output values, pellet weight, and thus the drug release, can be further influenced by the speed/number of knives. This can be shown by the performance of a test with a formulation of Kollidon®SR and Metformin (50:50) at different pelletizer speeds. The settings for the trial were the following:

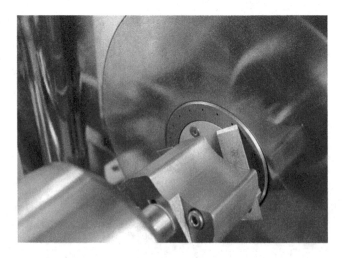

FIGURE 9.9 Knife head of LMP 18 2.0.

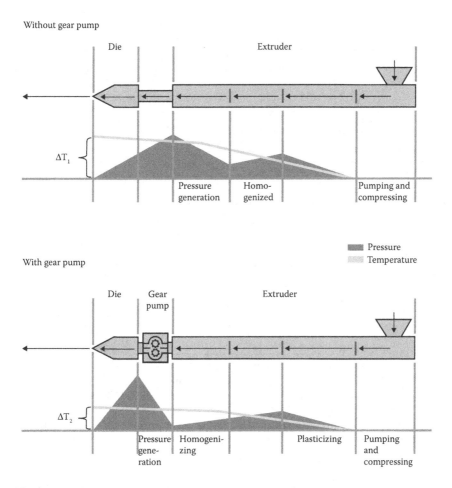

FIGURE 9.10 Influence of gear pump on melt pressure and temperature.

- Feed rate: 0.5 kg/h
- Die: 20 × 1.0 mm
- Number of knives: 2
- Pelletizer speed: 500–1000 rpm

Figure 9.12 demonstrates that with increasing pelletizer speed, the weight of one single pellet decreases, resulting in a faster drug release and vice versa. As continuous manufacturing is a preferred manufacturing methodology in the pharmaceutical industry, the pelletizer is ideally suited to facilitate this practice.

9.9 DIE DESIGN ISSUES

Die design is the subject of another chapter in this book. Therefore, only an overview specifically relating to the pelletization process is provided. Regardless of the style of pelletizer, the same basic design principles apply.

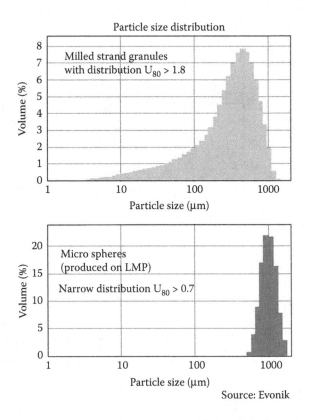

FIGURE 9.11 Comparison of particle size distribution of pellets made with an LMP compared to strand granules.

Pelletizers, just like any other extrusion process, require a quality extrudate. Given this concept, the die design becomes a critical part of the total system design. In the case of all dies, there are a few criteria that need to be recognized in order for the die to function properly.

All products do not exhibit the same level of "die swell." The term "die swell" is used when a product increases in diameter as it exits the hole from the high-pressure internal area to the atmospherical area outside (see Figure 9.13).

For an air quench pelletizer, the die swell calculation is much more critical because a drawdown of the product is not possible. Therefore, die swell must be recognized as a critical parameter during the design phase of the die hole geometry to make the correct pellet geometry.

The pressure distribution across the face of the die is an important design consideration. In a strand die, the comparison of pressure readings from the holes in the center of the die, when compared with the pressure readings at the outside holes, should be held at ±2%. A die with a higher differential of pressure will exhibit a higher flow in the center of the die when compared with the outermost strand flow. Given that the feedrolls of the pelletizer will pull all of the strands at the same lineal rate, the

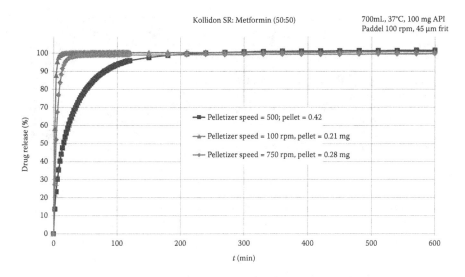

FIGURE 9.12 Drug release of a Kollidon® SRMetformin mixture (5050).

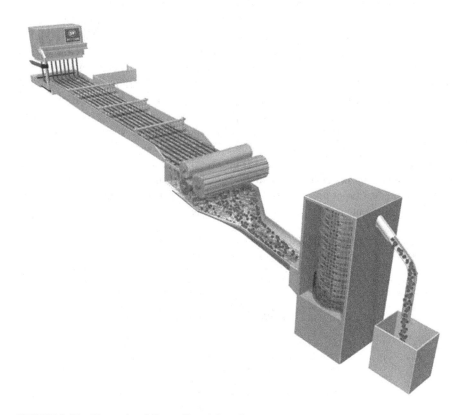

FIGURE 9.13 Example of die swell and drawdown.

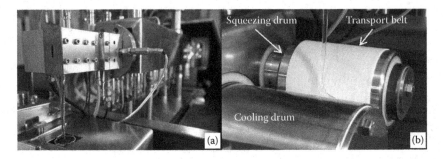

FIGURE 9.14   Melt drops into cooling drum (a) and squeezing drum (b).

outside strands will be a smaller finished diameter than those that were produced by the center of the die. This variation will show up in the final pelletized products as a range of bulk density due to the changes in volume from one pellet to another.

9.10   CHILL ROLL AS A NOVEL METHOD FOR COOLING AND MILLING OF PHARMACEUTICAL PRODUCTS

Another technology is available to cool the melt and facilitate particle size reduction. While the mixing and melting take place in the usual steps on a corotating twin-screw extruder, the hot melt exits the extruder and drops onto a cooled drum (Figure 9.14a).

After exiting the extruder, the product is squeezed between two drums (Figure 9.14b), the cooling drum and the squeezing drum. The gap between the drums is adjustable so that the melt thickness is variable. A transport belt mounted on the squeezing drum pressurizes the melt onto the cooling drum to allow maximum heat transfer. In general, the final product temperature is between 20°C and 40°C, and due to the rapid cooling, most of the polymers become brittle and break down to smaller fragments. These fragments are then transported to a pin breaker, where they are further reduced in size (Figures 9.15 and 9.16).

The result is a product shape called "flakes." Depending on desired flake size, different pin breaker types are available, which include a pin crusher and a teeth crusher. If smaller fragments are desired, a teeth crusher is useful; otherwise a pin crusher is

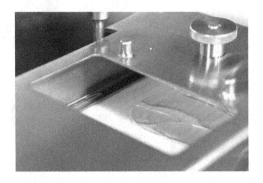

FIGURE 9.15   Transport of cooled polymer melt to the crusher.

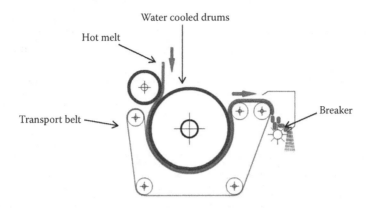

FIGURE 9.16 Visualization of the chill roll performance.

used. Depending on the end product requirements, the flakes can be further processed through, for example, milling and tableting. Therefore, an integration of a mill is possible so that the flakes can be milled in-line (Figure 9.17). Different mills are available that are used for different particle sizes. A conical sieve mill can be integrated for sizes up to 150 µm, while a hammer mill can be used for smaller sizes, down to 50 µm.

The main influencing parameter for this process is the viscosity of the melt, as it determines the handling at the product inlet to the cooler. Usually the melt viscosity after the extrusion process allows the product to be squeezed into a thin product layer between the rolls. Another important parameter is the specific heat capacity. The specific heat capacity determines the amount of heat that will be extracted from the product and will mainly determine the final product temperature. The smaller the heat capacity of a polymer, the higher the temperature difference between the melt and end product. The temperature of the chill roll has a less pronounced effect on the final product temperature compared to the heat capacity but also will influence the

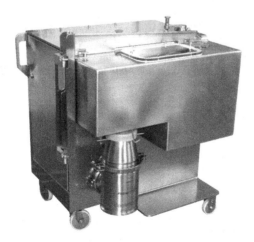

FIGURE 9.17 Chill roll (CCRM-PH) with integrated mill (BBA Innova).

cooling rate. Additional factors that affect the cooling rate are the speed of the drums (residence time) and the gap between the rolls (thickness of the product).

Materials of construction are very important to guarantee FDA conformity and to avoid product sticking to the belt.

This production method is a lean production method, allowing a process from powder to powder.

9.11 SUMMARY

Pelletization and size reduction via chill rolls with pin breakers are established technologies in plastics for a wide variety of materials and applications. Accordingly, almost every technical challenge presented by the pharmaceutical industry has been addressed at some level for plastics and can be successfully applied to manufacture an FDA product. The main issue faced today is for users to convince machine suppliers to downsize existing equipment and to implement the necessary machinery modifications as dictated for use in a good manufacturing practices environment.

The evolution of continuous processing via single-screw and twin-screw extruders in the medical device and pharmaceutical industries has already made this—to a significant degree—a reality.

BIBLIOGRAPHY

1. Progelhof RC, Throne JL. *Polymer Engineering Principles*. Cincinnati, OH: Hanser Gardner, 1993:427.
2. Sansone LF. Strand Cooling. Extrusion Solutions v 2.0 CD. SPE Extrusion Division 2001.
3. Dietz W. A cooling time model for plastics processing operations. *Polymer Engineering and Science* 1978; 18:13.
4. Sisfleet WL, Dinos N, Collier JR. Unsteady-state heat transfer in a crystalline polymer. *Polymer Engineering and Science* 1973; 13:10.
5. Herrmann H, ed. *Granulieren von Thermoplastichen Kunstoffen*. VDI-Verlag GMBH Düsseldorf.
6. Shoemaker P. Leistritz Training Workshop, June 2002.
7. Hartung H, Gryczke A, Kircher W, Gao X. *Investigation of a New Chill Roll with Integrated Mill for Hot-Melt Extrusion with Soluplus*.
8. Hartung H. *Latest Developments in Producing Micro Pellets*.
9. Schmotzer HJ. *Lean HME Production Method with Extruder, Chill Roll, Mill*.

10 Extended-Release Dosage Forms Prepared Using Twin-Screw Extrusion

Bo Lang, Xin Feng, and Feng Zhang

CONTENTS

10.1 INTRODUCTION

Extensive research has been pursued with extended-release drug delivery systems. The advantages of such systems over traditional dosage forms include less frequent dosing, improved patient compliance, and more stable blood levels of the drug, which can significantly increase the efficacy and reduce the side effects of the drug substance (Welling and Dobrinska 1987). Recent advances in the field of drug delivery have resulted in the precise control of the level and location of drug delivery in the body. In addition, lower doses of medication to the patient are needed (Langer 1998). Polymeric and hydrophobic lipid matrices for oral delivery and medical implants have been some of the most common approaches for achieving extended drug release profiles. Polymers and hydrophobic lipids can be used as both binders and retardants. The most widely used processes to manufacture extended-release oral dosage forms include the wet granulation, dry granulation, and direct compression techniques. The wet granulation process is both a labor- and equipment-intensive technique involving several unit operations. Excipients such as binders are required to facilitate processing. The direct compression and dry granulation techniques are subject to content uniformity and segregation problems during the tableting process. Poor compactibility of the tablet excipients or the drug substance may introduce additional problems into the compaction process.

Twin-screw extrusion technology is one of the most common processing techniques in the plastic and food industries. After 100 or so years of usage, the well-characterized nature of the twin-screw extrusion process lends itself to ease of scale-up and process optimization, while also affording benefits of continuous manufacturing and adaptability to process analytical technology in an ever-changing regulatory and fiscal environment. What is occurring today for pharmaceuticals, with regard to the implementation of extrusion technology to increase efficiencies and save costs, is analog to what occurred 80 or so years ago in the plastics and food sectors of industry as batch processes were replaced by continuous manufacturing alternatives for reasons that are now obvious. For over two decades, the importance of "continuous processing" in the pharmaceutical industry has also been recognized. The potential for better in-process control to improve product quality and the reduction of capital investment and labor costs have made twin-screw extrusion worthy of consideration as a pharmaceutical process. Table 10.1 contains a list of commercial drug products manufactured by a twin-screw extrusion process approved by the U.S. Food and Drug Administration (FDA).

In this chapter, twin-screw extrusion processes are categorized into melt extrusion and wet granulation. The melt extrusion process is further categorized into extrusion preparing polymer-based oral dosage forms, extrusion preparing hydrophobic lipid and wax-based oral dosage forms, extrusion preparing polymer-based implants. Compared to the conventional manufacturing processes, the twin-screw extrusion process involves different mechanisms of matrix formation. As a result, twin-screw extrusion could be applied to prepare extended-release dosage forms with unique drug release characteristics and physical properties.

This chapter describes the drug release mechanism of extended-release dosage forms, and the application of the twin-screw extrusion process to prepare various extended-release dosage forms. The mechanisms for matrix formation during the extrusion process are discussed. The advantages and challenges of twin-screw processes are also presented.

10.2 MECHANISMS OF DRUG RELEASE FROM EXTENDED-RELEASE DRUG DELIVERY SYSTEMS

10.2.1 HYDROPHILIC MATRIX DRUG DELIVERY SYSTEM

Twin-screw extrusion has been widely reported for the manufacturing of hydrophilic matrix systems, such as a polyethylene oxide-based extended-release system (Zhang

TABLE 10.1
List of Commercial Extended-Release Products Manufactured Using Twin-Screw Extrusion Processes

Product Name	Active	Key Excipients	Indication	Dosage Form	Company	Year Approved
Zoladex®	Goserelin Acetate	D,L-lactic glycolic acids copolymer	Prostate cancer	Subcutaneous implant	AstraZeneca	1996
ZMAX®	Azythromycin	Glycerol behenate	Antibiotic	Oral granules	Pfizer	1996
NuvaRing®	Etonogestrel, Ethinyl Estradiol	Polyethylene vinyl acetate	Contraceptive	Vaginal ring	Merck	2001
Palladon®	Hydromorphone HCl	Eudragit RS® Ethylcellulose Stearyl alcohol	Pain	Oral tablet	Purdue Pharma	2004
Implanon®	Etonogestrel	Ethylene vinyl acetate	Contraceptive	Vaginal ring	Merck	2006
Ozurdex®	Dexamethasone	D,L-lactic glycolic acids copolymer	Macular edema	Ophthalmic implant	Allergan	2009
Nucynta ER®	Tapentadol HCl	Polyethylene oxide	Pain	Oral tablet	Depomed Inc.	2011
Opana ER®	Oxymorphone HCl	Polyethylene oxide	Pain	Oral tablet	Endo Pharmaceuticals	2011
Probuphine®	Buprenorphine	Polyethylene vinyl acetate	Opioid addiction	Subdermal implant	Titan and Braeburn Pharma-ceuticals	2016

and McGinity 1999, Crowley et al. 2002). Before further exploring the application of twin-screw extrusion in hydrophilic matrix systems, it is critical to have a comprehensive understanding of the drug release mechanism of such systems. The initial trial of utilizing hydrophilic polymers for extended-release purposes can be dated back to the 1960s (Christenson and Dale 1962, Huber et al. 1966). Since then, a variety of hydrophilic polymers have been investigated for this purpose, such as cellulose derivatives (hydroxypropyl methylcellulose, hydroxypropyl cellulose, hydroxyethyl cellulose); natural polymers (xanthan gum, guar gum, locust bean gum, sodium alginate); and other synthetic polymers (polyethylene oxide, carbomer, polycarbophil). In contrast to the conventional immediate-release tablets that disintegrate in an aqueous environment and release granules and primary active pharmaceutical ingredient (API) particles, hydrophilic matrix extended-release tablets do not disintegrate and retain the monolithic morphology after administration due to the polymer hydration and gelation on the tablet surface in an aqueous environment (Huber et al. 1966). The gel layer on the tablet surface controls water penetration into the tablet and the API molecule diffusion to the aqueous environment. The swelling phenomenon of the polymeric matrix is shown in Figure 10.1. Significant efforts have been devoted to revealing the drug release mechanism of hydrophilic matrix systems and have been reviewed elsewhere (Colombo 1993, Siepmann and Peppas 2001). Drug release from a hydrophilic matrix system is initiated from water penetration, which plasticizes the release-controlling polymer, causing polymer glass transition. Meanwhile, the dissolution of API particles will also happen during the water penetration process. Dissolved API molecules have a greater diffusion coefficient in the rubbery state polymer, and API diffusion will partially contribute to the overall drug release from a hydrophilic matrix system. In addition to drug diffusion, the erosion of swollen release-controlling polymer is another source of drug release, especially of compounds with low aqueous solubility in which the drug molecule diffusion is very limited due to the low concentration of solubilized drug in the matrix and the low

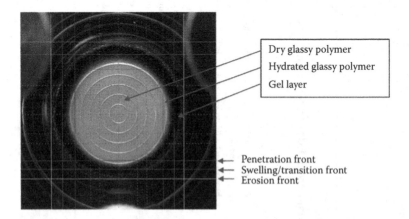

FIGURE 10.1 Swelling of a hydrophilic matrix tablet after water exposure. (Reprinted from Ferrero, C., D. Massuelle and E. Doelker (2010). *Journal of Controlled Release* 141(2): 223–233. With permission.)

concentration gradient between the tablet matrix and external aqueous environment. Besides the diffusion and erosion mechanism, the overall drug release of a hydrophilic matrix system may also be affected by several other factors. Taking diffusion area as an example, the surface area of an intact tablet is well defined by the tooling geometry and the tablet thickness. During matrix tablet dissolution, the polymer swelling will significantly affect the tablet geometry and surface area, leading to a varying tablet diffusion surface area and a varying drug release rate. Another example is the drug diffusion coefficient in the rubbery state polymer matrix. To simplify the modeling of a drug release profile from a matrix system, the drug diffusion coefficient is usually considered as a constant (Higuchi 1961). However, the ratio of water vs. polymer across the gel layer may not be a constant (Baumgartner et al. 2005). A higher percentage of water may be observed in the external portion of the gel layer and a higher percentage of polymer may be observed in the inner portion of the gel layer. The water level gradient across the gel layer may lead to a drug diffusion coefficient gradient that will further complicate the modeling of a drug release profile.

The Higuchi equation was derived and published back in 1961 to predict the drug release profile from a diffusion-controlled planar matrix system, followed by many other studies to predict the drug release profile from matrix systems with different system geometries (Higuchi 1961, Ritger and Peppas 1987a,b, Lee 2011).

$$\frac{Mt}{A} = \sqrt{Dt\left(2C_o - C_s\right)C_s}$$

where Mt is the cumulative amount of drug released at time t, A is the contact surface area, C_0 is the initial drug concentration, C_s is the solubility of the drug in the polymer matrix, and D is the diffusion coefficient of the drug in the polymer matrix.

A linear relationship was predicted between the percentage of drug release and the square root of time in a diffusion-controlled matrix system. However, the derivation of the Higuchi equation requires several assumptions, such as a constant diffusion coefficient and negligible polymer swelling and dissolution (Higuchi 1961, Siepmann and Peppas 2001, Siepmann and Peppas 2011). As described in the previous paragraph, those assumptions may be violated during the dissolution of a matrix tablet; therefore, caution should be exercised when directly applying the Higuchi equation to a hydrophilic matrix sustained release system. Besides the Higuchi equation, several other equations have also been proposed, such as the semiempirical power law equation (Ritger and Peppas 1987a,b, Siepmann and Peppas 2001). The diffusional exponent may provide insight into the underlying drug release mechanism from the matrix system (Ritger and Peppas 1987a,b, Peppas and Sahlin 1989). The original articles may be referred to for more detailed information.

10.2.2 Hydrophobic Matrix Drug Delivery System

Melt-extruded hydrophobic matrix systems have been adopted in some extended-release systems such as extended-release tablets and implants (Costantini et al. 2004, Almeida et al. 2011, Helbling et al. 2014). Due to the low glass transition temperature, polyethylene vinyl acetate has been used in recent years as a matrix polymer for hydrophobic matrix drug delivery systems (Almeida et al. 2011). In contrast to the hydrophilic matrix system, a hydrophobic matrix system contains a release-controlling polymer that is neither soluble nor swellable in an aqueous environment. Therefore, the drug release mechanism in a hydrophobic matrix system is predominantly drug diffusion. A few research articles have been published to model the drug release profile from extended-release implants comprising hydrophobic matrix polymers (Helbling, Cabrera et al. 2011, Helbling, Luna et al. 2011). In general, the basic assumptions in the Higuchi equation are valid, and the drug release is affected by the dosage form geometry. The drug release profile predicted from the model matches very well with the experimental data (Helbling, Cabrera et al. 2011, Helbling, Luna et al. 2011).

10.2.3 MEMBRANE-CONTROLLED DRUG DELIVERY SYSTEM

Besides hydrophilic and hydrophobic matrix systems, membrane-controlled extended-release systems are another category of extended-release system. Coextrusion technology has been reported to yield the laminar extrudate comprising a drug-loaded core and a release-controlling excipient surface layer (Oliveira et al. 2014, Vynckier et al. 2014a,b, Laukamp et al. 2015). Such extrudate may be considered as a membrane-controlled extended-release system and the drug release mechanism of a coated multiparticulate system may help understand the release mechanism of a coextruded laminar extrudate. A number of articles have been published to describe the release mechanism of membrane-controlled formulations. Depending on the mechanical strength and the composition of a drug-loaded core, the drug may be released by diffusion through an intact membrane or diffusion through membrane cracks (Lecomte et al. 2005). The two schemes of drug delivery mechanism from

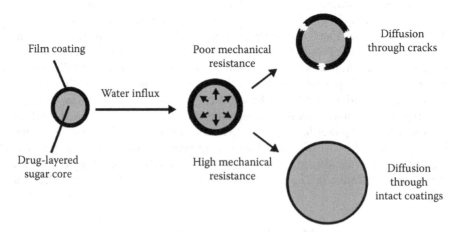

FIGURE 10.2 Schemes of drug release from membrane-controlled sustained release drug delivery system. (Reprinted from Lecomte, F. et al. (2005). *Pharmaceutical Research* 22(7): 1129–1141. With permission.)

membrane-controlled systems are summarized in Figure 10.2. When a membrane-controlled system is exposed to an aqueous environment, water will penetrate through the membrane and build up the hydrostatic pressure in the core. If the release-controlling membrane cannot withstand the hydrostatic pressure, membrane cracking will happen and the drug release will be dominated by diffusion through water-filled cracks. On the other hand, if the release-controlling membrane has a strong mechanical strength (i.e., greater elongation capacity and energy at break), the drug release mechanism will be dominated by drug diffusion through an intact membrane. Lecomte et al. investigated the drug release mechanism of Eudragit NE : Eudragit L coated pellets and ethylcellulose : Eudragit L coated pellets to elucidate the impact of polymer mechanical strength on the drug release mechanism (Lecomte et al. 2005). Due to its excellent mechanical strength, drug release from the Eudragit NE-based system is mainly driven by diffusion through an intact membrane. The poor mechanical strength of ethylcellulose-based membranes caused membrane cracking during water exposure, and the predominant drug release mechanism is considered to be diffusion through water-filled cracks (Lecomte et al. 2005). In addition to the membrane properties, the composition of the drug-loaded core also contributes to the drug release mechanism of membrane-controlled extended-release systems. Cuppok et al. investigated the drug release mechanism from Kollicoat SR : Eudragit NE coated sugar-based and microcrystalline cellulose-based pellets (Cuppok et al. 2011). Water uptake and polymer dissolution happened after exposing the polymer membrane to an aqueous environment. The authors proposed a membrane diffusion-controlled drug release mechanism and the drug release profile predicted by the model matched well with the dissolution data of coated microcrystalline cellulose pellets. However, the drug release rate from coated sugar sphere pellets is significantly greater than the predicted value, indicating the formation of cracks on the membrane and a mechanism shift from diffusion through an intact membrane to diffusion through cracks (Cuppok et al. 2011). Those findings from coated multiparticulate drug delivery systems may facilitate the design and development of twin-screw extruded extended-release formulations, especially the laminar extrudate from the coextrusion process.

10.3   TWIN-SCREW MELT EXTRUSION TO PREPARE ORAL DOSAGE FORMS

Extended-release oral dosage forms prepared using twin-screw melt extrusion could be categorized into two categories: a polymer-based matrix and a hydrophobic lipid and wax-based matrix. Detailed discussion of the formulation composition and manufacturing process used to prepare each type of matrix is presented in the following two subsections. The unique advantages of twin-screw melt extrusion over the conventional manufacturing processes to prepare these dosage forms are also discussed.

For polymer-based matrices, both hydrophilic and hydrophobic thermoplastic polymers have been used. Other components are also included in the formulations to modulate drug release, improve the processing conditions, or enhance the stability of the drug and excipients during processing. For a hydrophobic lipid and wax-based

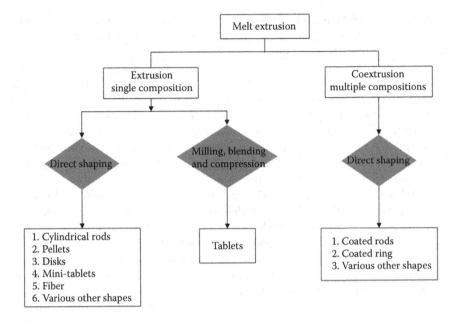

FIGURE 10.3   Melt extrusion for the preparation of various drug products.

matrix, water-insoluble lipid excipients are used. Because of the unique shaping capability of the melt extrusion processes, not only formulation composition but also the manufacturing process can be modified to achieve the desired drug release properties of the final dosage forms.

Depending on the extrusion setup and downstream processing, the manufacturing processes can be categorized into the following three types as shown in Figure 10.3:

1. Melt extrusion and shaping into final dosage forms
2. Coextrusion and shaping into final dosage forms
3. Melt extrusion, milling of extrudate, blending with extragranular excipients, and compression

10.3.1   POLYMER-BASED MATRIX

Polymeric materials are the most commonly used release retardants for extended-release oral dosage forms. Conventional manufacturing processes to prepare these dosage forms include direct compression, dry granulation and compression, high shear wet granulation and compression, and film coating. Please refer to Section 10.5 for twin-screw wet granulation. We will focus on the application of twin-screw extrusion in melt processing of extended-release dosage forms in this section.

Formulations for melt extrusion typically consist of the drug; thermoplastic polymer; drug release modifier such as pore formers; and processing aids such as the antioxidant, plasticizer, and lubricant. Melt extrusion is performed at 40 to 60°C above the glass transition temperature of the thermoplastic polymer, as a rule of thumb. Due to the heat conducted from the barrel and shearing by the rotating extruder screws, the thermoplastic polymer is transformed into its molten state during melt extrusion. Depending on the material miscibility and processing conditions, the drug and excipients could either be dissolved in or dispersed as individual particles in the thermoplastic polymer. After being pressurized through the die, melt extrudate could be directly shaped into final dosage forms. Depending on the shape of the die and downstream processes, the final product may take the form of a film, tablet, pellet, cylinder, or granule.

Because of the unique processing principles involved in the matrix formation during processing, twin-screw extrusion provides several processing advantages over conventional processes. The process has been applied to prepare (1) matrices of materials with poor compactibility, (2) dosage forms with lower porosity and higher mechanical strength, (3) dosage forms with unique drug release properties as the result of drug-polymer interactions during processing, and (4) dosage forms with layered structures and unique physical characteristics.

10.3.1.1   Formulation Composition

The twin-screw extrusion process has been successfully applied to prepare various extended-release drug-delivery systems. Commonly used water-insoluble and water-soluble polymers are summarized in Tables 10.2 and 10.3, respectively.

The matrix-forming polymer needs to be thermoplastic in order for the formulation to be processed using a twin-screw extruder. Drug release is primarily controlled by the properties of the matrix-forming polymer. The drug release modifier can either be dissolved into the matrix-forming polymer or simply dispersed as particles. Because melt extrusion is carried out at an elevated temperature, the degradation of the drug and excipients is a critical concern for the melt extrusion process. Processing aids such as antioxidants and thermal lubricants are present at

---

TABLE 10.2
Common Water-Insoluble Polymers for Melt Extrusion Process

Excipient	Trade Name	Tg (°C)	Tm (°C)	References
Ethylcellulose	Ethocel®	129–133	–	Vynckier et al. (2015), Vanhoorne et al. (2016)
Poly(vinyl acetate)	Sentry® Plus	32–36	–	Zhang and McGinity (2000), Shergill et al. (2016)
Poly(ethylene-co-vinyl acetate)	Elvax®	~ -25	40–100	Almeida et al. (2011), Sarraf et al. (2015)
Ammonio methacrylate copolymer—Type A	Eudragit® RL	63	–	Zhu, Shah et al. (2006), Quinten et al. (2012)
Ammonio methacrylate copolymer—Type B	Eudragit® RS	65	–	Zhu, Mehta et al. (2006), Tiwari et al. (2014))
Polyurethane	Pearlbond®	–70–10	50–75	Claeys et al. (2015)
Zein	N/A	150–180	–	Bouman et al. (2016)

TABLE 10.3
Common Water-Soluble Polymers for Melt Extrusion Process

Excipient	Trade Name	Tg (°C)	Tm (°C)	References
Hypromellose	Methocel®	170–180	–	Ma et al. (2013)
Poly(ethylene oxide)	PolyOx®	~ −55	62–67	Zhang and McGinity (1999), Bartholomaeus et al. (2012)
Starch	N/A	90–100 with 10% moisture	–	Kipping and Rein (2013)
Soy protein	N/A		–	Vaz et al. (2003)

a low level (<5%) in order to minimize the degradation of the drug and excipients during processing. Thermal lubricants have been used to facilitate the extrusion processing by reducing the melt viscosity of the polymer. Glycerol monostearate is the most commonly used thermal lubricant for pharmaceutical extrusion (Zhu et al. 2004).

Plasticizers are also used to lower the glass transition temperature of the matrix-forming polymer so that the extrusion process can be carried out at a lower temperature in order to minimize the degradation of formulation. Water has been used as a transient plasticizer when starch (Henrist et al. 1999), soy protein (Vaz et al. 2003), and zein (Bouman et al. 2015) were used as the matrix former. The water was removed during the extrusion process and secondary drying after extrusion. Conventional plasticizers including citric acid, citric acid esters, sebacic acid esters, and polyols are commonly used plasticizers. Some polymers or drugs with low glass transition temperatures can also act as plasticizers (Feng et al. 2016). The types and levels of plasticizers have been found to have no effect on drug release in some formulation matrices, while they have a significant effect on drug release in other matrices.

Drug release modifiers are present in the formulation to modulate drug release properties. Water-soluble polymers are commonly used to enhance the dissolution of melt-extruded matrices based on water-insoluble polymers. Polyethylene glycol and Tween 80 (Claeys et al. 2015) were used to increase the rate and extent of theophylline release from a polyurethane matrix. Polyethylene oxide was used to enhance the release of the drug from a polyethylene vinyl acetate-based matrix (Almeida et al. 2012). Xanthan gum was used to enhance the release of metoprolol tartrate from an ethylcellulose-based matrix (Quinten et al. 2011). Disintegrants dispersed in a polymer matrix have also been demonstrated to be an effective method to enhance the drug release of hydrophobic matrices. Low-substituted hydroxypropyl cellulose (L-HPC), a disintegrant, was used to improve the dissolution of metoprolol tartrate from an ethylcellulose matrix (Quinten et al. 2009). Without L-HPC, drug release was controlled by diffusion and the release rate slowed down over the course of dissolution. As shown in Figure 10.4, the presence of L-HPC resulted in a nearly zero-order drug release.

When the formulation matrix is based on water-soluble polymers, polymers with different viscosity grades and a mixture of different water-soluble polymers are

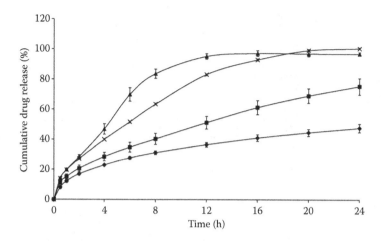

FIGURE 10.4 Influence of concentration L-HPC on drug release from injection-molded matrices. Mean dissolution profiles (±S.D.) of matrices (produced at 110°C) containing 30% MPT and variable L-HPC and EC4 concentrations. L-HPC concentration: (♦) 0%, (■) 20%, (×) 27.5%, and (▲) 35%. (Reprinted from Quinten, T. et al. (2009). *European Journal of Pharmaceutical Sciences* 37 (3–4): 207–216. With permission.)

common strategies to achieve different release profiles (Zhang and McGinity 1999, Ma et al. 2013).

10.3.1.2 Unique Dosage Forms Prepared Using Melt Extrusion

10.3.1.2.1 *Preparation of Matrix Containing Polymers of Poor Compactibility*

In conventional manufacturing processes, solid bridges are the mechanisms for the formation of matrices. When subjected to a compression force, drug and excipient particles undergo transitional packing. With an increase in the compression force and densification of the formulation composition, deformation occurs at the points of contact of drug and excipient particles. Ductile materials such as microcrystalline cellulose undergo plastic deformation, while brittle materials such as lactose undergo brittle fracture. Solid bridges are formed between particles when adjacent surfaces come into contact at the atomic level.

In contrast, the mechanism for matrix formation during the melt extrusion is quite different. When processed above their glass transition temperature at a high pressure, thermoplastic components of the formulation function as adhesive binders inside the extruder and are intimately mixed with other components. Thermoadhesive characteristics of polymeric drug release retardants are attributed to the formation of the matrix prepared by melt extrusion. Therefore, good compaction properties required for the matrix formation in a compression process are not necessary in the melt extrusion process.

As an example, polyethylene vinyl acetate and polyurethane are elastic materials that cannot be compressed. Extended-release matrix tablets containing these polymers as drug release retardants have been successfully prepared using the twin-screw melt extrusion process (Almeida et al. 2011, Claeys et al. 2015).

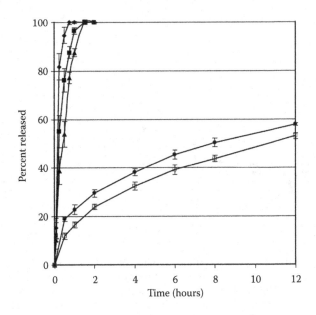

FIGURE 10.5 Influence of compaction force and extrusion temperature on guaifenesin release from matrix tablets prepared by direct compression and hot-melt extrusion containing 30% drug and 70% ethylcellulose using USP method II at 37°C and 50 rpm in 900 mL of purified water: (♦) direct compression, 10 KN; (■) direct compression, 30 KN; (▲) direct compression, 50 KN; (●) melt extrusion, 80, 85, 85, 90°C; (□) melt extrusion, 90, 105, 105, 110°C. (Reprinted from Crowley, M. M. et al. (2004). *International Journal of Pharmaceutics* 269(2): 509–522. With permission.)

10.3.1.2.2 Matrix of Lower Porosity and Better Control of Drug Release

Guaifenesin tablets containing ethylcellulose as a release retardant were prepared using both direct compression and melt extrusion processes. The extrudates were cooled to 50°C and manually cut into tablets. The dissolution profiles of tablets prepared by different processes are presented in Figure 10.5. Tablets prepared by melt extrusion exhibited a significantly slower drug release compared to those prepared by direct compression. Since ethylcellulose is not water soluble, the release of the drug was controlled by the porosity and tortuosity of the matrix. The porosity of the tablets was analyzed and the results are shown in Table 10.4. The melt-extruded matrix contained pores of smaller diameter and a more tortuous network. Therefore, drug release from the melt-extruded matrix was slower (Crowley et al. 2004). Sarraf et al. has demonstrated that key processing parameters including die temperature, shear rate, and die length can be used to modulate the pore structure of polyethylene vinyl acetate matrices in order to achieve different drug release properties (Sarraf et al. 2015).

10.3.1.2.3 Matrix of High Mechanical Strength

During melt extrusion, the polyethylene oxide-based formulation matrix is melted and pressurized inside the extruder barrel. As a result, the melt-extruded matrix

TABLE 10.4

Medium Pore Radius, Percentage Porosity and Tortuosity of Matrix Tablets Prepared by Direct Compression and Melt Extrusion Containing 30% Guaifenesin and 70% Ethylcellulose Measured Before and After Dissolution Testing

Processing conditions	Median pore radius (Å) Before	After	Percent porosity Before	After	Tortuosity Before	After
"Fine" ethyl cellulose (325–80 mesh)						
DC 10 kN	529 ± 24		4.1 ± 0.3		4.7 ± 1.1	
DC 30 kN	476 ± 26		3.8 ± 0.2		6.0 ± 0.6	
DC 50 kN	475 ± 17		3.1 ± 0.2		6.9 ± 0.9	
HME 80, 85, 85, 90°C	264 ± 8	575 ± 51	1.0 ± 0.2	8.1 ± 1.8	53.2 ± 8.1	4.7 ± 0.6
HME 90, 105, 105, 110°C	137 ± 6	521 ± 65	0.4 ± 0.2	7.8 ± 2.2	321 ± 22	5.2 ± 0.9
"Coarse" ethyl cellulose (80–30 mesh)						
DC 10 kN	1439 ± 42		6.5 ± 0.2		1.3 ± 0.7	
DC 30 kN	906 ± 23		5.7 ± 0.3		2.1 ± 0.6	
DC 50 kN	710 ± 25		5.2 ± 0.2		2.8 ± 0.5	
HME 80, 85, 85, 90°C	392 ± 11	642 ± 48	2.3 ± 0.4	8.7 ± 1.4	41.8 ± 5.5	4.4 ± 0.3
HME 90, 105, 105, 110°C	351 ± 13	588 ± 57	0.7 ± 0.1	8.0 ± 1.1	125 ± 16	5.0 ± 1.1

Source: Reprinted from Crowley, M. M. et al. (2004). *International Journal of Pharmaceutics* 269(2): 509–522. With permission.

Note: Each point represents the mean ± standard deviation, $n = 3$.

possesses stronger mechanical strength in comparison to the tablets prepared using a conventional tableting process. The abuse of prescription opioid drug products has been a growing problem in the United States. One of the most successful formulation strategies to deter this abuse is to prepare a dosage form with high physical strength to prevent crush and extraction. Both OPANA® ER extended-release oxymorphone hydrochloride tablets and NUCYNTA® ER extended-release tapentadol hydrochloride tablets are manufactured using INTACT™, a proprietary technology developed at Grünenthal GmbH (Bartholomaeus et al. 2012). Polyethylene oxide is used as the drug release retardant and matrix former. The manufacturing process consists of blending, extrusion, cooling, cutting, forming, and coating. The resulting PEO matrix tablet exhibits a breaking strength of greater than 500 N and could not be easily crushed by a mortar and pestle.

10.3.1.2.4 *Matrix Resistant to Alcohol-Induced Dose Dumping*

Extended-release tablets contain a higher amount of active ingredients than the immediate-release dosage tablets. Depending on the formulation composition, extended-release mechanisms could be compromised by the food and beverage taken by the

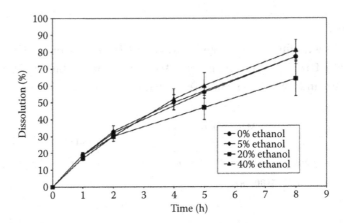

FIGURE 10.6 Dissolution profiles of verapamil release from the Meltrex® matrix over time, with increasing ethanol concentration in the dissolution medium. (Reprinted from Roth, W. et al. (2009). *International Journal of Pharmaceutics* 368(1–2): 72–75. With permission.)

patient. Concern over the alcohol-induced dose dumping has received a great deal of attention recently. Scientists at Abbvie have developed an innovative Meltrex® technology, in which extrudate is directly shaped. The technology has been applied to manufacture verapamil extended-release tablets that are resistant to alcohol-induced dose dumping (Roth et al. 2009). Both hypromellose and hydroxypropyl cellulose were used as the release retardants. As shown in Figure 10.6, the dissolution profiles of verapamil Meltrex® tablets, tested in 5 and 40% ethanol medium over 8 hours, did not significantly differ from the ethanol-free conditions ($P > 0.05$).

10.3.1.2.5 Matrix of Layered Structures

Downstream processing using a coextrusion die could be applied to combine extrudates from different extruders in various spatial arrangements in order to prepare a matrix of layered structure. Vynckier and his colleagues developed a coextrusion process to prepare a fixed-dose combination product of metoprolol tartrate (MPT) and hydrochlorothiazide (HCT). MPT was present in the extended-release core containing both polyethylene oxide of 1,000,000 Dalton molar mass and ethylcellulose as a release retardant. HCT was present in the immediate-release outer layer containing polyethylene oxide of 100,000 Dalton molar mass. Coextrusion was carried out using two corotating twin-screw extruders. A cylindrical coextrudate strand was cut into cylinder-shaped matrices with extended-release cores and immediate-release coating on the side (Figure 10.7) (Vynckier et al. 2014a,b). The same extrudate could also be guided between a pair of chilled pressurized rolls that contain tablet-shaped cavities, yielding tablets with a diameter of 8 mm and a thickness of 5 mm (Figure 10.8) (Vynckier et al. 2015).

10.3.1.2.6 Amorphous Solid Dispersions for Bioavailability Enhancement

Since melt extrusion is conducted at an elevated temperature, poorly water-soluble drugs could be solubilized in the polymeric matrix to prepare extended-release

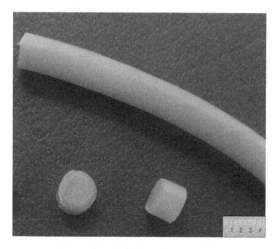

FIGURE 10.7 Image of co-extruded mini-matrices with a 2-mm length. Core diameter 3 mm and coat thickness 0.5 mm. (Reprinted from Vynckier, A. K. et al. (2014a). *International Journal of Pharmaceutics* 464(1–2): 65–74; Vynckier, A.-K. et al. (2014b). *Journal of Pharmacy and Pharmacology* 66(2): 167–179. With permission.)

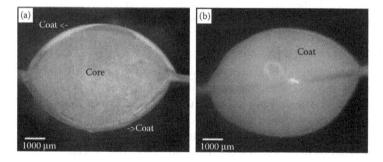

FIGURE 10.8 Cross section (a) and side view (b) of a calendared tablet with extended-release core and immediate-release coat. (Reprinted from Vynckier, A. K. et al. (2015). *European Journal of Pharmaceutics and Biopharmaceutics* 96: 125–131. With permission.)

dosage forms with enhanced dissolution properties. Shergill et al. has developed extended-release tablets containing amorphous disulfiram (Shergill et al. 2016). The drug was solubilized in a polymer matrix consisting of poloxamer and hypromellose. The extended-release tablets provided improved chemical stability in acidic media, improved solubility, and extended drug release.

10.3.1.2.7 Gastroretentive Dosage Forms

The formulation composition is subjected to elevated temperature and pressure inside the extruder barrel. Different foaming agents could be incorporated in the formulation. As the extrudate exits the die, the foaming agent will evaporate off and create a porous structure that will float in an aqueous medium. Ethanol introduced via in-line liquid injection (Vo et al. 2016), sodium bicarbonate (Fukuda et al. 2006),

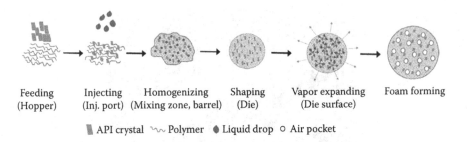

Feeding	Injecting	Homogenizing	Shaping	Vapor expanding	Foam forming
(Hopper)	(Inj. port)	(Mixing zone, barrel)	(Die)	(Die surface)	

API crystal Polymer Liquid drop o Air pocket

FIGURE 10.9 The mechanisms for the formation of porous structure during melt extrusion. (Reprinted from Vo, A. Q. et al. (2016). *European Journal of Pharmaceutics and Biopharmaceutics* 98: 108–121. With permission.)

and calcium phosphate dihydrate (Nakamichi et al. 2001) have been used as the foaming agent. The mechanism for the formation of the foamed structure is presented in Figure 10.9.

Malode and his colleagues incorporated sodium bicarbonate into the formulation matrix (Malode et al. 2015). The extrusion process was designed to minimize foaming. When the extrudate came into contact with the simulated gastric fluid, gas generated through the reaction between sodium bicarbonate and hydrochloric acid was trapped in the polymer matrix, enabling the floating of the matrix.

10.3.1.2.8 3D Printed Dosage Forms

The unique advantages of the melt extrusion process are its ability to produce dosage forms of various geometries and densities. These advantages were enhanced to a perfect level when coupling the extruder with 3D printing technology. Zhang and his colleagues combined fused deposition modeling in three-dimensional (3D) printing with hot-melt extrusion (HME) technology to facilitate additive manufacturing, in order to fabricate tablets with enhanced extended-release properties in a continuous process. They found extruded filaments prepared using binary polymer blends of HPMC E5 and EC N14 with HPC EF and LF, Soluplus®, or Eudragit® L100 can be printed well by the printer (Zhang et al. 2016). Goyanes studied the effect of geometry on drug release from 3D printed tablets with cube, pyramid, cylinder, sphere, and torus shapes. The filaments for the 3D printer were manufactured by hot melt extrusion. The data indicated that drug release from the tablets was not dependent on the surface area but instead on the ratio of surface area to volume (Goyanes et al. 2015).

10.3.1.3 Effect of Drug-Polymer Interaction on Drug Release

Because melt extrusion is conducted at elevated temperatures, the interactions between different components are likely to take place. A hydroxypropyl cellulose-based hydrophilic matrix was processed using a melt extrusion process. Theophylline and ibuprofen were used as the model compounds. Due to the solubilization of theophylline in a polymer matrix, the dissolution of theophylline from the melt-extruded matrix was faster than that from a directly compressed matrix

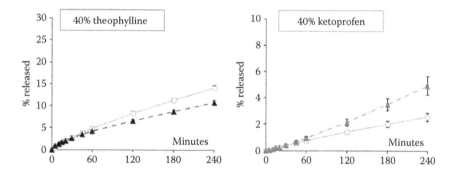

FIGURE 10.10   Release profiles of directly compressed (dotted line) and melt-extruded (solid line) hydroxypropyl cellulose matrices containing theophylline or ketoprofen. (Reprinted from Loreti, G. et al. (2014). *European Journal of Pharmaceutical Sciences* 52: 77–85. With permission.)

(Figure 10.10). The opposite effect of the extrusion process on drug release was observed with Ketoprofen. Ketoprofen release from the melt-extruded matrix was actually slower than that from the directly compressed matrix. This was attributed to the increased hydrophobicity of the matrix as a result of the solubilization of the hydrophobic ketoprofen. In a zein-based matrix processed using a melt extrusion process, the more hydrophobic the drug was, the lower the percentage of drug dissolved in the zein matrix (Bouman et al. 2016).

10.3.2   HYDROPHOBIC LIPID AND WAX–BASED MATRIX

Hydrophobic lipids and waxes have been used to prepare various extended-release dosage forms. The manufacturing processes are conducted either with the assistance of organic solvents or at an elevated temperature. When organic solvents are used, these hydrophobic excipients are dissolved in the solvents, which are then removed during the processing. High shear granulators and fluid bed granulators have traditionally been used to carry out processing at the elevated temperatures. Compared to a high shear granulator and a fluid bed granulator, a twin-screw extruder offers the following advantages: (1) more consistent product quality as a result of continuous manufacturing, (2) more efficient melting, (3) shorter exposure to thermal stress, and (4) more options of downstream processing to prepare dosage forms of various geometry.

Hydrophobic lipid excipients used for melt extrusion include (1) fatty acid and its salt, (2) glycerol fatty acid ester, (3) hydrogenated oils, and (4) wax. The properties of these excipients and representative examples are summarized in Table 10.5. These materials are semicrystalline with melting points ranging between 40 and 120°C. Melt extrusion of hydrophobic lipids and waxes is preferably conducted below the melting points of these hydrophobic materials. Under these processing conditions, the formulation compositions are only partially melted and softened so that the extrudates possess proper rheological properties for downstream processing.

TABLE 10.5
Hydrophobic Lipids and Waxes Melt Extruded to Prepare Extended-Release Dosage Forms

Excipient Types	Examples	Melting point (°C)	References
Fatty acid and its salt	• Stearic acid • Calcium stearate	• 69–70 • 149–160	Liu et al. (2001), Roblegg et al. (2011), Patil et al. (2015)
Glycerol fatty acid ester	• Glycerol distearate[a] • Glycerol behenate[b] • Glycerol trimyristate[c]	• 50–65	Prapaitrakul et al. (1991), Liu et al. (2001), Reitz and Kleinebudde (2007), Stankovic et al. (2013), Vithani et al. (2013), Islam et al. (2014), Vithani et al. (2014)
Hydrogenated oils	Hydrogenated vegetable oil	• 60–65	
Wax	• Microcrystalline wax • Carnauba wax • White wax	• 50–110	De Brabander et al. (2003), Quintavalle et al. (2008), Hasa et al. (2011)

[a] Precirol ATO 5 manufactured by Gattefosse.
[b] Compritol 888 ATO manufactured by Gattefosse.
[c] Dynasan 114 manufactured by Peter Cremer.

10.3.2.1 Design of Formulation Composition to Modulate Drug Release

Drug release from a melt-extruded hydrophobic matrix is controlled by Fickian diffusion. The percentage of drug release is proportional to the square root of dissolution duration. As a result, the drug release rate decreases with the progress of the dissolution process. Therefore, it is challenging to achieve complete drug release. Formulation strategies to enhance the drug release include increasing the ratio of drug to hydrophobic excipients and adding hydrophilic excipients as pore formers.

Incorporation of water-soluble excipients with a low melting point as pore formers is a common strategy to enhance drug release and to ensure complete release. Fatty acids matrix disks comprising the drug substance and glycerol fatty acids were prepared by Prapaitrakul using a melt extrusion and molding process (Prapaitrakul et al. 1991). The drug release rate from the disks could be modulated by incorporating PEGylated glycerol fatty acid, which are freely water soluble. Both glycerol fatty acids and PEGylated glycerol fatty acids were melted during the extrusion. It was reported that the higher the percentage of the PEGylated glycerol fatty acid, the faster the drug release. Glyceryl monostearate (GMS) and tributyl citrate (TBC) were incorporated into the pelletized melt extrudate containing acetaminophen crystals dispersed in a calcium stearate matrix in order not only to improve the processing conditions, but also to increase the dissolution rate of acetaminophen (Roblegg et al. 2011). The effect of GMS and TBC was different. At a 5% level, TBC reduced the extrusion torque by about 50%, while 5% GMS had no effect on the processing conditions. Due to the rapid cooling after extrusion, GMS was present in the extruded pellets in an α polymorph, which has water-soluble and emulsifying properties. Acetaminophen release was accelerated due to the formation of pores at the pellet surface following the solubilization of GMS. Increased dissolution rate was also observed when TBC was present in the formulation at 5%. When the level of GMS was increased to 10%, there was no further change in dissolution rate due to the formation of a denser calcium stearate matrix.

De Brabander applied the melt extrusion process to prepare extended-release ibuprofen tablets using microcrystalline wax. A binary mixture of microcrystalline waxes and ibuprofen was melt extruded. The extrudates were then milled and compressed into tablets. The release of ibuprofen was accelerated by incorporating starch with different swelling and disintegration properties (De Brabander et al. 2000). Microcrystalline wax is composed of a mixture of straight-chain and branched saturated alkanes obtained from petroleum. Depending on the chain length and degree of branch, various microcrystalline waxes of different melting points are available. Slower ibuprofen release was observed for wax with a higher melting point (De Brabander et al. 2000).

10.3.2.2 Design of Manufacturing Processes to Modulate Drug Release

Hydrophobic lipids and waxes are known to exist in different polymorphs. These polymorphs differ in physicochemical properties such as melting points, hydrophobicity, and water solubility. Since the excipients are melted during the melt extrusion process, the processing conditions could have a significant impact on the drug release properties of the final dosage forms by affecting the polymorph of these excipients. Studies have been conducted to investigate the impact of degree of melting, which is

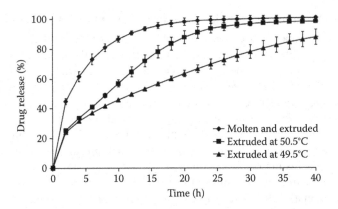

FIGURE 10.11 The effect of barrel temperature on theophylline release from extrudate rods consisting of glyceryl trimyristate. (Reprinted from Reitz, C. and P. Kleinebudde (2007). *European Journal of Pharmaceutics and Biopharmaceutics* 67(2): 440–448. With permission.)

controlled by the processing temperature, on drug release properties. An extended-release lipid matrix consisting of sodium naproxen and Compritol® 888 ATO was melt extruded with a "cold" (10°C below the melting point of Compritol®) or a "hot" (15°C above the melting point of Compritol®) process condition. No significant difference was observed in the drug release rate between the samples processed at these two temperatures (Vithani et al. 2014). The processing temperature was found to significantly impact the drug release rate of the glyceryl trimyristate matrix (Reitz and Kleinebudde 2007). The dissolution profiles of extrudate processed at different temperatures are shown in Figure 10.11. When the formulation was processed above the melting point of glyceryl trimyristate, the extrudate was more porous, resulting in faster drug release.

This unique feature of the melt extrusion process has been utilized to develop dosage forms of different shapes and with layered structures to modulate drug release. Application of the coextrusion process to apply hydrophobic wax as the coating to achieve extended release has been investigated. This process has been used to prepare cylinder-shaped carbamazepine extrudates consisting of a matrix core and hydrophobic wax coating (Laukamp et al. 2015). Even though a ram extruder was used in this study, a twin-screw extruder is more suited for this process. The lateral surface of the core was coated, while both bases of the core were exposed. The images of the extrudate are presented in Figure 10.12. The core consisted of carbamazepine dissolved in a mixture of PEG 1,500, PEG 2,000, and poloxamer 188. The hydrophobic coating consisted of wax only. Drug release through the coating was completely inhibited and the drug was released only in one dimension via the bases of the cylinder. As shown in Figure 10.13, carbamazepine was released at a constant rate following the burst at the beginning of the dissolution testing.

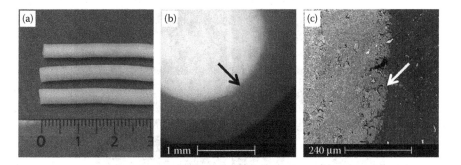

FIGURE 10.12 Photograph (a), light microscope image (b), and scanning electron microscope image (c) of the wax-coated extended-release carbamazepine extrudate. Arrow indicates the interface of core and coat. (Reprinted from Laukamp, E. J. et al. (2015). *European Journal of Pharmaceutics and Biopharmaceutics* 89: 357–364. With permission.)

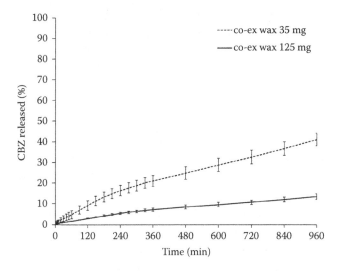

FIGURE 10.13 In vitro release of carbamazepine from the wax-coated coextrudates (co-ex wax) of different masses; 5 mm in diameter of extrudate; the weight ratio between wax coating and core is 3 to 1. (Reprinted from Laukamp, E. J. et al. (2015). *European Journal of Pharmaceutics and Biopharmaceutics* 89: 357–364. With permission.)

Hasa and his coworkers conducted an interesting study to prepare theophylline extrudates of various helical and cylindrical shapes to tailor different release characteristics (Hasa et al. 2011). The extrudates consisted of theophylline and microcrystalline wax at various ratios. Images of extrudates of various geometries are presented in Figure 10.14. Even though the extrusion process was conducted using a ram extruder in this study, the manufacturing process could be readily carried out using a twin-screw extruder. The effect of the geometry on the drug release properties is presented in Figure 10.15.

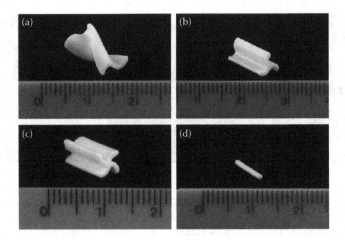

FIGURE 10.14 Image of (a) two-blades, (b) three-blades, (c) four-blades extrudate, and (d) cylindrical extrudate. (Reprinted from Hasa, D. et al. (2011). *European Journal of Pharmaceutics and Biopharmaceutics* 79(3): 592–600. With permission.)

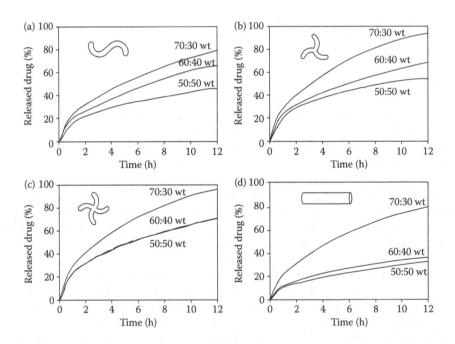

FIGURE 10.15 In vitro theophylline dissolution profiles of extrudates of various geometries. (Reprinted from Hasa, D. et al. (2011). *European Journal of Pharmaceutics and Biopharmaceutics* 79(3): 592–600. With permission.)

10.4   TWIN-SCREW MELT EXTRUSION TO PREPARE IMPLANTS

Besides the manufacturing of oral extended-release dosage forms, melt extrusion has also been applied to the manufacturing of extended-release implants. The feasibility of the melt extrusion process for producing implants has been demonstrated by a few commercially available implants such as Zoladex® (polylactic-co-glycolic acid–based implant), NuvaRing® (polyethylene vinyl acetate-based implant), Ozurdex (polylactic-co-glycolic acid–based implant), and the recently approved Probuphine® (polyethylene vinyl acetate–based implant).

There are several research articles discussing melt-extruded implants. The coextrusion of polyethylene vinyl acetate (EVA) for extended-release vaginal rings of etonogestrel and ethinyl estradiol has been evaluated in the literature (van Laarhoven et al. 2002a). The two APIs were mixed and extruded with EVA 28. Due to the high solubility of the two APIs in EVA 28, melt extrusion rendered the core composition in which the two APIs were molecularly dispersed. The subsequent coextrusion of core composition and EVA 9 rendered coaxial fiber comprising drug-EVA 28 core and EVA 9 release-controlling membrane. The drug release profile from a coextruded EVA ring can be affected by several factors, such as the drug loading in the core, the melt extrusion process parameters, and the storage conditions (van Laarhoven et al. 2002a,b).

In another study conducted by Clark et al., the melt extrusion process was investigated to produce polyether urethane-based extended-release vaginal rings (Clark et al. 2012). An antivirus agent, UC781, was extruded with polyether urethane (PU) at different drug loading ranging from 2% to 10%. PU was selected because of the high API solubility in this polymer. Results indicated that the chemical stability of UC781 was significantly improved in the melt-extruded amorphous solid dispersion compared to an aqueous solution. The PU-based hot-melt extruded rings showed good mechanical properties in terms of the minimal ring stiffness change during storage. The authors also reported the significant impact of drug loading on the physical and chemical stability of hot-melt extruded UC781/PU rings. At 10% drug loading, recrystallization of UC781 on the surface of the extrudate was observed. As a result, 7.5% drug loading was more preferred due to the desired physical and chemical stability.

As a biodegradable polymer, polylactic-co-glycolic acid (PLGA) has been extensively studied as a matrix polymer of extended-release dosage forms. U.S. patent 8034366 B2 and U.S. patent 9192511 B2 disclosed the preparation of PLGA-based implants by hot-melt extrusion. Micronized dexamethasone was blended with 50:50 PLGA ester and 50:50 PLGA acid. The powder mixture was extruded, yielding extended-release PLGA-based extrudate. The content uniformity of the extrudate was improved by a double extrusion process, in which the extrudate from the first-step extrusion was pelletized and processed by the second-step extrusion, yielding the dexamethasone intravitreal implants. It was reported that the potency variation of a dexamethasone implant can be significantly reduced from the initial range of 94.6% to 107.0% to the final range of 98.9% to 101.5% by adopting the double extrusion process.

10.5 TWIN-SCREW WET GRANULATION TO PREPARE ORAL DOSAGE FORMS

Historically, pharmaceutical wet granulation was predominantly conducted by either high shear wet granulation or fluid bed granulation. As a continuous and versatile process, twin-screw extrusion has been explored as an alternate technology for conventional batch wet granulation over the last decade. A scheme of the twin-screw wet granulation process is shown in Figure 10.16.

For the continuous wet granulation process using a twin-screw extruder, a powder blend is fed into the beginning of the extruder. Binders can be fed individually, in a powder blend, or as a predissolved solution or foam. Different from the granulation process in a high shear or fluid bed granulator, wetting, nucleation, agglomeration, and breakage may happen in sequence along the extruder in a much shorter time within a twin-screw extruder (Dhenge et al. 2012a,b). In conventional granulation processes, nucleation happens when the binder solution reaches the powder bed during a granulation process. The method by which the binder solution is applied (by spraying vs. drop-wise addition) can change the droplet size of the binder solution and therefore determines the mechanism of granulation. In the twin-screw extrusion processes, when the binder solution is fed as liquid drops into the extruder through a liquid nozzle, the droplet size is usually much larger than the powder particle. The "immersion" mechanism dominates, transforming the powder particles into "big, wet, loose lumps" (Dhenge et al. 2012a,b). In most cases, this nucleation phase takes place in the conveying screw element region. When the agglomerates reach the kneading elements, they are sheared, compressed, deformed, and fractured.

Keleb et al. investigated the application of the twin-screw extrusion process in the wet granulation of lactose (Keleb et al. 2002). In that study, twin-screw extrusion was compared with a conventional high shear wet granulation process. The screw configuration was designed to include two mixing elements. A number of lactose monohydrate granulation batches were manufactured by twin-screw extrusion and high shear wet granulation at different water and binder levels. The authors reported that twin-screw extrusion requires a smaller amount of granulating liquid to yield granules with desired properties compared to high shear wet granulation. Moreover, it was proven

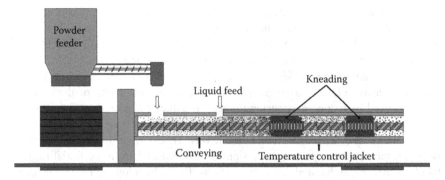

FIGURE 10.16 Scheme of a twin-screw wet granulation process. (Reprinted from Seem, T. C. et al. (2015). *Powder Technology* 276: 89–102. With permission.)

to be feasible to granulate lactose monohydrate without any binder by a twin-screw extrusion process but not high shear wet granulation process, indicating that twin-screw extrusion is an effective granulation process for particle size enlargement.

Quite a few studies were conducted to elucidate the impact of the screw configuration on the twin-screw wet granulation process. Djuric et al. studied the twin-screw wet granulation process of lactose monohydrate on a Leistritz twin-screw extruder using different screw configurations (Djuric and Kleinebudde 2008). A total of six different screw configurations were compared to investigate the effect of mixing elements (kneading element vs. combing mixer element) and conveying elements with different pitch distances on the lactose monohydrate granule properties. As expected, the granules became less porous and less friable when switching from a conveying element-only configuration to a screw configuration containing a kneading element. Combing mixer elements yielded granules with intermediate properties. Meanwhile, the authors also found that conveying element pitch distance has an impact on granule properties. Conveying elements with a 40-mm pitch distance were reported to yield granules with fewer large lumps and fines. The authors attributed this phenomenon to the relatively poor and inconsistent material conveying capacity of the low pitch distance conveying element, which could potentially cause nonuniform material wetting and agglomeration, thereby forming more fine particles and large lumps.

In another study, Thompson et al. investigated the effect of screw configuration on lactose monohydrate granulated by Kollidon aqueous solution (Thompson and Sun 2010). Data suggested that both the screw configuration and the screw fill level affect the granulation process. Similar to the results reported by Djuric et al. the addition of a kneading element and combing element reduced the level of fine particles in the granules compared to a screw configuration that only contained a conveying element. Besides the level of fine particles, the screw configuration also affected the granule morphology. A conveying-element-only screw configuration yielded granules with more spherical morphology. The addition of a combing element produced round-to-oblong granules with a larger particle size. A screw configuration with a kneading element yielded very unique ribbon-shaped granules. The screw fill level has also been demonstrated to have a significant impact on granule properties. The level of fine particles produced by a conveying-element-only screw configuration can be reduced by increasing the level of screw fill from 30% to 70%. This phenomenon may be attributed to a more frequent particle collision and a greater extent of granule growth in a high screw fill level.

Scientists have proposed several possible mechanisms by which channel fill level can affect the granules' morphology, strength, and particle size distribution. Gorringe et al. conducted studies to use the channel fill level in defining a design space for the wet granulation process with a twin-screw extruder. Interestingly they found that very similar particle size distributions can be obtained at the same φ (total volumetric fraction of the conveying element channels filled with powder) with the same material and screw configuration but radically different solid feed rates and screw speeds. The data also showed strong correlations of granule particle size distribution and the granule morphology trends with φ, though the sensitivity of these correlations appears to depend on the screw configuration (Gorringe et al. 2017).

To elucidate the granule growth mechanism in the twin-screw extrusion process, Dhenge et al. conducted a study on two different screw configurations and used colored tracer granules to visualize the granule growth, breakage, and dry powder adsorption (Dhenge et al. 2012a,b). The tracer study clearly demonstrated that the conveying element has a very limited contribution to granule breakage, as most of the tracer granules remained intact after mixing with uncolored granules and passing through the conveying zones. In contrast to the conveying element, the kneading element rendered mosaic granules containing both a colored tracer portion and an uncolored regular granule portion. Furthermore, the authors collected granule samples at each individual screw zone and characterized granule properties such as granule size, morphology, and mechanical strength. Large and spherical granules were observed in the conveying zone. Those granules showed very limited mechanical strength. Moving into the kneading zone and the downstream zones, much smaller granules with irregular shape were obtained and the granule mechanical strength was significantly improved. All those experiments indicated that granule growth in the conveying zone is mainly driven by powder coalescence. Meanwhile, the kneading element mainly contributed to granule breakage and granule consolidation.

Recently, a few studies have been conducted to investigate the impact of different types of mixing elements on granule properties (Sayin et al. 2015, Vercruysse et al. 2015). Vercruysse et al. reported the application of tooth mixing elements (TME) and screw mixing elements (SME) in twin-screw wet granulation (Vercruysse et al. 2015). Lactose monohydrate was granulated by water alone without any other binder on a ConsiGma-25 unit. A wide and multimodal granule size distribution was observed in a conveying-element-only screw configuration. The addition of a kneading element rendered a narrower granule size distribution but also generated a significant amount of large granules. Combining a kneading element with a mixing element, especially the SME, tended to produce granules with a narrow granule size distribution and a suitable average granule size (i.e., d_{50}) for tableting. Compared to a screw configuration containing SME, the addition of TME on the screw may impose a more significant impact on the torque because the TME inherently has a very limited conveying capacity. In another study, Sayin et al. investigated the effect of distributive mixing elements (DME) on the twin-screw wet granulation process (Sayin et al. 2015). Different from a number of studies using lactose monohydrate as a model granulation system, this article reported the granulation of a powder mixture system relevant to a conventional immediate-release formulation (i.e., lactose monohydrate, microcrystalline cellulose, hydroxypropylmethyl cellulose, and croscarmellose sodium). The multimodal granule size distribution rendered from a conveying-element-only screw configuration was attributed to the heterogeneous water distribution in the powder mixture. It was proposed that the DME behaved as a chopping section to break the overwetted large lumps from the conveying element and created the newly generated wet surface, facilitating the layering of undergranulated dry powders. Granules produced by a screw configuration containing DME exhibited several favored properties such as monomodal size distribution, spherical granule morphology, and relatively high granule porosity.

It is well known to the formulation scientists that extended-release formulation containing a significant amount of high viscosity/high molecular weight water-soluble polymers tends to exhibit a very sharp granulation end point in a high shear wet granulation process, causing a very narrow process window. Recently the potential application of twin-screw extrusion in the granulation of extended-release formulation was explored by a few groups (Thompson and O'Donnell 2015, Vanhoorne et al. 2016). Thompson et al. studied twin-screw wet granulation of an extended-release formulation containing hydroxypropylmethyl cellulose (Methocel K4M), Kollidon SR, lactose monohydrate, and microcrystalline cellulose (Thompson and O'Donnell 2015). The formation of twisted noodle-like granules ("rolling" effect) was observed from a standard screw configuration containing a conveying element and a kneading element. The noodle-like granules cannot be fluidized properly during fluid bed drying, thereby causing challenges in the downstream processes. The authors conducted a systemic study to elucidate the root cause of the "rolling" effect. It was observed that the formation of noodle-like granules happened in the conveying element right after the kneading element. Therefore, the authors proposed that the noodle-like granules were generated by material compaction between the screw tip and the barrel surface. In an immediate-release formulation without a high level of high viscosity polymers, the compacted material tends to have low mechanical strength and will break and convert back to granules with regular shape. The high viscosity/high molecular weight polymer enhances the mechanical strength of the noodle-like granules and prevents them from breakage, leading to the undesired "rolling" effect. Because the "rolling" effect mainly happened in the conveying element right after the kneading element, the authors hypothesized that the "rolling" effect may be mitigated by deliberately controlling the screw configuration and placing the nonconveying element at the very end of the screw. Experimental data proved this hypothesis and this screw configuration yielded granules with a more regular shape.

In another study, Vanhoorne et al. investigated the twin-screw wet granulation of metoprolol tartrate extended-release formulation containing 20% active ingredient, 20% hydroxypropylmethyl cellulose (90SH-4000, substitution type 2208), and 60% filler (lactose monohydrate alone or lactose monohydrate/starch 1:1 mixture) (Vanhoorne et al. 2016). Compared to the extended-release wet granulation formulation reported by Thompson et al., Vanhoorne's formulations did not contain microcrystalline cellulose. Since microcrystalline cellulose could absorb a significant amount of water, formulation reported by Thompson et al. required a higher level of water during granulation compared to the current formulations (a 0.25 liquid to solid ratio in Thompson's article, with 0.1 and 0.08 in Vanhoorne's formulations with and without starch as a filler, respectively). Meanwhile, wet granulation of the current extended-release formulations did not yield noodle-like granules even by adopting the undesired screw configuration reported by Thompson et al. To further understand the findings, the authors conducted twin-screw wet granulation on Thompson's formulation using similar screw configuration at different liquid to solid ratios. It was observed that the formation of noodle-like granules was more significant at high liquid to solid ratio conditions (L/S = 0.26 and 0.29) but not at low water conditions (L/S = 0.16). Therefore, the authors concluded that it is not only the screw configuration but also the formulation and water level that affect the morphology of granules of extended-release formulation processed by twin-screw wet granulation. A design of experiments (DoE) study was also performed to elucidate the impact of twin-screw extrusion process parameters (i.e., extrusion temperature, screw speed, and feeding rate) on granule properties. An optimized twin-screw extrusion system yielded extended-release tablets with the desired mechanical properties and highly reproducible dissolution properties, demonstrating that twin-screw wet granulation is a viable approach to manufacture extended-release formulation.

10.6 CONCLUSIONS

The feasibility of the twin-screw extrusion process as a platform for extended-release dosage forms has been demonstrated by a number of commercially available products. The twin-screw extrusion process renders versatile drug delivery systems including hydrophilic matrix, hydrophobic matrix, and membrane-controlled systems. The versatility of this process enables its application on compounds with different properties and drug delivery needs. From a dosage form perspective, twin-screw extrusion has been proven to be able to produce a variety of dosage forms, including oral tablets, oral granules, subcutaneous implants, ophthalmic implants, and vaginal rings.

Twin-screw extrusion has demonstrated several unique advantages compared with many other technologies and can be used to overcome certain drug delivery hurdles, such as the low compactibility of high polymer loading tablets and the alcohol-induced dose dumping. Due to the low porosity and unique binding mechanism, twin-screw melt extrusion has been used to manufacture tablets with high mechanical strength that are resistant to mechanical crushing, which is in particular critical for extended-release pain medications. For thermally liable compounds, twin-screw wet granulation offers an alternate continuous process compared with conventional high shear wet granulation. As a process with demonstrated commercial success, we expect twin-screw extrusion to gain more attention in the future for the development of extended-release dosage forms.

REFERENCES

Almeida, A., S. Possemiers, M. N. Boone, T. De Beer, T. Quinten, L. Van Hoorebeke, J. P. Remon and C. Vervaet (2011). Ethylene vinyl acetate as matrix for oral sustained release dosage forms produced via hot-melt extrusion. *European Journal of Pharmaceutics and Biopharmaceutics* 77(2): 297–305.

Almeida, A., L. Brabant, F. Siepmann, T. De Beer, W. Bouquet, L. Van Hoorebeke, J. Siepmann, J. P. Remon and C. Vervaet (2012). Sustained release from hot-melt extruded matrices based on ethylene vinyl acetate and polyethylene oxide. *European Journal of Pharmaceutics and Biopharmaceutics* 82(3): 526–533.

Bartholomaeus, J. H., E. Arkenau-Maric and E. Galia (2012). Opioid extended-release tablets with improved tamper-resistant properties. *Expert Opinion on Drug Delivery* 9(8): 879–891.

Baumgartner, S., G. Lahajnar, A. Sepe and J. Kristl (2005). Quantitative evaluation of polymer concentration profile during swelling of hydrophilic matrix tablets using 1H NMR and MRI methods. *European Journal of Pharmaceutics and Biopharmaceutics* 59(2): 299–306.

Bouman, J., P. Belton, P. Venema, E. van der Linden, R. de Vries and S. Qi (2015). The development of direct extrusion-injection moulded zein matrices as novel oral controlled drug delivery systems. *Pharm Res* 32(8): 2775–2786.

Bouman, J., P. Belton, P. Venema, E. van der Linden, R. de Vries and S. Qi (2016). Controlled release from zein matrices: Interplay of drug hydrophobicity and pH. *Pharmaceutical Research* 33(3): 673–685.

Christenson, G. L. and L. B. Dale (1962). Sustained release tablet. US Patent 3065143 A.

Claeys, B., A. Vervaeck, X. K. D. Hillewaere, S. Possemiers, L. Hansen, T. De Beer, J. P. Remon and C. Vervaet (2015). Thermoplastic polyurethanes for the manufacturing of highly dosed oral sustained release matrices via hot melt extrusion and injection molding. *European Journal of Pharmaceutics and Biopharmaceutics* 90: 44–52.

Clark, M. R., T. J. Johnson, R. T. Mccabe, J. T. Clark, A. Tuitupou, H. Elgendy, D. R. Friend and P. F. Kiser (2012). A hot-melt extruded intravaginal ring for the sustained delivery of the antiretroviral microbicide UC781. *Journal of Pharmaceutical Sciences* 101(2): 576–587.

Colombo, P (1993). Swelling-controlled release in hydrogel matrices for oral route. *Advanced Drug Delivery Reviews* 11(1): 37–57.

Costantini, L. C., S. R. Kleppner, J. McDonough, M. R. Azar and R. Patel (2004). Implantable technology for long-term delivery of nalmefene for treatment of alcoholism. *International Journal of Pharmaceutics* 283(1–2): 35–44.

Crowley, M. M., F. Zhang, J. J. Koleng and J. W. McGinity (2002). Stability of polyethylene oxide in matrix tablets prepared by hot-melt extrusion. *Biomaterials* 23(21): 4241–4248.

Crowley, M. M., B. Schroeder, A. Fredersdorf, S. Obara, M. Talarico, S. Kucera and J. W. McGinity (2004). Physicochemical properties and mechanism of drug release from ethyl cellulose matrix tablets prepared by direct compression and hot-melt extrusion. *International Journal of Pharmaceutics* 269(2): 509–522.

Cuppok, Y., S. Muschert, M. Marucci, J. Hjaertstam, F. Siepmann, A. Axelsson and J. Siepmann (2011). Drug release mechanisms from Kollicoat SR:Eudragit NE coated pellets. *International Journal of Pharmaceutics* 409(1–2): 30–37.

De Brabander, C., C. Vervaet, L. Fiermans and J. P. Remon (2000). Matrix mini-tablets based on starch/microcrystalline wax mixtures. *International Journal of Pharmaceutics* 199(2): 195–203.

De Brabander, C., C. Vervaet and J. P. Remon (2003). Development and evaluation of sustained release mini-matrices prepared via hot melt extrusion. *Journal of Controlled Release* 89(2): 235–247.

Dhenge, R. M., J. J. Cartwright, M. J. Hounslow and A. D. Salman (2012a). Twin screw granulation: Steps in granule growth. *International journal of pharmaceutics* 438(1): 20–32.

Dhenge, R. M., J. J. Cartwright, M. J. Hounslow and A. D. Salman (2012b). Twin screw wet granulation: Effects of properties of granulation liquid. *Powder technology* 229: 126–136.

Djuric, D. and P. Kleinebudde (2008). Impact of screw elements on continuous granulation with a twin-screw extruder. *Journal of pharmaceutical sciences* 97(11): 4934–4942.

Feng, X., A. Vo, H. Patil, R. V. Tiwari, A. S. Alshetaili, M. B. Pimparade and M. A. Repka (2016). The effects of polymer carrier, hot melt extrusion process and downstream processing parameters on the moisture sorption properties of amorphous solid dispersions. *Journal of Pharmacy and Pharmacology* 68: 692–704.

Ferrero, C., D. Massuelle and E. Doelker (2010). Towards elucidation of the drug release mechanism from compressed hydrophilic matrices made of cellulose ethers. II. Evaluation of a possible swelling-controlled drug release mechanism using dimensionless analysis. *Journal of Controlled Release* 141(2): 223–233.

Fukuda, M., N. A. Peppas and J. W. McGinity (2006). Floating hot-melt extruded tablets for gastroretentive controlled drug release system. *Journal of Controlled Release* 115(2): 121–129.

Gorringe, L. J., G. S. Kee, M. F. Saleh, N. H. Fa and R. G. Elkes (2017). Use of the channel fill level in defining a design space for twin screw wet granulation. *International Journal of Pharmaceutics* 519(1): 165–177.

Goyanes, A., P. R. Martinez, A. Buanz, A. W. Basit and S. Gaisford (2015). Effect of geometry on drug release from 3D printed tablets. *International journal of pharmaceutics* 494 (2), 657–663.

Hasa, D., B. Perissutti, M. Grassi, M. Zacchigna, M. Pagotto, D. Lenaz, P. Kleinebudde and D. Voinovich (2011). Melt extruded helical waxy matrices as a new sustained drug delivery system. *European Journal of Pharmaceutics and Biopharmaceutics* 79(3): 592–600.

Helbling, I. M., J. A. Luna and M. I. Cabrera (2011a). Mathematical modeling of drug delivery from torus-shaped single-layer devices. *Journal of Controlled Release* 149(3): 258–263.

Helbling, I. M., M. I. Cabrera and J. A. Luna (2011b). Mathematical modeling of drug delivery from one-layer and two-layer torus-shaped devices with external mass transfer resistance. *European Journal of Pharmaceutical Sciences* 44(3): 288–298.

Helbling, I. M., J. C. D. Ibarra and J. A. Luna (2014). The optimization of an intravaginal ring releasing progesterone using a mathematical model. *Pharmaceutical Research* 31(3): 795–808.

Henrist, D., R. A. Lefebvre and J. P. Remon (1999). Bioavailability of starch based hot stage extrusion formulations. *International Journal of Pharmaceutics* 187(2): 185–191.

Higuchi, T (1961). Rate of release of medicaments from ointment bases containing drugs in suspension. *Journal of Pharmaceutical Sciences* 50(10): 874–875.

Huber, H. E., L. B. Dale and G. L. Christenson (1966). Utilization of hydrophilic gums for the control of drug release from tablet formulations I. Disintegration and dissolution behavior. *Journal of Pharmaceutical Sciences* 55(9): 974–976.

Islam, M. T., M. Maniruzzaman, S. A. Halsey, B. Z. Chowdhry and D. Douroumis (2014). Development of sustained-release formulations processed by hot-melt extrusion by using a quality-by-design approach. *Drug Delivery and Translational Research* 4(4): 377–387.

Keleb, E. I., A. Vermeire, C. Vervaet and J. P. Remon (2002). Continuous twin screw extrusion for the wet granulation of lactose. *International Journal of Pharmaceutics* 239(1–2): 69–80.

Kipping, T. and H. Rein (2013). A new method for the continuous production of single dosed controlled release matrix systems based on hot-melt extruded starch: Analysis of relevant process parameters and implementation of an in-process control. *European Journal of Pharmaceutics and Biopharmaceutics* 84(1): 156–171.

Langer, R. (1998). Drug delivery and targeting. *Nature* 392(6679 SUPPL.): 5–10.

Laukamp, E. J., A. K. Vynckier, J. Voorspoels, M. Thommes and J. Breitkreutz (2015). Development of sustained and dual drug release co-extrusion formulations for individual dosing. *European Journal of Pharmaceutics and Biopharmaceutics* 89: 357–364.

Lecomte, F., J. Siepmann, M. Walther, R. J. MacRae and R. Bodmeier (2005). pH-sensitive polymer blends used as coating materials to control drug release from spherical beads: Elucidation of the underlying mass transport mechanisms. *Pharmaceutical Research* 22(7): 1129–1141.

Lee, P. I (2011). Modeling of drug release from matrix systems involving moving boundaries: Approximate analytical solutions. *International Journal of Pharmaceutics* 418(1): 18–27.

Liu, J. P., F. Zhang and J. W. McGinity (2001). Properties of lipophilic matrix tablets containing phenylpropanolamine hydrochloride prepared by hot-melt extrusion. *European Journal of Pharmaceutics and Biopharmaceutics* 52(2): 181–190.

Loreti, G., A. Maroni, M. D. Del Curto, A. Melocchi, A. Gazzaniga and L. Zema (2014). Evaluation of hot-melt extrusion technique in the preparation of HPC matrices for prolonged release. *European Journal of Pharmaceutical Sciences* 52: 77–85.

Ma, D. C., A. Djemai, C. M. Gendron, H. M. Xi, M. Smith, J. Kogan and L. Li (2013). Development of a HPMC-based controlled release formulation with hot melt extrusion (HME). *Drug Development and Industrial Pharmacy* 39(7): 1070–1083.

Malode, V. N., A. Paradkar and P. V. Devarajan (2015). Controlled release floating multiparticulates of metoprolol succinate by hot melt extrusion. *International Journal of Pharmaceutics* 491(1-2): 345–351.

Nakamichi, K., H. Yasuura, H. Fukui, M. Oka and S. Izumi (2001). Evaluation of a floating dosage form of nicardipine hydrochloride and hydroxypropylmethylcellulose acetate succinate prepared using a twin-screw extruder. *International Journal of Pharmaceutics* 218(1–2): 103–112.

Oliveira, G., M. A. Wahl and J. F. Pinto (2014). Delivery of drugs from laminar co-extrudates manufactured by a solvent-free process at room temperature. *Journal of Pharmaceutical Sciences* 103(11): 3501–3510.

Patil, H., R. V. Tiwari, S. B. Upadhye, R. S. Vladyka and M. A. Repka (2015). Formulation and development of pH-independent/dependent sustained release matrix tablets of ondansetron HCl by a continuous twin-screw melt granulation process. *International Journal of Pharmaceutics* 496(1): 33–41.

Peppas, N. A. and J. J. Sahlin (1989). A simple equation for the description of solute release. III. Coupling of diffusion and relaxation. *International Journal of Pharmaceutics* 57(2): 169–172.

Prapaitrakul, W., O. L. Sprockel and P. Shivanand (1991). Release of chlorpheniramine maleate from fatty-acid ester matrix disks prepared by melt-extrusion. *Journal of Pharmacy and Pharmacology* 43(6): 377–381.

Quintavalle, U., D. Voinovich, B. Perissutti, E. Serdoz, G. Grassi, A. Dal Col and M. Grassi (2008). Preparation of sustained release co-extrudates by hot-melt extrusion and mathematical modelling of in vitro/in vivo drug release profiles. *European Journal of Pharmaceutical Sciences* 33(3): 282–293.

Quinten, T., Y. Gonnissen, E. Adriaens, T. De Beer, V. Cnudde, B. Masschaele, L. Van Hoorebeke, J. Siepmann, J. P. Remon and C. Vervaet (2009). Development of injection moulded matrix tablets based on mixtures of ethylcellulose and low-substituted hydroxypropylcellulose. *European Journal of Pharmaceutical Sciences* 37(3–4): 207–216.

Quinten, T., T. De Beer, F. O. Onofre, G. Mendez-Montealvo, Y. J. Wang, J. P. Remon and C. Vervaet (2011). Sustained-release and swelling characteristics of xanthan gum/ethylcellulose-based injection moulded matrix tablets: In vitro and in vivo evaluation. *Journal of Pharmaceutical Sciences* 100(7): 2858–2870.

Quinten, T., G. P. Andrews, T. De Beer, L. Saerens, W. Bouquet, D. S. Jones, P. Hornsby, J. P. Remon and C. Vervaet (2012). Preparation and evaluation of sustained-release matrix tablets based on metoprolol and an acrylic carrier using injection moulding. *Aaps Pharmscitech* 13(4): 1197–1211.

Reitz, C. and P. Kleinebudde (2007). Solid lipid extrusion of sustained release dosage forms. *European Journal of Pharmaceutics and Biopharmaceutics* 67(2): 440–448.

Ritger, P. L. and N. A. Peppas (1987a). A simple equation for description of solute release I. Fickian and non-Fickian release from non-swellable devices in the form of slabs, spheres, cylinders or discs. *Journal of Controlled Release* 5(1): 23–36.

Ritger, P. L. and N. A. Peppas (1987b). A simple equation for description of solute release II. Fickian and anomalous release from swellable devices. *Journal of Controlled Release* 5(1): 37–42.

Roblegg, E., E. Jager, A. Hodzic, G. Koscher, S. Mohr, A. Zimmer and J. Khinast (2011). Development of sustained-release lipophilic calcium stearate pellets via hot melt extrusion. *Eur J Pharm Biopharm* 79(3): 635–645.

Roth, W., B. Setnik, M. Zietsch, A. Burst, J. Breitenbach, E. Sellers and D. Brennan (2009). Ethanol effects on drug release from Verapamil Meltrex (R), an innovative melt extruded formulation. *International Journal of Pharmaceutics* 368(1–2): 72–75.

Sarraf, A. G., S. Cherkaoui, O. Jordan, R. Gurny and E. Doelker (2015). Controlled drug release from melt-extrudates through processing parameters: A chemometric approach. *International Journal of Pharmaceutics* 481(1–2): 9–17.

Sayin, R., A. El Hagrasy and J. Litster (2015). Distributive mixing elements: Towards improved granule attributes from a twin screw granulation process. *Chemical Engineering Science* 125: 165–175.

Seem, T. C., N. A. Rowson, A. Ingram, Z. Y. Huang, S. Yu, M. de Matas, I. Gabbott and G. K. Reynolds (2015). Twin screw granulation - A literature review. *Powder Technology* 276: 89–102.

Shergill, M., M. Patel, S. Khan, A. Bashir and C. McConville (2016). Development and characterisation of sustained release solid dispersion oral tablets containing the poorly water soluble drug disulfiram. *International Journal of Pharmaceutics* 497(1–2): 3–11.

Siepmann, J. and N. A. Peppas (2001). Modeling of drug release from delivery systems based on hydroxypropyl methylcellulose (HPMC). *Advanced Drug Delivery Reviews* 48(2–3): 139–157.

Siepmann, J. and N. A. Peppas (2011). Higuchi equation: Derivation, applications, use and misuse. *International Journal of Pharmaceutics* 418(1): 6–12.

Stankovic, M., H. de Waard, R. Steendam, C. Hiemstra, J. Zuidema, H. W. Frijlink and W. L. J. Hinrichs (2013). Low temperature extruded implants based on novel hydrophilic multiblock copolymer for long-term protein delivery. *European Journal of Pharmaceutical Sciences* 49(4): 578–587.

Thompson, M. R. and K. P. O'Donnell (2015). 'Rolling' phenomenon in twin screw granulation with controlled-release excipients. *Drug Development and Industrial Pharmacy* 41(3): 482–492.

Thompson, M. R. and J. Sun (2010). Wet granulation in a twin-screw extruder: Implications of screw design. *Journal of Pharmaceutical Sciences* 99(4): 2090–2103.

Tiwari, R., S. K. Agarwal, R. S. R. Murthy and S. Tiwari (2014). Formulation and evaluation of sustained release extrudes prepared via novel hot melt extrusion technique. *Journal of Pharmaceutical Innovation* 9(3): 246–258.

Vanhoorne, V., B. Vanbillemont, J. Vercruysse, F. De Leersnyder, P. Gomes, T. D. Beer, J. P. Remon and C. Vervaet (2016). Development of a controlled release formulation by continuous twin screw granulation: Influence of process and formulation parameters. *International Journal of Pharmaceutics* 505(1–2): 61–68.

van Laarhoven, J. A. H. v., M. A. B. Kruft and H. Vromans (2002a). In vitro release properties of etonogestrel and ethinyl estradiol from a contraceptive vaginal ring. *International Journal of Pharmaceutics* 232: 163–173.

van Laarhoven, J. A. H., M. A. B. Kruft and H. Vromans (2002b). Effect of supersaturation and crystallization phenomena on the release properties of a controlled release device based on EVA copolymer. *Journal of Controlled Release* 82(2–3): 309–317.

Vaz, C. M., P. van Doeveren, R. L. Reis and A. M. Cunha (2003). Soy matrix drug delivery systems obtained by melt-processing techniques. *Biomacromolecules* 4(6): 1520–1529.

Vercruysse, J., A. Burggraeve, M. Fonteyne, P. Cappuyns, U. Delaet, I. Van Assche, T. De Beer, J. P. Remon and C. Vervaet (2015). Impact of screw configuration on the particle size distribution of granules produced by twin screw granulation. *International journal of pharmaceutics* 479(1): 171–180.

Vithani, K., M. Maniruzzaman, I. J. Slipper, S. Mostafa, C. Miolane, Y. Cuppok, D. Marchaud and D. Douroumis (2013). Sustained release solid lipid matrices processed by hot-melt extrusion (HME). *Colloids and Surfaces B-Biointerfaces* 110: 403–410.

Vithani, K., Y. Cuppok, S. Mostafa, I. J. Slipper, M. J. Snowden and D. Douroumis (2014). Diclofenac sodium sustained release hot melt extruded lipid matrices. *Pharmaceutical Development and Technology* 19(5): 531–538.

Vo, A. Q., X. Feng, J. T. Morott, M. B. Pimparade, R. V. Tiwari, F. Zhang and M. A. Repka (2016). A novel floating controlled release drug delivery system prepared by hot-melt extrusion. *European Journal of Pharmaceutics and Biopharmaceutics* 98: 108–121.

Vynckier, A. K., L. Dierickx, L. Saerens, J. Voorspoels, Y. Gonnissen, T. De Beer, C. Vervaet and J. P. Remon (2014a). Hot-melt co-extrusion for the production of fixed-dose combination products with a controlled release ethylcellulose matrix core. *International Journal of Pharmaceutics* 464(1-2): 65–74.

Vynckier, A.-K., L. Dierickx, J. Voorspoels, Y. Gonnissen, J. P. Remon and C. Vervaet (2014b). Hot-melt co-extrusion: Requirements, challenges and opportunities for pharmaceutical applications. *Journal of Pharmacy and Pharmacology* 66(2): 167–179.

Vynckier, A. K., H. Lin, J. A. Zeitler, J. F. Willart, E. Bongaers, J. Voorspoels, J. P. Remon and C. Vervaet (2015). Calendering as a direct shaping tool for the continuous production of fixed-dose combination products via co-extrusion. *European Journal of Pharmaceutics and Biopharmaceutics* 96: 125–131.

Welling, P. G. and M. R. Dobrinska (1987). *Controlled Drug Delivery: Fundamentals and Applications.* New York, Marcel Dekker, Inc.

Zhang, F. and J. W. McGinity (1999). Properties of sustained-release tablets prepared by hot-melt extrusion. *Pharmaceutical Development and Technology* 4(2): 241–250.

Zhang, F. and J. W. McGinity (2000). Properties of hot-melt extruded theophylline tablets containing poly(vinyl acetate). *Drug Development and Industrial Pharmacy* 26(9): 931–942.

Zhang, J., X. Feng, H. Patil, R. V. Tiwari and M. A. Repka (2016). Coupling 3D printing with hot-melt extrusion to produce controlled-release tablets. *International Journal of Pharmaceutics* 519, 186–197. http://dx.doi.org/10.1016/j.ijpharm.2016.12.049

Zhu, Y., N. H. Shah, A. W. Malick, M. H. Infeld and J. W. McGinity (2004). Influence of a lipophilic thermal lubricant on the processing conditions and drug release properties of chlorpheniramine maleate tablets prepared by hot-melt extrusion. *Journal of Drug Delivery Science and Technology* 14(4): 313–318.

Zhu, Y. C., K. A. Mehta and J. W. McGinity (2006). Influence of plasticizer level on the drug release from sustained release film coated and hot-melt extruded dosage forms. *Pharmaceutical Development and Technology* 11(3): 285–294.

Zhu, Y., N. H. Shah, A. W. Malick, M. H. Infeld and J. W. McGinity (2006). Controlled release of a poorly water-soluble drug from hot-melt extrudates containing acrylic polymers. *Drug Development and Industrial Pharmacy* 32(5): 569–583.

11 Shape Extrusion— Extruded Implantable Drug Delivery Devices
Materials, Applications, and Processing

Tony Listro and Bob Bessemer

CONTENTS

11.1 INTRODUCTION

Oral drug delivery of many active pharmaceutical ingredients (APIs) such as hormones, pain relief medications, and antibiotic medications may have side effects that are unintended in addition to achieving the desired therapeutic effect of the dose delivered. These side effects can range from nausea to unexpected death. One way to minimize, or potentially eliminate, these unintended side effects is to deliver the drug locally. Shape extrusion or injection molding can be used to make dosage forms for local drug delivery. By their very nature, polymers are readily shaped into numerous

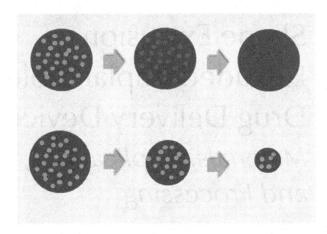

FIGURE 11.1   Graphical depiction of diffusion controlled and erodible matrix drug delivery systems.

geometries. Shape extrusion is an extension of hot melt extrusion (HME) that leverages the shapeability of polymers to produce specific, customized dosage forms.

At a high level, polymers can deliver drugs through one of two mechanisms: diffusion controlled and erodible matrix. A graphical description of the diffusion controlled and erodible matrix mechanisms is shown in Figure 11.1. Diffusion controlled drug delivery involves the diffusion of the drug through a polymer matrix over time. Through this process the polymer remains intact while the drug is gradually deployed to the therapeutic site. This can be achieved either by encapsulating the drug in a polymer shell or coating or by distributing the drug throughout a non-degradable, or biodurable, polymer matrix. Erodible matrix implants are produced through the encapsulation or distribution of the drug in an erodible polymer, such as a water soluble or bioresorbable polymer. As the polymer erodes in the body, the drug is released.

In addition to the pharmaceutical polymers that are used in HME for oral dosage forms (Polyvinylpyrrolidone [PVP], cellulosics, and acrylics), the polymers that are used in the shape extrusion of drug delivery implants and devices consist of bioresorbable and biodurable polymers. Examples of bioresorbable polymers include polylactic acid (PLA), polyglycolic acid (PGA), polycaprolactone (PCL), polydiaxanone (PDO), and various copolymers. Biodurable polymers are used to produce diffusion controlled implants. Biodurable polymers include low density polyethylene (LDPE); ethylene co-vinyl acetate (EVA, at various VA levels); and polyurethanes.

11.2   EXTRUDED SHAPES AND FORMS

The types of shapes that can be produced by extrusion include fibers, rods, pellets, tubes, sheets or films, and profiles. Profile shapes are less common in drug delivery applications, although a profile may be a useful means to control the release of an API by varying the surface area through geometrical variations in the extrudate. For example, fins or ribs can be incorporated into a sheet for a transdermal patch, or on a drug loaded fiber for an implant. Theoretically, this profile shape would have more surface area than a similar geometry without these features and therefore exhibit a different drug release rate than an extrudate without these features.

11.2.1 COEXTRUSION

Any of the shapes mentioned previously can accommodate multiple melt streams to produce coextruded shapes. Coextrusion allows for the incorporation of multiple polymer layers to achieve a desired effect. Both diffusion controlled and erodible matrix dosage forms can be made by coextrusion. Any of the shapes previously mentioned can be made using coextrusion. One such device made by the coextrusion process is Nuvaring®. Here, a natural EVA copolymer is coextruded as a permeable skin layer over a drug loaded core. The core contains a progestogenic steroid compound and an estrogenic steroid compound in an EVA polymer matrix. The two layers are coextruded in rod form, cut to length, and then welded into a circular ring. The steroid compounds are released through the skin layer in a fixed physiological ratio whereby the skin acts as a rate controlling membrane. Coextrusion can afford modulated drug release through polymer selection and by varying the drug loading level in each of the coextruded layers. For example, theoretically a construct could have a fast dissolving outer layer and a slower releasing inner layer. Bioresorbable polymers are particularly useful in this respect since many of these polymers offer a broad range of molecular weights and corresponding resorption times.

11.2.2 FIBERS

Drug loaded polymers can be shaped into fibers that can be wound or spooled and then cut to specified lengths required to achieve the appropriate dose of API for the application. The fibers can be cut short so that they can be loaded into a syringe and injected to the site of drug delivery inside the body. Fibers can be used in dental applications delivering very high drug loads to the site of action. Also, the drug loaded polymeric fiber can be used as a suture offering both mechanical functionality and drug delivery. Fibers can be woven into a mesh or various constructs and geometries. The mechanical properties of the woven construct are influenced by the design of the weave, the dimensions of the fiber(s) used, the inherent properties of the polymer, drug loading level, and other excipients in the formulation.

11.2.3 PELLETS

An example of a drug loaded pellet is reported by Beall, et al. Pellets were comprised of clonidine HCl and a biodegradable polylactic acid polymer to form a dose of approximately 300 micrograms. In vitro elution was carried out by placing three clonidine HCL loaded pellets in 2 mL of a phosphate-buffered saline solution (pH 7.4) at 37°C. Cumulative drug elution is plotted as a function of time and displayed in Figure 11.2. Sustained release of clonidine HCL was observed over 98 days. Elution of 56% of the drug was released in the first 28 days, followed by a much slower drug release (29% of clonidine HCL) over the remainder of the test.

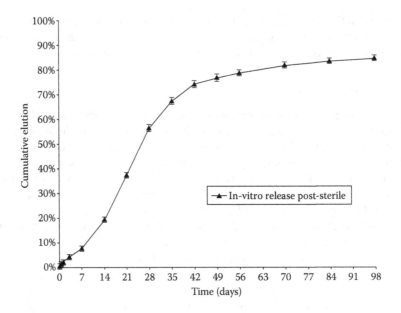

FIGURE 11.2 In vitro elution of clonidine HCL from a biodegradable drug depot.

11.2.4 FILMS

The manufacturing techniques for films include hot melt extrusion and solvent casting. Solvent casting involves dissolving the polymer/drug formulation in a solvent and casting the solution on a roll to produce the film. One of the key advantages of HME is that it is a solvent-free process. Films used for drug delivery and implantable applications can be manufactured in various widths. Thicknesses of 0.0012 to 0.0394 in. (0.03 to 1.00 mm) are typical. Drug eluting films are used for localized delivery in applications such as postoperative therapy wraps. Fast dissolving drug delivery films are used for transdermal, transmucosal, and buccal patches.

11.2.5 TUBES

Implantable and drug delivery tubes can be made from a wide range of biocompatible polymers to meet specific application requirements. Single lumen tubing, made of only one material are most common for implants. An example of a tube extruded from a drug loaded EVA formulation and then converted into a ureteral stent is shown in Figure 11.3. The polymer formulation comprises 13% ketorolac in an EVA polymer matrix. Ureteral stents are used to maintain urinary flow to the bladder after uretoscopy. The procedure is quite painful and the idea is to incorporate ketorolac as a pain medication to be delivered locally.

11.2.6 ORAL DRUG DELIVERY

Direct extrusion of a solid oral dosage form can be made using HME. Abbott's Kaletra, an anti-HIV oral medication, is manufactured using HME whereby the components

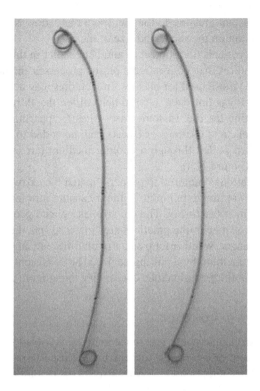

FIGURE 11.3   Ureteral stent made with a drug loaded EVA polymer.

are melt blended in a twin-screw extruder and the melt stream is then shaped directly into a tablet using a calendaring system. Another example where HME is utilized to shape an extrudate that is then shaped into a finished dosage form is the INTAC® formulation platform for abuse deterrent systems from Gruenthal. Here, the formulation is melt mixed using HME, and a rod is formed directly off the extruder. The rod is cut in-line to a specified length. Cut rods are then fed into a tablet press to form a tablet that may then be coated to produce the finished dosage form.

11.3   EXTRUSION PROCESSING FOR QUALITY AND REPEATABILITY

Any pharmaceutical product demands strict process control and validation, and the latest extrusion equipment and processing techniques have been enhanced in order to make extrusion more scientific. A better relationship has been established between the variables of the process and their potential effect on size, shape, and many physical properties as well. These scientific process developments can be used when processing active biomedical ingredients into shapes.

Twin-screw extruders are commonly used in pharmaceutical applications because of their ability to mix and convey solids, liquids, or gases. It is imperative that the extruder provides a thoroughly mixed, devolatilized, and thermally homogenous melt stream at a constant pressure to the die. From there, downstream equipment is used to form and maintain the shape and size of the part.

Dies for pharmaceuticals (the subject of another chapter in this book) often operate at lower temperatures than conventional plastic processes and do not necessarily need heaters, such as those used for plastics. In fact, dies may actually have cooling passages for water or gas (nitrogen, etc.) to help stiffen the extrudate and maintain the shape upon exiting the die. In some cases, dies for pharmaceuticals often use specialized tool steels, and coatings or inserts may be added to minimize sticking. The extrudate is then pulled through a cooling medium (air or water) and cut or wound as required (Figure 11.4).

Careful consideration is required to properly match the extruder screw design to the material so as to optimize pumping without causing unwanted material issues, such as burning or melt fracturing. The die size, associated geometry, materials of construction, and even machining practices are "material specific."

Most shape extrusions, whether for plastics or pharmaceutical products, are pulled through the cooling medium by a pulling device. The consistent drawing or pulling of the extrudate from the extrusion die is necessary to maintain a consistent size.

11.3.1 COOLING AND CONVEYING

The basic "free" extrusion process, where the material is cooled in air or water without the use of vacuum or associated tooling, can be used to extrude many shapes and materials, whether solid or hollow. An extrusion die or another material-shaping

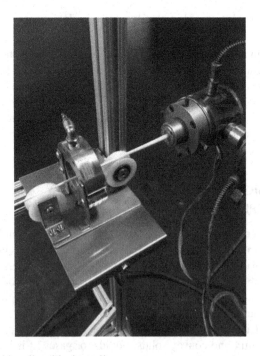

FIGURE 11.4 Tubing die with air cooling.

fixture is located at the exit of the extruder, similar to the pelletizing process (which is explained in another chapter). Depending on the material and throughput rate, the die shape will be somewhat larger than the final product dimensions and, as the extrudate is pulled from the die, "drawdown" will reduce it to the proper dimensions. This drawdown effect makes it possible to use a gauging system to measure critical dimensions and then automatically vary the puller speed to maintain size.

For complex shapes, and especially for hollow structures, vacuum calibration tooling is placed in a substantially closed-to-atmosphere cooling tank connected to a vacuum-generating device, such as a liquid ring vacuum pump or regenerative vacuum blower (Figure 11.5). This creates a cooling chamber with lower than atmospheric pressure. The pressure differential between the tank and the inside of a hollow extrusion exerts an outward pressure that holds the still-molten hollow extrusion against the walls of the calibration tooling, maintaining its shape while it cools. The length of the tool depends on the material and the production rates. The vacuum level can be manually controlled or, for better process control, automatically controlled using a feedback device, such as a laser gauge that measures the outside dimensions of the product. These calibration tools may also serve to smooth the outside surface of the extrudate.

11.3.2 Cooling/Sizing in a "Dry" Environment

If the extrudate does not need to be drawn from the die for sizing, a simple conveyor can be used to support and to convey the part from the die. For years in the plastic industry, air racks were used to cool profiles, especially in small production runs. These cooling tables, which typically are between 1 and 10 m (3.3 to 33 ft) in length, can include a series of forming guides (Figure 11.6) to support the profile or rod as it is cooled. A series of fans and air nozzles are used to enhance cooling. These air-cooling tables achieve a more gradual cooling rate and a controlled temperature transfer. Slower cooling can prevent the developments of voids in the material caused

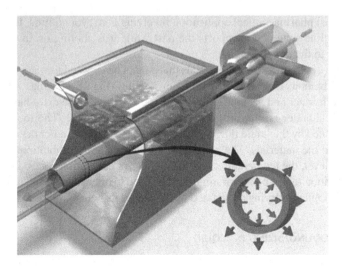

FIGURE 11.5 Vacuum calibration tooling.

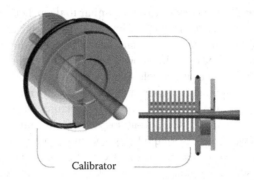

FIGURE 11.6   Forming guides.

by differential shrinkage, which occurs when the outside surface is cooled rapidly but the center remains molten for a longer time.

A belt-type conveyor (Figure 11.7) is the most basic cooling method for pharmaceutical products. They can be made of a solid material approved by the Food and Drug Administration (FDA) or a screen-type material, which allows cooling and/or drying from all sides. This can be especially important when extruding a pharmaceutical formulation that is very wet in order to facilitate flow. Screen materials would be stainless steel or plastic for ease of wash-down. Air-cooling fans can be positioned both above and below the extrudate for cooling and/or drying prior to cutting or further processing. If necessary, a heating hood can be mounted over the conveyor to enhance the drying or conditioning of the material. Conveyor speed must be matched to the flow of the profile. In some cases, a loop control device, either a dancer or ultrasonic device, senses the loop of the extrudate and outputs a signal to control the speed of the conveyor. In this way, even very delicate materials can be conveyed without distortion or breakage. The length of the conveyor depends on the rate of production and the material properties.

In a typical pharmaceutical application involving conveyor cooling, the conveyor matches the line speed and supports the part while it is cooling or, in some cases, drying prior to the next operation.

Extrusion of pharmaceutical materials that cannot be exposed to water requires dry vacuum calibration. Dry vacuum calibration tooling (Figure 11.8) has internal passages for both water and vacuum so that water never contacts the extrudate. This kind of vacuum calibrator is typically constructed of stainless steel. The tooling will be chilled or heated by the liquid flowing through it so the cooling and/or drying rates can be tailored to the materials. The controls associated with the calibration tool include the vacuum level, the temperature, and the number of calibration zones. Downstream of the calibration tool, a conveyor might still be used to offer support and as an area for additional cooling or drying as dictated by the materials being processed.

11.3.3   COOLING/SIZING IN LIQUID

In plastics extrusion, it is very typical to use a water tank as the cooling medium. The extrudate is either immersed within the tank or sprayed with a fine, atomized mist

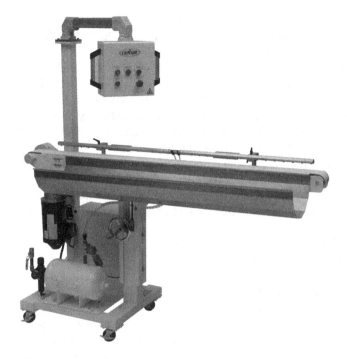

FIGURE 11.7   Belt-type conveyor.

to enhance cooling rates. The length of these cooling tanks is dependent on the rate of extrusion and how quickly the extrudate will release the heat (measured in British thermal units [BTUs]) generated during extrusion.

In some medical extrusion processes, deionized water is used within the cooling tank to minimize contamination. The tank is constructed of 316 stainless steel, including all fittings and valves, as the deionized water will quickly corrode bronze or copper.

A closed-loop water-circulation system maintains consistent temperature within the cooling tank. A water pump with stainless-steel housing and impeller is typically used in combination with filtration capable of removing pyrogens (dead germ bodies) from the water. The filtered water passes through a nickel-braised 316-stainless-steel

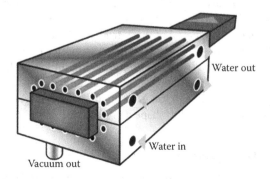

FIGURE 11.8   Enhanced dry calibration tooling, radiator water intercooling.

heat exchanger, which is connected to a chiller system. This way, the process-water circuit is a closed system and it does not flow through the chiller. Pumps and tooling may be disassembled for cleaning.

In some cases, the "coolant" in the tank may need to be heated to facilitate a more gradual cooling process, so the same closed-loop isolation of process water is used in temperature control units. A 316-stainless-steel immersion heater is used to heat the water and an automatic modulating valve, controlled by a programmable logic controller (PLC) using feedback from a thermocouple in the cooling or vacuum tank, is used to maintain the setpoint temperature.

If the extrudate is hollow and is able to make contact with water, "wet" vacuum-sizing tooling may be used. As with dry calibration, a vacuum causes the hollow part to expand outward against the tooling walls while the material is setting up. The difference lies in the fact that the wet tooling is in the tank, surrounded by cooling water (Figure 11.5).

11.3.4 TAKEOFF DEVICES

If the extrudate is being drawn down from the extrusion die, the takeoff is a critical component in maintaining product size. In addition to a precision mechanical design, the motor drive (discussed in another chapter) is extremely important. For pharmaceutical applications, servomotors directly coupled to the puller belts or wheels are preferred because they eliminate the error that can be caused by the more complicated linkage systems required. If more torque or speed is required, a sealed-for-life in-line planetary reducer is used. Servo drives utilize a serial operator interface to control speed and/or position. The most basic takeoff would be a roller or multiple rollers used above the conveyor to hold the pharmaceutical profile against the conveyor (Figure 11.9). This option applies only a minimal pulling force. Obviously, these rollers would be made of 316 stainless steel or another FDA-approved material. Wheel pullers have historically been used for applications in the extrusion of plastics and rubber, where only two points of contact are required with minimal pulling force. Most applications using wheel pullers involve small-diameter flexible medical tubing. The pinching action of the rolls can be used to maintain an internal air pressure for a tube.

Belt pullers are much more common (Figure 11.10). They consist of an upper and a lower boom or conveyor track, which, when closed on the profile, applies traction and pulling force. The length of these belts varies depending on the pulling force required and the potential of the extrudate to deform. Typical units utilize belts that are 150–300 mm (6 to 12 in.) in length; shorter or longer belts are also available. Poly-V belts, timing belts, and flat belts are all available and supplied in FDA-approved materials, such as natural rubber and nitriles of various durometers. In some cases, high-temperature or low-sticking belt coverings, such as silicone, are used. Belts can also be contoured to shape a product during the pulling phase.

11.3.5 CUT-TO-LENGTH DEVICES

If the pharmaceutical extrusion needs to be cut to length, this is accomplished in-line with rotary-knife cutters, which can be mounted at the die face or downstream after

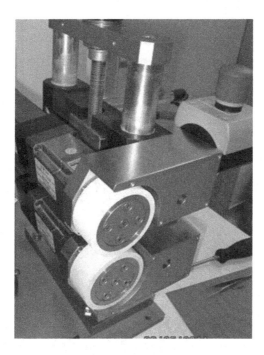

FIGURE 11.9   Roller style takeoff system.

controlled cooling/drying takes place. In some pharmaceutical extrusion applications, the upstream cutter die is actually the extruder die. Die-face cutting may be considered if the material has enough structure and density. This is the simplest extrusion method and requires no cooling or sizing after the die prior to cutting to length. A simple photo eye can be used to input length information and activate the cut cycle. A conveyor can be used to support the part during and after the cut, and to convey it to the next operation.

Rotary-knife cutters are popular for cutting rubber and plastics, especially since the introduction of servomotor drive technology (Figure 11.11). Because they can cut simply, cleanly, and quickly, these units are ideal for many pharmaceutical applications. A blade is mounted to a disc, which is driven by a servomotor. Cutter bushings support the extrudate while the blade passes between them to make the cut. The bushings and all components coming in contact with the product are constructed of stainless steel. An advantage of this design is that instead of the material being removed, as with a toothed saw blade, it is actually displaced by the blade. In some cases, residual heat in the extrudate can allow material displacement without fracturing. Many different shapes of blades are available to allow chopping or slicing of different materials. Different edge geometries and materials can enhance cut quality and blade life. To minimize material sticking to the blade or bushings, lubricant materials such as isopropyl alcohol may be used to minimize particulate generation.

Rotary-knife cutters operating in an on-demand mode, where an input signal initiates a single cut cycle, commonly make up to 350 cuts/min. Alternatively, rotary-knife cutters can operate in a continuous, or flywheel, mode. One or more blades are

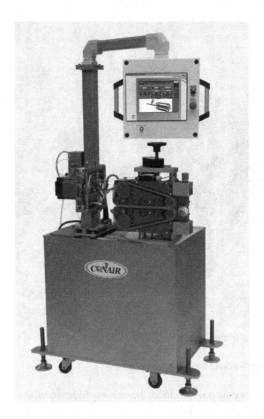

FIGURE 11.10   Belt puller takeoff system.

attached to a speed-controlled wheel that rotates at a constant speed. The diameter of the wheel directly relates to the blade velocity and is typically sized to minimize interruption. In this mode, 12,000 cuts/min or more are possible.

Typically, brushless servomotors are used to cycle the rotary-knife blade. Servomotors are fully sealed units, supplied with stainless-steel shafting, and they operate cleanly and quietly. If higher cutting torque is required, an in-line planetary reducer may be coupled directly to the servomotor. On-demand cutting modes use input devices such as timers, encoder counters or photosensors to activate a single revolution of the blade, which cuts the extrudate in the middle of the revolution. In continuous-cutting mode, the speed of the wheel is slaved to the puller speed at a set ratio. Thus, even if the puller speed is changed, the cut length remains constant.

The rotary-knife cutter, which is placed downstream of the puller, requires a consistent delivery of material, so the consistency of the puller speed directly affects cut-to-length tolerances (Figure 11.12). The rigidity of the material being extruded dictates how close the puller and the cutter are positioned. If the material is very flexible, they should be close together to ensure consistent feeding. In some cases, cryogenics may be required to stiffen the material to allow more consistent feeding and, thus, cut-to-length precision. With rigid materials, more distance between the puller and the cutter will allow the extrudate to deflect momentarily as the blade passes through it.

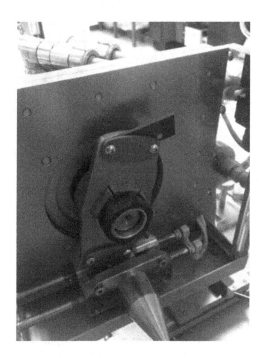

FIGURE 11.11   Rotary knife cutter.

Regardless of whether the cutter is set in on-demand or flywheel mode, the face of the bushings, between which the cutting blade passes, must be properly maintained to minimize particulate generation caused by scratches or wear (Figure 11.13). Think of the surfaces of the blade and the bushings as a pair of scissors, which must be clean and sharp to prevent material being pulled down between the surfaces, tearing it and/or generating particulates. Often, a blade-wipe system is used to clean the blade between cuts and to lubricate it to minimize sticking. A blade wipe may consist of a piece of absorbent material sandwiched between stainless steel plates, with a controlled drip system keeping it wet. The cutter guard itself may include a tray of water or alcohol so that the blade passes through it during each the cutting cycle. This is the simplest and often the best method of lubricating the blade. With some materials, however, lubrication may actually make the sticking problem worse. However, cryogenics can be used to stiffen the material and minimize sticking in the bushings or on the blade.

11.3.6   DISCHARGE CONVEYERS

Similar in design to the cooling/drying conveyers mentioned earlier, discharge conveyors are commonly used to support the part during and after cutting and also to remove the cut part in a controlled manner (Figure 11.14). It is typical for the speed of this conveyor to be 10%–15% faster than the line speed to create a part separation. In many cases, an automatic ejection system is incorporated into the conveyor to eject or divert parts off to the side for batching or boxing. To coordinate the ejection

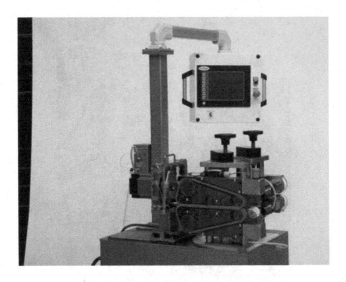

FIGURE 11.12   Puller/cutter system.

system with the rest of the line, a delay and duration signal can be generated from the cut signal. It is also possible to use in-line gauging equipment to signal the ejection system to automatically separate out-of-specification parts.

11.3.7   COIL WINDING

Coil winders, which are positioned in-line to make reels of relatively flexible extrusions, are common in the plastic and rubber extrusion industry, and they can be easily modified and applied to pharmaceutical extrusion applications (Figure 11.15).

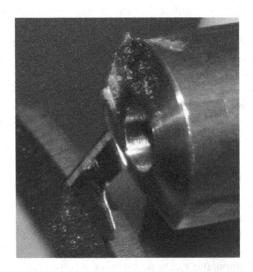

FIGURE 11.13   Close-up of rotary knife cutter and bushings with particulate buildup.

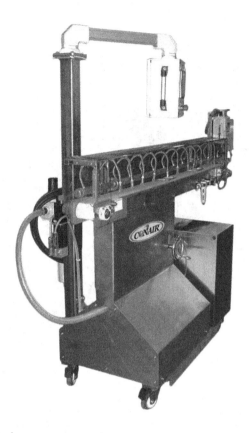

FIGURE 11.14 Discharge conveyor system.

These reels can be designed to accommodate a single width of material (like a row of tape) or multiple rows side by side up to 750 mm (30 in.) wide.

A collapsible coiling head can allow for coreless reels. The collapsible head supports extrudate as it is wound. Once the desired length is attained, the coiled material is strapped or shrink-wrapped to maintain the reel when the collapsible head is removed. Collapsible heads are common in medical or pharmaceutical applications, with the head itself being constructed of FDA-approved plastics or 316 stainless steel.

These in-line winders must be controlled to follow the extrusion-line speed. Mechanical dancers or noncontact (ultrasonic) loop-control devices can be used to monitor and control the speed of the winder so tension on the extruded material is minimized. Medical and pharmaceutical operations typically use a noncontact loop control, with a stainless-steel tray below the loop to prevent contamination in case the loop reaches the floor.

Servo-driven level-wind units are available to ensure even layering of the extruded material on the reels or collapsible heads. These units are easily set for different widths of material or shapes. Often, guides are used to enhance the consistency of the layering of material to minimize crossover or, in some cases, prevent the layers from touching one another.

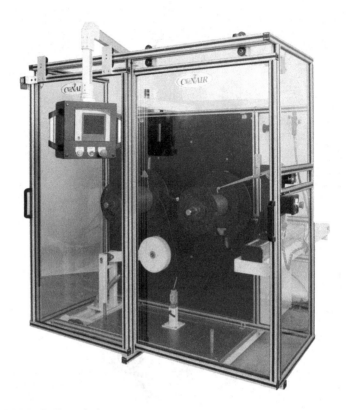

FIGURE 11.15   In-line winder.

As with belt pullers, servo drives are preferred for medical or pharmaceutical applications. With stainless-steel shafting and totally sealed housings, winders are well suited to wash-down. Of course, all exposed surfaces should be stainless steel and easily cleaned.

Much of the current plastic extrusion downstream technology can be applied to pharmaceutical shape extrusion. The extrusion industry has always been quick to respond to new markets and will continue to work with users in the pharmaceutical industry to customize equipment as required for a general pharmaceutical product installation. As in medical or food applications, the processes and equipment that have historically been used for plastic extrusion can be easily modified for pharmaceutical applications.

REFERENCE

Beall DP, Deer TR, Wilsey JT, Walsh AJL, Block JH, McKay WF, Zanella JM, Tissue distribution of clonidine following intraforaminal implantation of biodegradable pellets: potential alternative to epidural steroid for radiculopathy, *Pain Physician* 2012, 15:E701–E710.

12 Film, Sheet, and Laminates

Bert Elliott and Brian Haight

CONTENTS

12.1 INTRODUCTION

One of the largest volume processes for extrusion within the plastics industry is the production of sheets and films. Many products are needed in sheet form, or at least start out as a sheet and undergo postprocessing afterward. Common examples are roll roofing, packaging films, flexible printing plates, filtration membranes, agricultural films and tarps, frozen dinner trays (thermoformed from sheets), building insulation, kitchen countertops, battery separators, various sheets for electronics applications, interior and exterior panels for automobiles, photographic and x-ray films, etc.

As with most extrusion equipment used in the pharmaceutical industry, the sheet and film processing machinery is almost all derived from units designed for processing plastics. Even though many of the pharmaceutical applications are new, this has a real benefit in that the machine designs are well proven from 40 years or so of fine-tuning these devices for plastics processes. One problem that may arise, however, is that most pharmaceutical sheets and films are typically much narrower in a transverse direction than high-volume plastic products. The most common application of sheet/film downstream equipment is for product packaging for medical and pharmaceutical products. Another application is for transdermal drug delivery systems where an active ingredient is intimately mixed with a carrier and applied to a substrate.

12.2   BASIC CONCEPTS

Most melt extrusion systems are generally thought of as having an imaginary separation line, immediately after the extruder (where the extrudate will emerge from the die). The first half of the system (the portion with the extruder) is considered the upstream or melt processing section. The second half of the system is the downstream or takeoff section. This chapter will deal primarily with the downstream section.

In designing or selecting a transdermal downstream system, it is best to start with the end product and work backward. The desired physical properties of the solid dosage form will dictate the configuration of the downstream system. Some important parameters are as follows:

- *Extrusion throughput rate:* This is typically expressed in kilograms per hour.
- *Finished product width:* This is in the transverse direction, or across the web.
- *Product thickness:* Products less than 0.005 in. are generally referred to as films, while products thicker than 0.005 in. are considered sheets.
- *Product tolerances:* This will usually be expressed as a + or – figure, such as +0.002 or –0.002 in. For instance, if the product target thickness is 0.040 in., with a tolerance of +0.002 or –0.002 in., the extrudate can be anywhere in the range of 0.038–0.042 in. and still be acceptable. Tolerances should be arrived at very carefully. For instance, in the example above, merely changing the ±0.002 in. tolerance to ±0.001 in. could significantly increase the complexity and cost of the machinery.
- *Sheet characteristics:* Flexible, rigid, or semiflexible.
- *Final product of the system:* Will the product be wound up on a core or cut in lengths and stored flat?
- *Line speed:* Line speed is usually expressed in feet per minute and is determined by the extrusion throughput rate, die width and gap, material-specific gravity, etc. Most products will only process with good stability within a certain range of line speed. Either too slow or too fast will be unstable and uncontrollable.
- *Web path:* The web path is the route the material and any substrate will take from the die exit all the way to the end of the line. In designing this path, it is important to take into consideration the properties of the product as it moves through the path (e.g., as it cools, does the sheet become too stiff to

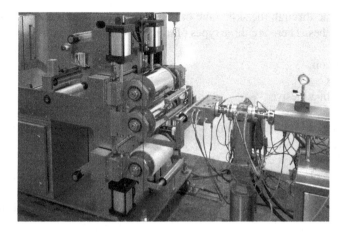

FIGURE 12.1 Close-up gear pump, film/sheet die, and stack/lamination system.

make an "S" wrap around a roll?). Typically, it is best to work out the web path with the equipment manufacturer's input, as they may have experience with similar processes.

- *Type of drive system:* Because the rolls directly determine the product thickness, speed control is critical. The rolls should be driven by a variable-speed motor, and have a closed-loop feedback drive giving +0.5% or –0.5% speed regulation or better. This can be accomplished with either a d.c. or a.c. motor drive. The latest a.c. flux vector drives have an advantage because of their tremendously wide speed range (1000:1 turndown ratio in some cases). The d.c. drives typically have a 10:1 or 20:1 turndown ratio. The motor will typically drive the roll through a gear reducer to achieve the proper roll speed range.
- *Gear pump integration:* A gear pump can be used at the discharge of the extruder, to provide a more stable flow and adequate pressure to the die. This is particularly advantageous with a twin-screw extruder, whose outlet pressure may be inherently inconsistent. In almost every case, significantly tighter product dimensional tolerances will be attained when using a gear pump, as compared to a system without an outlet pump. A system using a gear pump requires a computer control system, as the pump inlet pressure must be controlled to a setpoint. The computer has a pressure control algorithm, which automatically modulates the feeder and screw revolutions per minute (rpm) setpoints to keep the pump inlet pressure under stable control (Figure 12.1) (1).

12.3 PROCESSES AND SUBPROCESSES

12.3.1 Transdermal Drug Delivery Systems

One common pharmaceutical application using extrusion is transdermal drug delivery systems (TDDS), which are alternatives to more classic drug delivery systems such as tablets, capsules, or even injections. Transdermal delivery is a noninvasive method of drug delivery where the medication is delivered into the body over a period of time through the skin. One of the most common examples of TDDS are nicotine patches. There are three types of transdermal constructions (2):

1. Reservoir
2. Matrix
3. Drug-in-adhesive

These systems typically contain adhesive material, a rate-controlling membrane, backing materials, a reservoir vehicle, and a release liner (Figure 12.2). In the reservoir and matrix–type systems, the adhesive component is simply there to keep the system in place on the skin and has no further function. In the drug-in-adhesive system, the drug is actually incorporated into the adhesive and is much more critical to the overall function of the system (3). Ideal properties of TDDS include (4):

* Shelf life—up to 2.5 years
* Patch size—less than 40 cm^2
* Dose frequency—between once daily and once per week
* Skin reaction—nonirritating
* Drug release properties—consistent pharmacokinetic and pharmacodynamic profiles over time

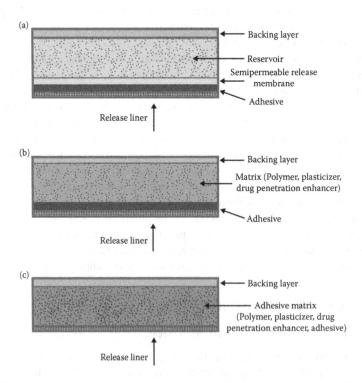

FIGURE 12.2   (a) Reservoir type; (b) matrix type; (c) drug-in-adhesive type. (From Bala, Rajni. et al. *International Journal of Pharmaceutical Investigation* 3.2 (2013): 67.)

TABLE 12.1
Polymers Found in Different TDDS Sections

	Adhesive		Release			
Backing	Polymer	Additive	Surface	Base	Membrane	Matrix
PET	Natural rubber	Tackifier, oil	Silicone (polydimethyl-	PET	Polyurethane	Eudragit E100
PET/EVA laminate	SIS rubber	Tackifier, oil	siloxisane + silicone resin)	Al foil	PE	PVP
PET nonwoven fabric	Polyisobutylene	Isobutylene oligomer		PE/Al laminate	EVA	HPMC
PP nonwoven fabric	Silicone gum	Silicone resin		PE/glassine laminate	Ethyleneproplene rubber	HPC
PET woven fabric	Polyacrylic acid	Water, glycerin		PE/paper laminate	Cellulose acetate	PEG
Al/PE laminate					Isotactic propylene	Kollidon

Source: Christie A. *Film and Sheet Conference 97,* Somerset, NJ, 1997.

Because of the nature of the system itself, polymer selection is extremely important for efficacy and functionality of the TDDS. All components, with the exception of the reservoir TDDS [typically a liquid suspension (2)], are made of polymers. Therefore, selecting the right polymer will be the direct cause of properties like adhesion to skin, compatibility with skin, drug release rate, duration of release, formulation stability, etc. Common polymers used for transdermal systems can be found in Table 12.1.

Traditionally, matrix and drug-in-adhesive forms of TDDS have been manufactured through solvent casting, but hot-melt extrusion has several advantages over this method. Solvent casting includes long processing time, high costs, and environmental concerns (5). On the other hand, extrusion is a continuous, cost-effective mixing process that does not use harmful solvents. It can increase solubility, absorption, and efficacy of poorly soluble drugs through the creation of a solid dispersion (6). Extrusion is also not only limited to creating the drug matrix and drug-in-adhesive, but it can create all parts of the TDDS using a film line with the polymers listed above. Implementing the various film manufacturing methods and techniques discussed in this chapter, it is simple to see that extrusion is a versatile option when it comes to this dosage form (Table 12.2).

12.3.2 DISSOLVABLE FILMS

Initially developed in the 1970s to deal with swallowing difficulties (7), dissolvable oral thin films have become popular in recent years due to their ease of use and convenience. They are most commonly manufactured through solvent casting or

TABLE 12.2
Advantages and Disadvantages of Dissolvable Films

Advantages (6)	Disadvantages (6)
Convenient dosing and administration	Difficult to package and preserve long term
Rapid action and controllable release	More expensive to manufacture than tablets
Bypass the gastrointestinal tract	Only small dosages can be administered
Enhanced stability	Eating and drinking restriction after consumption

Source: Sharma, Deepak et al. *International Journal of Drug Delivery* 7.2 (2015): 60–75.

hot-melt extrusion. There are several unique applications for this technology in the pharmaceutical, food, and cosmetic industries, including the following (8):

Edible Oral Films (Food): Edible oral films can be used in a variety of ways: breath fresheners, oral hygiene strips, candy strips, caffeine and energy strips, and vitamin and nutritional strips. The most well-known product causing widespread knowledge of dissolvable films was released in 2002, the Listerine Breath Fresheners created by Pfizer (7).

Films and Soaps (Cosmetic): Soaps and face masks are two common applications for dissolvable films in the cosmetic industry. They both allow convenient and clean ways to apply messy ingredients to skin. Similar to single-layer dermal films, these are applied to wet skin. Moisturizers, antimicrobials, cleansing agents, etc. can all be added to the film to give the necessary properties.

Dermal, Sublingual, and Buccal Films (Pharmaceutical): Dermal applications of dissolvable films are typically associated with bandages and treatments for skin diseases. The films can either be incorporated into transdermal films as the skin contact layer or stand-alone films where they are able to control the release of the drug (antimicrobials, anti-inflammatory, etc.) through the skin. Depending on the polymer selection, polymer solubility in water, and drug loading, the rate can be adjusted. Single-layer dissolvable films are applied to wet skin, causing the film to adhere and dissolve into the skin where it then dries, protects, and releases the drug. It can then be washed off with water as needed.

Dissolvable films for drug delivery are most commonly used either under the tongue (sublingual) or along the inside of the cheek (buccal) using hydrophilic polymers that have mucoadhesive properties (9). Mucoadhesion is "commonly defined as the adhesion between two materials, at least one of which is a mucosal surface" (10). Some common polymers that are used in these films include hydroxyethyl cellulose (HEC), hydroxypropyl cellulose (HPC), hydroxypropylmethyl cellulose (HPMC), poly(vinylpyrrolidone) (PVP), and poly(ethylene oxide) (9). Typically, water-soluble films will dissolve or disintegrate within one min (11). The technology has become an alternative to liquids, tablets, and capsules for patients with difficulty swallowing or a fear of choking, as well as a method to bypass the first pass effect (7).

12.3.3 PROCESSES FOR MAKING FILM (LESS THAN 0.005 IN. THICK)

For making thin continuous films out of a polymer-based material, there are two main processes: blown film and cast film.

12.3.3.1 Blown Film

A blown film is named as such because the polymer is actually "blown" into a balloon-like shape using internal air pressure. This inflation is performed as the material exits a round die orifice shaped like an annular ring and is accomplished under precisely controlled conditions in order to give a uniform film thickness. The extruded bubble is cooled by an outside stream of cool air supplied by an external blower. These are all performed continuously as the bubble is being pulled upward vertically within a tower framework. At the top of the tower, the film is completely cooled and is then progressively collapsed into a flat film "tube" (there are two layers at this point, having collapsed the two sides of the bubble flat), so it can be wound up into a roll (Figure 12.3).

A blown film can produce very strong thin films because it causes a biaxial orientation in the material as it is blown into the bubble shape. Orientation is a phenomenon that occurs within many polymer-like materials when they are stretched at a certain temperature, causing the long molecular chains to line up, or be oriented in a specific direction rather than just random directions. A common example is plastic garbage bags, which are only 0.0005 in. thick but are remarkably strong in all directions because they have been biaxially oriented.

Unfortunately, a blown film does not work with many materials—the critical parameter being the melt strength. Low-viscosity polymers, or polymers which do not have enough melt strength to maintain a film when blown, are not viable.

12.3.3.2 Cast Film

To make a cast film, a die is mated at the discharge end of the extruder to spread the melted material (or fluid) out into a thin "melt curtain" of uniform thickness. This type of die is referred to as a cast film die and is commonly available in widths from four in. up to any width desired. Note that the finished film will generally be narrower than the width of the die opening because of "neckdown." Neckdown is caused because the roll speed will typically be adjusted so that it is actually pulling the film

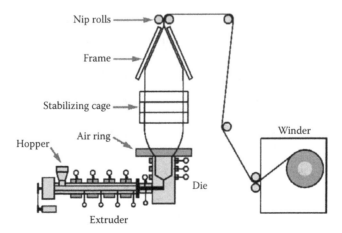

FIGURE 12.3 Blown film schematic.

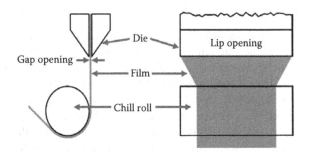

FIGURE 12.4 Cast film drawdown.

away from the die. For instance, a die with a 10-in. opening may yield an 8.5-in. product width (see Figure 12.4).

A cast film is made by continuously "casting" a thin layer of material onto a rotating steel roll. The die is generally positioned either fully vertically (with the die lips pointing at the floor), or at a 45° angle. The roll surface is maintained at the desired temperature by pumping a liquid (typically water or oil) through the inside. Because the molten material is generally hot and solidifies onto the roll as it cools, the main function of the water is for cooling, although it may be used to preheat the roll during initial startup (Figure 12.5).

An essential feature of a well-designed cast film takeoff unit is the height adjustment mechanism. When the extruder is started up or purged, there must be a provision to move the casting roll from underneath the die to allow for collection of the extrudate. This requires lowering the takeoff unit, and either putting a temporary "chute" in the way or rolling the unit away from the extruder. When it is time to thread up the line and to produce the final film, the roll must be raised up into position close to the die lips. This mechanism may be a manual hand crank on a very small unit, or fully motorized on a larger machine. Production units typically use a motorized height adjustment.

12.3.3.3 Orienting

A cast film is typically oriented in the machine direction [machine direction orientation (MDO)] only. To biaxially orient cast film requires an immensely complex and

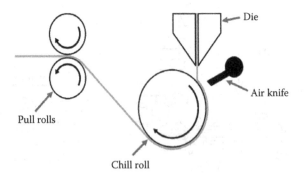

FIGURE 12.5 Cast film process.

expensive system called a tenter frame takeoff that heats and stretches the film after it has been cooled. The MDO is generally accomplished by having a separate motor drive on the pull roll station, so that the film can be stretched while moving along the web path. This will make a film that is very strong in the machine direction, but with normal strength in the transverse direction. Common examples of this in consumer-type goods are wrapping and strapping tapes (13).

12.3.3.4 Roll Design

The film casting roll is the key to the whole process. First of all, it must have the correct surface finish to impart the desired surface characteristics to the film. This may be a supersmooth mirror chrome for a glossy film, a medium mirror chrome, or a matte or other textured finish. Chrome plating has been used traditionally in the plastics industry because it offers excellent hardness and wear resistance. Rolls can also be fabricated from various grades of stainless steels but are made mostly from 400 series stainless steel because of both weldability and hardenability.

The required roll diameter will be dictated from the throughput rate and the line speed. It is important to note that the roll is a heat exchanger, and therefore its capacity is proportional to its surface area. A casting roll that will handle 200 kg/hr will have to have a much larger diameter than one designed for 20 kg/hr. Also, the line speed must be considered because the material is leaving the die in a molten state and must be completely solidified by the time it leaves the roll. There will be a certain residence time required for the film to be in contact with the roll, and this, in conjunction with the line speed, will dictate the minimum diameter of the roll.

In order to remove heat from the roll surface and to maintain it continuously at the desired temperature, the internal geometry of the roll must be designed properly. A simple single-shell roll will allow a liquid to be pumped through the interior of the roll, but the heat exchange is inefficient, and the roll surface temperature can vary considerably from end to end. This is because there is no predetermined path for the water to take—it is only flowing in a random pattern, and at a slow velocity. This type of design is generally not deemed appropriate for pharmaceutical products.

The optimum roll construction is called the "double-shell, spiral baffled" roll. A film casting roll has a thin outer shell to optimize heat transfer capabilities to cool the product. *Double shell* refers to the second roll shell within the inside of the main roll shell, with a gap of typically 10 mm between the two shells. *Spiral baffled* refers to the fact that within this annular space, there is a helical barrier welded in place. This forces the coolant to flow only within the spiral channel, keeping it along the inner wall of the main roll shell. Because this channel has a small cross-sectional area, the water flows at a higher velocity, making convection more efficient (Figure 12.6).

12.3.3.5 Pull Rolls and Slitter

After the film leaves the main casting roll, the rest of the process is very straightforward. The film generally goes through a set of rubber-covered nip rolls, and from there to a winder. Note that film made with most materials will have an "edge bead," meaning that the outer edges of the film will be thicker than the middle. For some

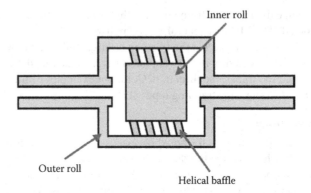

FIGURE 12.6 Double-shell, spiral baffled roll.

materials and purposes, the effect is not noticeable and can be used as is with the edge bead on.

If the edges must be slit off, the slitter station would typically be located after the nip rolls, and prior to the winder. Depending on the type of film (and type of winder), this may require another set of nip rolls after the slitter. Slitters for films can usually use simple fixed razor knives, unless there is a laminated substrate layer that is difficult to slit, in which case a motorized rotary blade system may be required.

12.3.3.6 Laminations

A film casting unit can also be outfitted with one or more unwind stations to cast the film onto a substrate. The position of the unwind must be chosen by taking into account the proposed web path to bring the substrate into the casting roll at the correct place to allow adhesion. In general, there are only two possibilities, with the unwind shaft being either above or below the casting roll. Sometimes a front rubber nip roll is necessary to apply nip pressure to the substrate/film to gain proper adhesion strength (Figure 12.7).

Unwind designs can range in sophistication depending on the tension control accuracy required. To determine the tension needed, the substrate properties must be evaluated carefully. If it is a strong, thick substrate that is not stretchy, the equipment will work with a fairly wide range of tensions. On the other hand, if the substrate web is thin and weak, or will wrinkle easily, then it is important to have a better control of tension to successfully laminate.

An unwind shaft must have a brake mechanism to apply drag to the shaft to produce tension in the substrate web. The simplest type of brake is mechanical, using a friction drum or disc applied either with a hand adjuster or pneumatically. A smoother braking drag can be attained using a magnetic particle brake, where the drag is varied by changing the voltage to the brake. With any system, it is important to determine if a manually set drag is acceptable, as this type will not automatically "taper" or compensate for the change in substrate roll diameter. This is required because as the material is unwound from the payoff, the roll diameter gets smaller and smaller—changing the actual web tension.

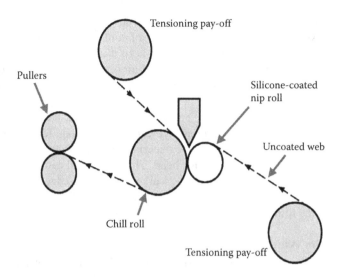

FIGURE 12.7 Typical lamination line.

The optimum arrangement is where there is an automatic taper compensation for changes in the roll diameter. This is usually done by having the web make an approximately 90° turn over an idler roll that is supported on load cells, so it is always measuring the force on the idler roller. This force signal is fed back to a controller, which has a closed loop to the brake control. In this way, the operator enters a tension setpoint, and the control modulates the brake to maintain this tension, regardless of the substrate roll diameter.

Another hardware issue to be considered is how to affix the substrate roll onto the unwind shaft. There are various methods, depending on how often there is a need to change the rolls, and how quickly this operation must be done. Most substrates are supplied on three-in. Interior diameter (ID) plastic cores. Cone collars are a simple, tried-and-true method of holding the core, but are not convenient if the core changes occur often or quickly while running. Air chucks are a better choice for production applications. An air chuck uses compressed air to inflate a rubber bladder within the shaft, which expands aluminum "leaves" or "buttons" to grab the core. With an air chuck, the operator merely presses a switch to either release or grab the core, which permits easy, rapid changeovers.

A final bit of hardware that may be needed is a transverse adjustment for each unwind. This is necessary if the edge alignment of your product is important. The transverse adjustment is usually accomplished by having the unwind mounted to a carriage on linear bearings, with a simple threaded rod and manual handwheel for adjustment back and forth.

12.3.3.7 Air Knives and Edge Pinners

Sometimes a condition can develop on the main casting roll immediately downstream of the die, where a layer of air gets continuously trapped in between the film and the roll surface. This entrapped air will cause a reduction in heat transfer, and the finish of the film will suffer as a result. One device to alleviate this problem is an air knife. An air knife puts out a "curtain" of cool air about the same width as the film, which is directed against the film to keep it in contact with the roll. On a small unit, air knives are generally compressed-air operated. In addition to keeping the film pressed against the roll, the air knife also provides some auxiliary cooling of the opposite side of the film.

Edge pinners are similar devices, but instead of a curtain, these devices emit a "point" jet of compressed air. There are typically two jets, one for each edge. The reason edge pinners are used is that some materials may have heavy flow at the outer ends of the die, producing a thick edge bead. This edge bead can then lift the film off the roll surface or cause alternating "scalloping" on the edge. The jet of air is directed to pin the edge down against the roll surface, thus improving the overall uniformity of the film.

12.3.3.8 Film Winders

As with unwinds, there are many different types of winders. Probably the single most important concern is the required winding tension. Some films require very delicate tension held within a tight tolerance range; otherwise, wrinkles will result. For these types of films, an automatic taper tension control system is necessary. Other important parameters are:

- the diameter of the wound roll,
- the weight of the final roll,
- whether a cantilevered design is possible,
- the winding feet per minute and
- the method for core changeovers.

12.3.3.9 Spreader Rolls

Thin films of many materials have a tendency to wrinkle and to "bunch together" when under tension. The film can even "fold over" in places, making it impossible to wind into a uniform roll. The solution to most of these problems is to use a spreader roll. A spreader roll is designed to continuously pull the film from the center out to both edges. There are many different designs of these rolls from various manufacturers. Some are rubber covered and warped into a curve (a "banana roll"), and others may be aluminum or stainless steel with helical grooves cut into the roll.

The other factor that must be decided is where to put the spreader roll.

Spreader rolls are typically used just prior to the winder, but others may be placed in the web path depending on the intended process.

12.3.4 PROCESSES FOR MAKING SHEET

12.3.4.1 Sheet Takeoff Machines

Many of the same comments noted above for cast film also apply to sheet extrusion. Sheet extrusion also uses a flat-type die, and water- or oil- cooled rolls to form the product. In general, sheet equipment is of a heavier construction than film machinery, as the roll nip forces are much higher. Sheet also tends to run at much slower line speeds because the product is thicker. Many sheet products run in the range of 1–30 ft/min.

Sheet takeoff units are made in several different configurations, with the main ones being vertical stack, 45° canted stack, and horizontal stack (referring to the positions of the main cooling rolls). Vertical and canted stacks can be either "upstacks" or "downstacks," which refer to which direction the web is going to move away from the die. Some products will run equally well on any of these configurations, but sometimes a material will be much easier to run on a particular type of machine. For instance, a low-viscosity material may not have enough melt strength to work well with a vertical stack because the melt curtain will sag in between the die and the primary roll nip. For this type of material, either a canted or horizontal stack will work better, as the material can fall by gravity right into the roll nip (Figures 12.8 and 12.9).

A major design criterion that must be answered when specifying a sheet takeoff is the required nip force of the rolls to "squeeze" the materials to make the product. This is defined in pounds per linear inch (PLI). The design of the rolls, bearings, and frame of the takeoff machine depends greatly on the rated PLI. A light-duty machine would typically be capable of 150–200 PLI. A medium-duty unit would typically be rated for 350–400 PLI, and a high-PLI machine would be in the 700–1000 range (Figure 12.10).

As a general rule, low-melt viscosity materials will not need much PLI force, while tougher, higher molecular weight materials will need more. If the machine does not have enough PLI, the rolls will be pushed open by the melted material, with the end result being inconsistent gauge control (because the roll arms are not being held firmly against the gap stops). The best approach is to test the materials on an existing takeoff unit to determine the required PLI for the application.

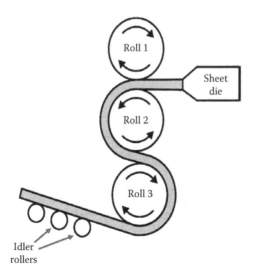

FIGURE 12.8 Sheet takeoff downstack.

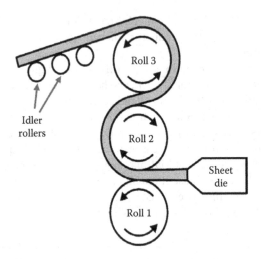

FIGURE 12.9   Sheet takeoff upstack.

12.3.4.2   Sheet Dies

A sheet die looks similar to a cast film die from the outside. Both take a round melt input and distribute it into a melt curtain of uniform thickness and desired width. The sheet die will usually need a wider range of gap openings, however, as the product may range from 0.010 to 0.125 in. or more. Sheet dies are offered in light-duty and heavy-duty designs, with the choice depending on the internal pressure expected.

Lip gap adjustment mechanisms for almost all modern dies are of the flex lip type (Figure 12.11). Flex lip means that a row of bolts is used to adjust the lip by flexing a thin section of steel within the die. One feature that is different from a cast film die is that a sheet die very often has a choker bar, particularly to run thicker products.

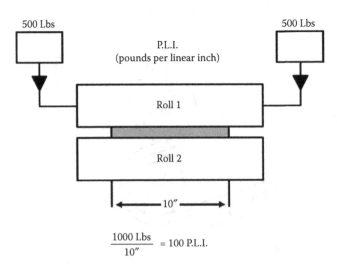

FIGURE 12.10   Example PLI.

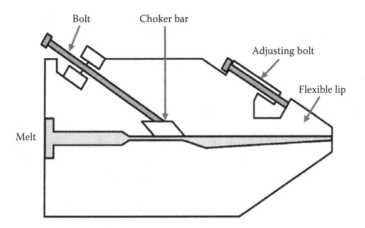

FIGURE 12.11   Flexible lip sheeting die.

A choker bar is a moveable dam inside the preland area, which can be adjusted to reduce the gap in the preland. This serves to increase the pressure within the distribution manifold, improving the uniformity of the melt curtain.

Flex lip mechanisms are offered in a few different designs also. The simplest type is called "push only" because the adjuster bolts can just push on the lip to close it down to a smaller gap. A more complex lip adjustment design is "push–pull," meaning that the adjuster bolt can both push and pull the lip.

The most sophisticated and expensive lip adjustment method is an automatic die (or auto die, for short). This is a system using a noncontact thickness scanner located in the downstream web path, near the pull rolls, where the sheet is fully cooled. The scanner traverses the full width of the sheet back and forth continuously while running and takes very precise thickness measurements. Most scanners today use a radioactive material that emits beta or gamma rays. These thickness measurements are collected in a computer, which correlates them to the transverse position of the measuring head. The software for these systems is very sophisticated, providing a multitude of real-time statistical process control data in addition to the thickness profile. The bolt adjustment controls automatically adjust the die lip to correct it.

This is generally done via special heated bolts in place of the normal lip adjustment bolts (14).

12.3.4.3   Sheet Slitters
Sheets generally always have an edge bead on both sides, which often must be slit off. Thinner sheet gauges in flexible materials may use a simple razor slitter, identical to the unit described above for film. Heavier gauge sheets or tough materials will usually need a powered shear or score cut slitter.

12.3.4.4   Web Guiding
Web guiding is a term used to describe a feature to either manually or automatically guide the sheet to keep it centered on the rolls as it progresses along the web path. This is necessary with a web that tends to walk off to one side. Web guiding may

not be necessary with a relatively short web path from die to winder. As this path gets longer with more and more stations in between, web guiding may become necessary. The most sophisticated systems use an edge sensor (typically a photo eye), which picks up the direction the edge is drifting toward. This is fed back to a motor-controlled pivoting idler roll carriage that can skew the sheet one way or the other.

12.3.4.5   Roll Temperature Control

Rolls are maintained at a desired temperature by circulating a liquid through the inside of the shell. This liquid is generally either water with some additives, such as ethylene glycol or oil. Water may be used with pressurization up to about 100°C; above this temperature, oil must be used. Oil is less desirable for a few reasons:

1. The thermal conductivity of oil is only about 60% that of water, meaning heat transfer is less efficient.
2. Oil is very messy when there is a leak or a rotary union must be taken apart.
3. Most heat transfer oils degrade over time at elevated temperatures, so the oil must be changed at certain intervals.
4. Oil pumps and temperature control units generally require more maintenance than water units.

Whether water or oil is used, temperature control units are required for each independent "zone" of control. With a roll stack with three rolls, it is possible to operate all three from a common temperature control unit, but this results in the same temperature for all three rolls, which may be detrimental to the process. A more flexible setup would be to have an independent unit for each roll, allowing individual temperature set points for each roll (Figure 12.12). Each unit will have a heat exchanger for cooling, so that even if it is an oil unit, a source and a return of cooling water must be supplied.

12.3.4.6   Sheet Processing Tips

Like many extrusion processes, there are many nuances that result in a successful operation. An issue that can have a significant effect on the sheet properties is the

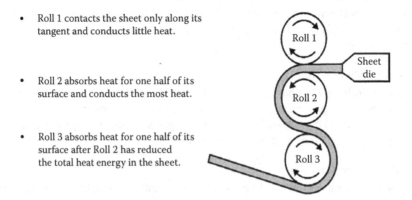

- Roll 1 contacts the sheet only along its tangent and conducts little heat.

- Roll 2 absorbs heat for one half of its surface and conducts the most heat.

- Roll 3 absorbs heat for one half of its surface after Roll 2 has reduced the total heat energy in the sheet.

FIGURE 12.12   Differential temperature control.

degree of "drawdown." Drawdown is simply the linear speed of the takeoff rolls relative to the linear speed of the melt curtain exiting the die. If these speeds were exactly matched, the sheet would be taken away at the same speed as the material coming out of the die. This can be done with some materials, but very often this is not the most stable way to run. Because the melt curtain has no "melt tension" on it, the sheet may wander and not cool in a uniform way, resulting in poor gauge control. Because the rolls are just "kissing" the sheet, surface contact may be lost from time to time, which also may cause an uneven surface texture.

Many materials process best with the takeoff rolls running a little faster than the material exiting the die. This provides a definite drawdown to the product, meaning it will be both thinner and narrower (necked down) than the die lip dimensions. So this has to be taken into consideration when setting up the die lip gap. For instance, if a 0.050-in. product is desired, the die lips may be set to 0.065 in., with the product drawdown using roll speed.

Note that drawdown can create different physical properties in the sheet for machine direction versus transverse direction. The more the product is drawn, the greater this effect. Drawdown can be used to optimize the material properties. For instance, some rigid materials—when run with excessive drawdown—will be very strong in one direction, and easily crack if flexed in the other direction.

It is important to note that the roll gap is not necessarily set to the exact dimension as the final product gauge. This again is highly material dependent. Because the sheet is still cooling inside as it leaves the primary nip, it may either continue to swell or expand, or it may contract upon subsequent cooling. This even depends somewhat on what meters-per-minute speed range is operated. The correct gap is generally arrived at by performing test runs with known roll gap settings and by checking the gauge of the cooled sheet.

The opposite condition of drawdown is to run what is called a "rolling bank" (Figure 12.13). This effect is created when the rolls are run at a slightly slower linear speed than the melt curtain is exiting the die. This causes a "pool" of molten material to build up continuously in the primary nip gap. Because of the surface friction of the rolls, this pool tends to roll over itself continuously, hence the term rolling bank. The rolling bank is a pool of excess material, so one benefit is that it

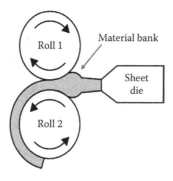

FIGURE 12.13 Rolling bank.

ensures that the nip gap is 100% filled, making for good contact between the rolls and the sheet.

Running a rolling bank can be a delicate balancing act. If the pool is too large, it will cause excessive forces on the rolls, which can actually cause damage to the steel face of the roll. A large rolling bank may also induce residual stresses into the sheet product or cause visible arc lines in the sheet examined under a light. The decision to process with a rolling bank is another decision that is material dependent. Some materials with a certain melt viscosity and elasticity run very well this way; others do not (15).

12.4   GMP REQUIREMENTS

As mentioned in Section 12.1, almost all of these types of equipment are derived from units designed for the plastics industry. For each machine built for a pharmaceutical customer, the manufacturer may be building 100 units for plastics processors. Various machinery builders have different degrees of experience with pharmaceutical practices. Some are very familiar with the requirements, while others are not. The safest approach when purchasing a GMP machine system is to generate a detailed document of specifications for both mechanical and electrical components within the system (16).

The GMP considerations can have a significant effect on the cost of the equipment. For instance, one way to build the equipment is with material contact surfaces made of stainless steel and supporting frames and other noncontact parts of painted carbon steel (Figure 12.14). This is very cost effective and may meet your requirements. Another variation is to allow painted carbon steel below the process height and to require stainless steel above the process height (to prevent paint chips from accidentally falling into the material). Some GMP systems require everything to be

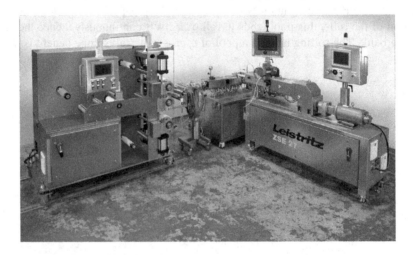

FIGURE 12.14   System for wound care, dissolvable films, and transdermal products.

fabricated from stainless steel, including machine bases and framework. This will involve significantly higher cost.

The level of finish expected on the rolls should also be specified, and in quantitative terms. It is far better to specify that the rolls will have a "finish of 0.8–1.5 in." than to merely say "mirror finish."

12.5 CONCLUSION

The technology to continuously produce a sheet or film is well proven, with literally thousands of installations in North America alone. Currently, the challenge is applying this well-proven technology to the pharmaceutical industry. Generally, this does not relate to design and process issues, but rather to "downsizing" the equipment and configuring the machinery for a GMP environment.

REFERENCES

1. Martin C. Using twin screw extruders to perform compounding with direct sheet extrusion of tpo formulations. *TPO RETEC*: Troy, MI, September 20, 1999.
2. Gungor, Sevgi et al. Plasticizers in transdermal drug delivery systems. *Recent Advances in Plasticizers* (2012): 91–112.
3. Kamiyama, Fumio, and Ying-shu Quan. Polymers in transdermal delivery systems. *Encyclopedia of Pharmaceutical Technology*. Ed. James Swarbrick. 3rd ed. Vol. 1. N.p.: n.p., 2007. 2925–2934.
4. Dhiman, Sonia et al. Transdermal patches: a recent approach to new drug delivery system. *International Journal of Pharmacy and Pharmaceutical Sciences* 3 (2011): 26–34.
5. Prodduturi, Suneela et al. Stabilization of hot-melt extrusion formulations containing solid solutions using polymer blends. *AAPS PharmSciTech* 8.2 (2007): E152–E161. PMC.
6. Keen, Justin M. et al. Investigation of process temperature and screw speed on properties of a pharmaceutical solid dispersion using corotating and counter-rotating twin-screw extruders. *J Pharm Pharmacol Journal of Pharmacy and Pharmacology* 66.2 (2013): 204–217.
7. Bala, Rajni, Sushil Khanna, Pravin Pawar, and Sandeep Arora. Orally dissolving strips: a new approach to oral drug delivery system. *International Journal of Pharmaceutical Investigation* 3.2 (2013): 67.
8. Hatton, Chris. Drug delivery: thin dissolving films begin to come of age. 4.1 (n.d.): 80–81. http://www.ipimedia.com/. International Pharmaceutical Industry.
9. Morales, Javier O., and Jason T. Mcconville. Manufacture and characterization of mucoadhesive buccal films. *European Journal of Pharmaceutics and Biopharmaceutics* 77.2 (2011): 187–199.
10. Shaikh, Rahamatullah, Thakur Raghu Raj Singh, Martin James Garland, A. David Woolfson, and Ryan F. Donnelly. Mucoadhesive drug delivery systems. *Journal of Pharmacy and Bioallied Sciences*. Medknow Publications, 2011. August 24, 2016. <http://www.ncbi.nlm.nih.gov/pmc/articles/PMC3053525/>.
11. Cilurzo, Francesco, Irma E. Cupone, Paola Minghetti, Francesca Selmin, and Luisa Montanari. Fast dissolving films made of maltodextrins. *European Journal of Pharmaceutics and Biopharmaceutics* 70.3 (2008): 895–900.
12. Sharma, Deepak, Daljit Kaur, Shivani Verma, Davinder Singh, Mandeep Singh, Gurmeet Singh, and Rajeev Garg. Fast dissolving oral films technology: a recent trend for an innovative oral drug delivery system. *International Journal of Drug Delivery* 7.2 (2015): 60–75.

13. Christie A. Machine direction orientation of thin films: properties and processes. *Film and Sheet Conference 97*, Somerset, NJ, December 9, 1997.

14. Cloeren PF. Getting the most out of your die system investment. *Film and Sheet Conference 97*, Somerset, NJ, December 9, 1997.

15. Lamont PR. Equipment and processing considerations for thin gauge PP sheet. *Film and Sheet Conference 97*, Somerset, NJ, December 9, 1997.

16. Martin C. Continuous mixing/devolatizing via twin screw extruders for drug delivery systems. *Interphex Conference*, Philadelphia, PA, March 20, 2001.

13 Melt Extruded Amorphous Solid Dispersions

Pinak Khatri, Dipen Desai,
Harpreet Sandhu, Atsawin Thongsukmak,
Gaurang Patel, Jaydeep Vaghashiya,
Wantanee Phuapradit, and Navnit Shah

CONTENTS

13.1 INTRODUCTION

Combinatory chemistry and high throughput screening are the principal components in new drug discovery. They reveal that more than 50% of newly identified active pharmaceutical ingredients (APIs) show superior lipophilicity and higher melting point. These two properties significantly affect the aqueous solubility of newly identified APIs (i.e., the APIs suffer from poor aqueous solubility) and thus result in poor bioavailability (Lipinski, 2000; Tiwari et al., 2016). This creates a big challenge for the pharmaceutical research and development scientist to develop a marketable drug formulation without compromising on the safety and efficacy. Further, the crystalline material consists of a lattice structure in which molecules are strongly held together by intermolecular bonds, making it more stable, but has a poor solubilization profile due to higher lattice energy. However, several methods can be used to improve the solubility, which include physical and chemical modification, particle size reduction, complexation, salt formation, co-crystallization, drug dispersion into the carrier matrix (solid dispersion and solid solution), and so forth (Savjani et al., 2012). In the last few decades, pharmaceutical scientists have shown an increasing interest in preparing a noncrystalline (amorphous) form of API. The amorphous material lacks a strong lattice structure (disordered) and thus it requires less energy to overcome the lattice structure. This results in improved dissolution rates and higher apparent solubility (Craig, 2002; Leuner and Dressman, 2000). The higher dissolution rate and kinetic solubility from the amorphous form may result in supersaturation of the API in the gastrointestinal fluid, increasing the bioavailability of poorly water-soluble compounds. However, the amorphous material possesses higher free energy, making them thermodynamically less stable (metastable state) and entropically driving them to a more stable crystalline state (i.e., they recrystallize on storage) (Hancock and Parks, 2000). Therefore, instead of a pure amorphous API, pharmaceutical scientists have tried to stabilize the amorphous form using other excipients, which has promoted the development of amorphous solid dispersions. An amorphous solid dispersion formulation is a single-phase system of API and stabilizing polymers. Successful development of amorphous solid dispersion mainly depends on the API properties, stabilizing polymer, and processing technology. The polymer provides the essential stabilization framework for the amorphous form of API, whereas the process provides the necessary energy to transform the crystalline physical mixture of API and polymer into a stabilized amorphous dispersion. Many processes such as spray drying (Patterson et al., 2007), co-precipitation (Shah et al., 2013), and mechanical and thermal processing technologies such as melt extrusion (Patterson et al., 2007) have been employed to achieve stabilized amorphous dispersions. In essence, all these technologies utilize two primary steps: uniform mixing of API with appropriate excipients or polymers, possibly at the molecular level, followed by instant quenching to essentially freeze the API-polymer matrix in a "stabilized amorphous form."

Hot-melt extrusion (HME) is being used as a preferred option in the development of solid dispersions as it offers various advantages over the other techniques, including solvent-free processing, suitability for continuous processing, no requirement of major downstream processing, and ease of scale-up. However, HME suffers from a need for a high processing temperature, which limits the use of temperature-sensitive molecules (thermolabile) and only select pharmaceutical polymers are thermally stable (Patil et al., 2016). HME technology can combine multiple unit operations, including material conveying, melting, mixing, devolatilization, pumping, and pressurization for shaping, into a single manufacturing process (Tadmor and Gogos, 2013; Todd, 1998a). The API, a polymer (carrier), and other excipients are fed either as a preblend or as an independent component, through a feeder; if needed, additional solids and/or liquids can be fed downstream. Solids are conveyed down the barrel length with the help of corotating or counterrotating screws. In most cases, conveying elements are used in the feed section to facilitate the feeding and conveying of solids, followed by melting with the aid of barrel temperature and kneading elements. Devolatilization may be needed, prior to pumping and pressurization, to remove air, moisture, or volatile contents from the melt. Short-pitched conveying elements can be used to pump the melt and build pressure before forcing it through a die to achieve the desired shape. After the material exits the die, the material is then cooled and subjected to downstream processes such as milling, pelletizing, or calendaring for desired profiling. In short, for melt extrusion, the mixing of components takes place as part of the extrusion process, and stabilization occurs as part of the downstream processing, where the extrudate is rapidly cooled by forced air, a water bath, chilled rolls, or other techniques (DiNunzio and Miller, 2013).

For amorphous solid dispersions by melt-extrusion technology, material properties of API and polymeric carriers, equipment designs, and processing conditions are strongly interrelated. Judicious selection of extruder design and optimization of processing conditions to suit the physicochemical and thermomechanical properties of materials are required for successful development and scale-up of amorphous solid dispersion systems.

Both single- and twin-screw extruders are widely used in food, plastics, and medical applications and have been investigated and utilized for pharmaceutical applications. Due to their efficient mixing, shorter processing time, and tighter residence time distribution, twin-screw extruders with fully intermeshing corotating designs have been widely used for development and manufacturing of amorphous solid dispersions (McCrum et al., 1997; Tadmor and Gogos, 2013). A detailed discussion of processing conditions and excipient selection criteria for HME technology is presented in later parts of this chapter.

13.1.1 CURRENT STATUS OF TECHNOLOGY

Melt extrusion technology is a very advanced and widely used for the manufacturing of plastic tubes, electric cables, pipes, plastic bags, pet products, snacks, cereals, infant formula, etc. (Singh et al., 2007). For the last two decades, the pharmaceutical industry has explored the utility of the HME process as an alternative "platform technology" to other pharmaceutical conventional techniques for manufacturing of the dosage form such as tablets, capsules, films, and implants for drug delivery via oral, transdermal, and transmucosal routes (Table 13.1) (Patil et al., 2016). In recent years, the tremendous growth and adaptation of this technology has been clearly evident by the number of research and review articles published in the public domain and the steady rise in the number of HME-based patents worldwide. The HME process has been primarily utilized to improve solubility and bioavailability of poorly soluble drugs (Serajuddin, 1999). Recently it has also been utilized to modify the drug release profile (controlled and target release) (Djuris et al., 2013) to develop abuse deterrent formulations of habit-forming substances (Maddineni et al., 2014) and to taste mask the bitter API, indicating that its application is not only limited to BCS Class II drugs.

As the melt extrusion technology has advanced within the pharmaceutical industry, pharmaceutical scientists and engineers have also started exploring mixing efficiency, process modularity, and temperature control aspects of melt extruders to develop continuous processes for conventional batch processes such as wet and melt granulation. On the same note, excipient manufacturers have initiated the development of special polymers, including, for example, BASF—Soluplus® (polyvinyl caprolactam-polyvinyl acetate-polyethylene glycol graft copolymer), Dow Chemical Company (DOW)—Affinisol® (hydroxypropylmethylcellulose acetate succinate [HPMCAS]), Ashland-Klucel™ (hydroxypropyl cellulose [HPC]), etc., to manufacture stabilized amorphous solid dispersions using melt extrusion technology.

Prior to extrusion, a thorough understanding about the physicochemical/thermal properties of the API as well as other excipients (especially polymers) is the key to a successful process. Moreover, process parameters such as screw design, screw speed, barrel temperature, and feed rate should be optimized in order to control the quality of the final product.

TABLE 13.1

Marketed Pharmaceutical Products Manufactured Using HME Process

Marketed Product

Name	API	Polymer	Role of HME	Indications
Lacrisert® (Merck)	No drug[a]	HPC	Shaped system—ophthalmic insert	Dry eye syndrome e.g., keratoconjunctivitis sicca
NuvaRing® (Merck)	Etonogestrel (11.4 mg) + Ethinyl estradiol (2.6 mg)	EVA	Shaped system—vaginal ring	Contraceptive
Implanon® (Organon)	Etonogestrel (68 mg)	EVA	Shaped system—implant	Contraceptive
Zoladex® (AstraZeneca)	Goserelin acetate (3.6 mg; 10.8 mg)	PLGA	Shaped system—implant	Prostate and breast cancer
Orzurdex® (Allergan)	Dexamethasone (0.7 mg)	PLGA	Shaped system—implant	Macular edema
Gris-PEG® (Pedinol Pharmacal Inc.)	Griseofulvin (125 mg; 250 mg)	PEG	Crystalline dispersion—tablet	Antifungal (ringworm infection)
Rezulin®* (Parke Davis)	Troglitazone (200 mg; 300 mg; 400 mg)	PVP	Amorphous dispersion—tablet	Antidiabetic
Noxafil® (Merck)	Posaconazole (100 mg)	HPMCAS	Amorphous dispersion—tablet	Antifungal
Cesamet® (Meda)	Nabilone (1 mg)	PVP	Amorphous dispersion—capsule	Nausea and vomiting associated with chemotherapy
Kaletra® (Abbott)	Lopinavir + Ritonavir (100 + 25 mg; 200 + 50 mg)	PVP-VA	Amorphous dispersion—tablet	Antiviral (HIV)
Norvir® (Abbott)	Ritonavir (100 mg)	PVP-VA	Amorphous dispersion—tablet	Antiviral (HIV)

(Continued)

TABLE 13.1 *(Continued)*
Marketed Pharmaceutical Products Manufactured Using HME Process

Marketed Product Name	API	Polymer	Role of HME	Indications
Onmel® (Merz)	Itraconazole (200 mg)	HPMC	Amorphous dispersion—tablets	Antiviral (HIV)
Eucreas® (Novartis)	Vildagliptin (50 mg) + Metformin HCl (850/1000 mg)	HPC	Melt granulation—film-coated tablet	Antidiabetic
Zithromax® (Pfizer)	Azithromycin (250 mg; 500 mg)	Pregelatinzed starch	Melt congeal	Antibiotic
Palladone™* (Purdue)	Hydromorphone (12 mg; 16 mg; 24 mg; 32 mg)	EC + ERS	Controlled release	Pain
Opana® ER (Endo)	Oxymorphone HCl (5 mg; 7.5 mg; 10 mg; 15 mg; 20 mg; 30 mg; 40 mg)	PEG	Controlled release	Pain
Isoptin SRE® (SOLIQS)	Verapamil HCl (240 mg)	HPC/HPMC	Shaped system—oval-oral tablets	Hypertension and angina pectoris
Covera-HS® (Pfizer)	Verapamil HCl (240 mg)	HPC	Melt granulation—film-coated tablet	Hypertension and angina pectoris
Nurofen Meltlets lemon® (Reckitt Benckiser Healthcare)	Ibuprofen (200 mg)	HPMC	Melt granulation—oral tablet	Analgesic

ª Insert-ocular lubricant (HPC-5 mg).
* Currently discontinued.
EVA = ethyl vinyl acetate, HPC = hydroxypropyl cellulose, HPMC = hydroxypropyl methylcellulose, HPMCAS = hydroxypropylmethylcellulose acetate succinate, PLGA = poly(lactic-co-glycolic acid), PVP-VA = polyvinyl pyrrolidone co-vinyl acetate, PEG = polyethylene glycol, PVP = polyvinyl pyrrolidone, EC = ethyl cellulose, ERS = Eudragit® RS.

13.2 THEORETICAL CONSIDERATION

Introduction of melt extrusion in the pharmaceutical industry has revolutionized the original concept of producing eutectic mixtures by the fusion method as reported by Sekiguchi and Obi in 1961 and Chiou and Riegelman in 1969. Advances in melt extrusion technology combined with more sophisticated process analytical technology (PAT) have helped evolve the understanding and classification of solid dispersions. In order to enhance solubility and bioavailability, particularly of the BCS Class II and IV drugs, the science of solid dispersions has expanded to include more complex systems including mixtures of polymers (binary/ternary polymer blends) or polymer-surfactant blends. As shown in Figure 13.1, the evolution of an amorphous system can be described in three major steps (Vasconcelos et al., 2007).

Simplistic two-component, one-phase models or the two-component, two-phase models originally described have evolved to include more complex structures (Laitinen et al., 2014; Vasconcelos et al., 2007). Specifically, for systems prepared using HME technology, a clear distinction is made between the solubility-driven and miscibility-driven solid dispersions. Although it is possible to predict, but almost impossible to determine the solubility of the drug in the polymer, the term "solubility-driven" solid dispersion is used to imply that a crystalline drug is dissolved in the molten polymer and that the solution state is maintained upon cooling. Due to the actual solubility of the drug in the molten polymer at storage temperature, the performance of a solubility- or miscibility-driven system could be very different. On the other hand, the term miscibility is used to imply that the amorphous drug is miscible with the polymer. Based on the nature of the matrix, the solid dispersion can be classified as follows: (a) simple eutectic systems, (b) amorphous API in a crystalline carrier, (c) amorphous API in an amorphous carrier, (d) solid solutions (API dissolved in a crystalline carrier in the solid state), and (e) glass solutions and glass suspension (API dissolved in an amorphous carrier) (Chiou

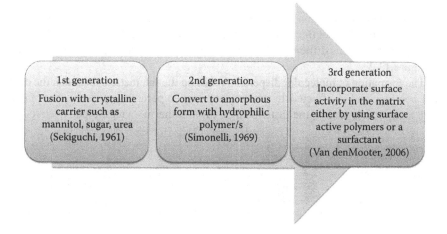

FIGURE 13.1 Evolution of solid dispersion. (Adapted from Vasconcelos, T., Sarmento, B., and Costa, P. (2007). *Drug Discovery Today*, 12(23–24), 1068–1075.)

and Riegelman, 1971). The solubility advantage of the amorphous solid dispersions depends on the ability of the drug substance to form an amorphous glass form and the stability of this amorphous form. From a theoretical perspective, the key formulation and process aspects that can affect the glass-forming ability and glass stability can be attributed to:

Inherent properties of the API: Melting temperature, glass transition temperature, critical crystallization temperature, and critical cooling rate (Laitinen et al., 2014; Vasconcelos et al., 2007)

Properties of the stabilizing polymer: Solubility or miscibility of the drug in polymeric systems as estimated by solubility parameters or thermal methods, including the melting point depression or Flory-Huggins interaction parameters, glass transition temperature of the solid glass, molecular weight, hygroscopicity, and surface activity (to stabilize the amorphous form during the dissolution in aqueous systems)

Processing conditions: From a hot-melt extrusion perspective, the processing conditions that can affect the nature of amorphous glass include extrusion temperature, molecular weight, melt viscosity of the polymer, shear, feed rate, physicochemical properties of the API and polymer, and cooling rate associated with postextrusion and downstream processing (milling and compaction)

Based on the interactions between the API and the polymer and the key operative mechanism in the formation of amorphous dispersion, the process can be classified into two major classes: miscibility region and solubility region. The key characteristics of each system and its implication in the development of the hot-melt extrusion process are described below.

13.2.1   TYPE I ASD (SOLUBILITY DRIVEN)

Analogous to solubility in a liquid state, the formation of ASD may be driven by the solubility of the drug in the molten polymer. Although the true definition of solubility in the solid state is difficult to discern, a simplistic view of such a system is shown in Figure 13.2.

The formation of molecular dispersion relies on the interactions between the drug and polymer and is affected by factors such as temperature, pressure, concentration, and particle size of the drug (solute). From a thermodynamic perspective, the

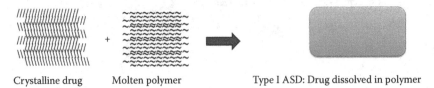

Crystalline drug   Molten polymer   Type I ASD: Drug dissolved in polymer

FIGURE 13.2   Simplified schematic of solubility driven Type I amorphous solid dispersion (ASD).

interaction between the drug and the polymer can be assessed as follows (Bellantone et al., 2012):

$$\Delta G_{ss} = \Delta G_{HC} + n_1 \Delta h_{1,M}\left(1 - \frac{T}{T_{1,M}}\right) + n_1\phi_2\chi RT + RT(n_1 ln\,\phi_1 + n_2\phi_2) \quad (13.1)$$

where ΔG_{ss} is the free energy of the solution, ΔG_{HC} is the energy required to heat and melt the crystalline drug, $\Delta h_{1,M}$ is the heat of fusion of the solute, ϕ_1 and ϕ_2 are the volume fraction of the drug and polymer, n_1 and n_2 denote the moles of the drug and polymer, χ is the interaction parameter, R is the gas constant, $T_{1,M}$ is the melting point of the drug, and T is the absolute room temperature. While $T_{1,M}$, ΔG_{HC}, and $\Delta h_{1,M}$ can be determined by differential thermal analysis, χ can be calculated by a solubility parameter method using the following expression:

$$\chi = \frac{v_1(\delta_1 - \delta_2)^2}{RT} + 0.34 \quad (13.2)$$

where δ_1 and δ_2 denote the solubility parameters for the drug and polymer, respectively, and v_1 denotes the molar volume of the drug. Solubility parameters can be calculated using one of the well-established group contribution methods (Shah et al., 2014). Molar volume can be determined by using a group contribution method or using commercially available software like ChemSketch Freeware (Advanced Chemistry Development Inc.) (Khatri, 2011). The factor 0.34 is an empirical factor and is used to improve the estimation. The solubility parameter is a composite factor that takes into account the van der Waal's forces of interaction (dispersion or dipole-dipole force) and hydrogen bonding. A lower difference in the solubility parameters leads to a smaller value of the interaction factor and eventually a lower and even negative free energy of the solution. Lower free energy of the solution implies a greater stability of the overall system. Therefore, matching the solubility parameter of the drug and polymer has often been used to select the optimum polymer to prepare ASD. An example of such a system is shown in Figure 13.3, where the drug's inherent solubility was determined in a hydrophilic polymer using this approach.

Processing conditions such as temperature, shear rate, and residence time can be used to maximize the rate and extent of solubilization during the hot-melt extrusion process. The bulk properties of the drug and excipients, particularly particle size, can also affect the rate of solubilization, as the drug dissolution can be enhanced by decreasing the particle size of the drug as described by the Noyes-Whitney equation (1891):

$$\frac{dM}{dt} = \frac{DA}{h}[C_s - C(t)] \quad (13.3)$$

where dM/dt is the rate of dissolution, D is the diffusion coefficient, A is the surface area of the dissolving particle, C_s is the saturation solubility, and $C(t)$ is the bulk drug concentration.

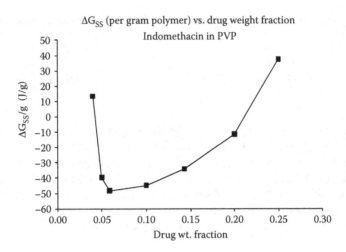

FIGURE 13.3 Estimation of drug's solubility in polymer using free energy of solution. (Adapted from Bellantone, R. A. et al. (2012). *Journal of Pharmaceutical Sciences*, 101(12), 4549–4558.)

The development of an HME process for such systems requires compatibility of the drug and polymer properties in the process. If a drug has high solubility in the molten polymer, then extrusion may be performed at a temperature below the melting point of the API. Similarly, if a drug acts as a plasticizer for the polymer, the processing temperature could be reduced below the melting point of the drug and may be beneficial if there are thermal stability concerns. Since the drug is dissolved in the polymeric carrier, the maximum drug loading is generally limited by the drug solubility in both the molten polymer and storage condition. By virtue of the high shear and temperature employed during the HME process, it may be possible to produce a supersaturated system; however, it is critical for the solution state to be maintained at room temperature. Therefore, cooling/quenching efficiency becomes a critical process parameter to be carefully evaluated during the development of the HME process.

As shown in Figure 13.1, other additives such as the plasticizer, surfactant, or flow aids may be added to the formulation to achieve or maintain higher solubility during processing and stability during dissolution. Due to the complexity of multicomponent systems, it may not be possible to discern the true nature of the dispersion; however, it is important to systemically evaluate its impact on the processing and performance of the drug product.

13.2.2 Type II ASD (Miscibility of Amorphous Drug in the Polymer)

The solid dispersions produced by uniformly mixing the amorphous drug in a molten polymer at high temperatures can provide single-phase systems. Some drugs may be solubilized in the polymer but most exist in a molecularly dispersed state. Depending on the drug-polymer interaction, drug loading, and processing conditions, the final product may vary from eutectic mixtures to solid solutions. The amorphous drug may be stabilized in the polymeric matrix by dispersion and/or hydrogen bonding forces. Therefore, favorable solubility parameters and Flory-Huggins interaction parameters are still important to develop a stable ASD. The glass solutions produced by mixing the amorphous drug with amorphous polymer are stabilized by the low mobility imparted by the high glass transition temperature of the polymer. From a practical perspective, because these systems allow higher drug loading, they may be more relevant. The key considerations from a drug loading and stability perspective are miscibility of the drug and polymer, the glass transition temperature, and the sensitivity of glass transition temperature to environmental stress (such as humidity). A simplified schematic of these systems is shown in Figure 13.4.

In addition to the favorable interactions, the two key parameters critical for achieving and stabilizing the amorphous form are a reduced glass transition temperature (K_T) and the critical cooling temperature.

The reduced glass transition temperature, as defined by Kauzmann, is the ratio of glass transition temperature and the melting point. A higher T_g/T_m ratio signifies higher viscosity and higher stability (Kauzmann, 1948). Similarly, the successful development of an ASD by an HME process also depends on the cooling rate. The critical cooling rate assessed either by isothermal time-temperature diagrams or a continuous cooling rate can be estimated as follows (Karmwar et al., 2011):

$$q_{crit}^n = \frac{T_m - T_n}{t_n} \tag{13.4}$$

where $q^n{}_{crit}$ is the critical cooling rate, T_m is the melting temperature, and T_n and t_n are the minimum temperature and time where amorphous form can still be achieved. Since accurate measurement of cooling rate is generally difficult and tedious, a simplified approach based on a differential scanning calorimetry (DSC) measurement was developed by Cabral et al., 2003 as shown below:

$$q_{crit}^n = \exp\left(A - \frac{B}{T_m^2}\right) \tag{13.5}$$

where A and B are the empirical constants obtained by linear regression.

In recent years, computational data mining has been developed as a theoretical approach to study the drug-excipient miscibility. Alhalaweh et al. (2014) have used this approach to predict the miscibility of a drug and several excipients, using

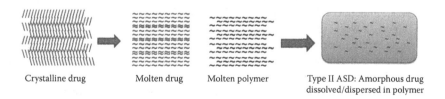

| Crystalline drug | Molten drug | Molten polymer | Type II ASD: Amorphous drug dissolved/dispersed in polymer |

FIGURE 13.4 Simplified schematic of miscibility-driven Type II ASD.

Hansen solubility parameters (HSPs) as the data set. The K-means clustering algorithm was applied to predict the miscibility of indomethacin with a set of more than 30 compounds based on their partial solubility parameters (dispersion forces, polar forces, and hydrogen bonding). The predictability of miscibility by the K-means algorithm correlated well with the DSC results, with an overall accuracy of 94%. It was also shown that the prediction accuracy was the same (94%) when the two-dimensional parameters or the hydrogen-bonding (one-dimensional) parameter was used. Therefore, the hydrogen-bonding parameter was a determining factor in predicting miscibility in such a set of compounds, whereas the dispersive and polar parameters had only a weak correlation. This approach is advantageous as it is easy to use and time and cost effective (Alhalaweh et al., 2014).

13.3 EXPERIMENTAL TECHNIQUES TO ESTIMATE DRUG CARRIER MISCIBILITY

Apart from the abovementioned theoretical approaches, some of the experimental techniques employed to estimate drug-carrier miscibility are as follows.

13.3.1 GLASS TRANSITION TEMPERATURE MEASUREMENT BY DIFFERENTIAL SCANNING CALORIMETRY

Glass transition temperature (T_g) has been used to determine the miscibility of binary or ternary drug-polymer systems. A single T_g indicates a one-phase system, i.e., miscibility between the components of the system. If two or more T_gs are observed, the system is said to be fully or partially separated into individual amorphous phases. Rumondor et al. (2009) showed that, while only one T_g was observed for felodipine-polyacrylic acid systems containing 70% or 90% indicating miscible systems, systems containing 30% or 50% polymer showed two distinct T_g events, which indicates the immiscibility of the two phases.

In spite of its widespread use to evaluate the miscibility in amorphous systems, this technique suffers from several drawbacks. Some of these drawbacks include the inability of traditional DSC to differentiate between the T_gs if there is a difference of less than 10°C between them and the inability to detect small domains (less than 30 nm) in the systems containing more than one amorphous phase; this may result in a failure of the technique in detecting separate T_g values. Moreover, with an increase in the temperature, the constant heating rate in a traditional DSC may alter the miscibility of the system. The detection of a single T_g above the T_g of the lowest individual component may give insufficient information about the number of amorphous phases present at ambient conditions (Meng et al., 2015).

It should, however, be noted that the T_g value of the drug-polymer system can also provide valuable information regarding the drug-polymer miscibility, as the deviation between experimental T_g and theoretically calculated T_g might be an indication of the molecular interaction between the drug and the polymer (Baird and Taylor, 2012; Papageorgiou et al., 2009). While investigating the miscibility of nimodipine-PVP systems by DSC, modulated temperature differential scanning calorimetry

(MTDSC), and other techniques, Papageorgiou et al. (2009) used the measured T_g values in the Gordon-Taylor equation and found that the k values are much higher than 1, indicating molecular interaction between the drug and the polymer.

13.3.2 MELTING POINT DEPRESSION METHOD

In this method, a DSC study is performed on drug-polymer physical mixtures, and the melting behavior of drug-polymer systems is compared to that of the pure drug. Generally, if the drug and the polymer are miscible, a significant melting point depression is observed due to the exothermic mixing. On the contrary, in an immiscible system, the melting point depression is negligible or absent, since the mixing is endothermic (Marsac et al., 2006). Absence of the melting endotherm peak of the drug may be due to the formation of a eutectic/monotectic mixture, solid solution, or solubilization of the drug in the molten carrier during thermal analysis (Khatri, 2011).

Polyethylene glycol and poloxamer have shown to form a eutectic mixture with ibuprofen (Greenhalgh et al., 1999; Law et al., 2002). Theoretically, the possibility of the formation of a monotectic or eutectic mixture can be estimated using the Schroder–Van Laar equation (Equation 13.6). According to this equation, the melting points of both components decrease with a decrease in their mole fractions. A plot of the melting point of individual components vs. their mole fraction is plotted and their point of intersection is taken as the eutectic point.

$$-LnX_1 = \left(\frac{\Delta H_f^m}{R} \right) \left(\frac{1}{T} - \frac{1}{T_1^\circ} \right) \tag{13.6}$$

where X_1 is the mole fraction of the drug, ΔH_f^m is the heat of fusion of the component, R is the universal gas constant, T is the absolute temperature, and T_1° is the melting point of the component.

If a higher drug-to-polymer ratio does not decrease the melting point of the drug from its original, then the possibility of the solid dispersion to be a eutectic/monotectic mixture can be ruled out. Due to the dissolution of the drug in the carrier melt, DSC provides less information on the physical nature of the drug in the solid dispersion. On the other hand, powder x-ray diffraction can provide valuable information on the physical nature of the drug in such cases (Khatri, 2011). Nair et al. (2002) have proposed melting of the crystalline carbamazepine in the carrier melt of PEG 6000.

13.3.3 MICRO-RAMAN MAPPING

Nowadays a lot of consideration is given to Raman spectroscopy for its application in drug development, especially in the preformulation stages. It allows chemical mapping of a material or system through depth analysis. Raman mapping has been extensively utilized in the study of the phase behavior of polymer-polymer systems (Keen et al., 2002). Confocal micro-Raman mapping was able to detect the nonuniform distribution of a drug on a microscopic level and the presence of crystals of nimodipine with sizes varying between 1 and several micrometers (Docoslis et al., 2007).

13.3.4 Solid-State NMR

In recent years, solid-state nuclear magnetic resonance (ssNMR) spectroscopy/ relaxometry, as a single and nondestructive technique, has been explored to deduce diverse and critical structural information of complex ASD formulations that are difficult to determine from other available techniques. Paudel et al. (2014) have summarized the recent findings on the application of ssNMR spectroscopy/relaxometry for the analysis of molecular mobility, miscibility, drug-carrier interactions, crystallinity, and crystallization in ASD. Amorphous solid dispersions of nifedipine and PVP were studied using ssNMR ^{1}H relaxation time measurements. It was observed that this technique could identify different phase homogeneities or inhomogeneities that are undetected by other complementary techniques like DSC (Yuan et al., 2013).

13.3.5 Atomic Force Microscopy

For several decades, atomic force microscopy (AFM) has been used to study the growth rates of a drug crystal within different polymer combinations in amorphous pharmaceutical formulations. In recent years, the capability of AFM has been utilized for determining the amorphous drug-polymer system miscibility. The ability of AFM to identify nanometer-sized grains enables it to measure/compare the homogeneity of amorphous drug-polymer systems at a nanoscale range.

13.3.6 Techniques Used in Combination

Combinations of AFM and Raman microscopy have been used to discriminate between homogeneously and heterogeneously mixed drug/polymer combinations. In combination with micro-Raman, TEM and SEM can be used to identify the morphology and particle size distribution of the API in the solid dispersion. It might also provide valuable information about the drug-polymer miscibility (Meng et al., 2015).

13.3.7 Film-Casting Technique

Parikh et al. (2015) demonstrated application of the film-casting technique to determine the drug-polymer miscibility and physical stability of the drug with various polymers in solid dispersion, especially those formed by HME. In this study, the solutions of the drug and the carrier were casted on glass plates using an Elcometer® model no. 3540 bird film applicator equipped with a 200-micron fitting in order to achieve uniform film thickness. Films containing the mixtures of itraconazole (ITZ) with various polymers like hydroxypropylmethylcellulose phthalate (HPMCP), Kollidon® VA 64, Eudragit® E PO, and Soluplus® were exposed to 40°C/75% relative humidity (RH) for 1 month and were then analyzed using DSC, powder x-ray diffractometry, and polarized light microscopy (PLM). It was found that ITZ had the highest miscibility with HPMCP, with miscibility at a drug-to-polymer ratio of 6:4 (w/w). The miscibility decreased with Soluplus® (miscible at 3:7, w/w, and a few microcrystals present at 4:6, w/w); Kollidon® VA 64 (2:8, w/w); and Eudragit® E PO (<1:9, w/w). Compared to DSC and powder x-ray diffractometry, PLM was found to be more sensitive to detect drug crystallization. Good correlation was observed between film-casting and hot-melt twin-screw extrusion with only a few deviations. For example, with ITZ-Soluplus® mixtures, HME at 4:6 (w/w) resulted in a single phase, whereas film casting showed the presence of few microcrystals. This may be attributed to the very high shear achieved using HME, which allows intimate mixing of the drug and polymer as well as the lesser specific surface of the melt extrudates than the films, which reduces the exposure of the API to moisture. HME of ITZ-Kollidon® VA 64 mixtures showed good correlation with the miscibility predicted by film casting. Therefore, it can be safely assumed that the film-casting technique is a conservative estimate of the physical stability of the drug-polymer melt extrudate, at least, at accelerated stability conditions (40°C/75%RH) of one month storage.

From a processing perspective, the key considerations for these systems include:

They may enable higher drug loading.
Processing temperature needs to be higher than the melting point of the drug, which may need to be optimized with respect to thermal stability.
Adequate shear rate is required to achieve uniform mixing.
Bulk excipient properties may not be critical as the mixing is occurring at temperatures above the T_m of the drug or T_g of the polymer.
Cooling rate plays an important role in quenching the desired state.
Glass transition temperature of the final ASD is critical for maintaining stability (Cabral et al., 2003).

13.4 PRACTICAL CONSIDERATIONS

Structurally, an amorphous solid dispersion is an amorphous drug entrapped by an inert carrier or polymeric matrix, acting as a stabilizer along with other excipients like surfactants that help in the stabilization. In case of HME, formulation processing aids such as plasticizers, glidant (to improve the flow property of the physical mixture), lubricant, antioxidants, surfactants, etc. are utilized in order to overcome the process challenges on a case-by-case basis.

13.4.1 Active Pharmaceutical Ingredients (API)

13.4.1.1 Suitability and Role of API

13.4.1.1.1 Melting Point of API

Because APIs are exposed to high processing temperature conditions during the extrusion process, they should be thermally stable at the desired processing temperature. Additionally, a temperature in excess of 200°C is very rare for HME applications for pharmaceutical use due to polymer degradation dictating that the drug under consideration should have a melting point less than 200°C and ideally between 120 and 150°C. As an exception, if the drug dissolves in the molten polymer, processing of higher melting point drugs for the formation of amorphous solid dispersion is feasible using HME (Albano et al., 2012). This can be determined by the absence of a melting endotherm peak of the drug by thermal cycling in DSC of the drug-polymer physical mixture (Forster et al., 2001) manufacturing process.

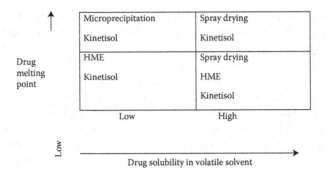

FIGURE 13.5 Factors to be considered to a select process for amorphous solid dispersion. (Adapted from Sandhu, H. et al. (2014). *Amorphous solid dispersions* (pp. 91–122) Springer.)

Figure 13.5 shows the key criteria relevant for the selection of a manufacturing process for the formation of amorphous solid dispersion and the choice of the manufacturing process.

13.4.1.1.2 Glass Transition Temperature of API

For a one-phase amorphous solid dispersion, the glass transition temperature (T_g) of the overall system is usually between the glass transition temperatures of the individual components (API and polymer) (Forster et al., 2001). Therefore, the higher the glass transition temperature of the API, the higher the glass transition temperature of the overall system, which will result in the reduced mobility of the drug molecule and will enhance the physical stability of the system. The Gordon-Taylor equation (Equation 13.7) and Fox equation (Equation 13.8) have been extensively used for predicting the glass transition temperatures of the resultant amorphous dispersion system based on glass transition temperatures, weight fractions, and densities of individual components, i.e., API and polymeric stabilizers.

$$T_{g,\text{mix}} = \frac{w_1 T_{g1} + K_{GT} w_2 T_{g2}}{w_1 + K_{GT} w_2} \tag{13.7}$$

where T_{g1} and T_{g2} are the glass transition temperatures of the drug and polymer, respectively, and w_1 and w_2 are their weight fractions.

$$K_{GT} = \frac{\rho_1 T_{g1}}{\rho_2 T_{g2}}$$

where ρ_1 and ρ_2 are the densities of two components.

$$\frac{1}{T_g} = \frac{w_1}{T_{g1}} + \frac{w_2}{T_{g2}} \tag{13.8}$$

is useful for approximate estimates of the value.

Based on these expressions, the glass transition of the drug and polymer mixed by HME will shift between the glass transition temperature of the drug and polymer.

During the preformulation screening, the glass transition temperature of the physical mixture of the drug and polymer should be determined by DSC using a heat-cool-heat cycle. The main endothermic peak during the first heating cycle represents the melting point of the drug (T_m), while the glass transition of the drug-polymer mixture (T_g) is observed during the second cycle. Based on the empirical evidence, a T_m/T_g ratio of 1.25 or lower is a good approximation for the stability of the amorphous system during long-term storage (Friesen et al., 2008).

In general, the storage temperature should be lower than the glass transition temperature of drug-polymer ASD (50°C or below) (Hancock et al., 1995). On the other hand, miscibility of the drug with the polymer does not guarantee chemical compatibility between the same. The compatibility of the drug and polymer needs to be evaluated at different storage conditions using appropriate stability indicating analytical methods.

13.4.1.1.3   Particle Size Distribution of API

Particle size distribution (PSD) of API is not expected to play a major role in terms of formulation aspects because the drug should miscible with the polymer in an ASD. However, PSD of crystalline API is critical from an HME processing point of view. PSD of the API can affect the blend uniformity of the preblend as well as the flow property during processing. Segregation of the drug and polymer while in the feed hopper can result in a drug remaining in crystalline form after HME processing. Apart from this, particle size of crystalline API can affect the processing temperature since smaller particles have faster dissolution in a molten polymer.

Li et al. (2015) have studied the effect of particle size on acetaminophen in Soluplus® as a polymer stabilizer. The acetaminophen was milled from its original average size (16 μm) to a reduced particle size average of 2 μm. These two sizes of acetaminophen were mixed with Soluplus® and tested with hot-stage microscopy to evaluate the effect of its particle size. As illustrated in Figure 13.6, the smaller particle size of acetaminophen can reduce both processing temperature and thermal impurity (Li et al., 2015).

13.4.1.1.4   Residual Solvents and Moisture Content

Since the residual solvents in an API evaporate due to the high processing temperature in HME, the volatile residual solvent is not a major concern. However, moisture can interfere with the hydrogen bonding of the polymer and solubilizer with API, especially with anhydrous API. As previously mentioned for residual solvents, higher processing temperatures may evaporate the residual moisture from the API; therefore, the risk of moisture content is relatively low. If present, the adsorbed moisture can lead to crystallization by plasticizing the polymer matrix and increasing the molecular mobility, displacing a drug substance from the bonding site on the polymer, or both.

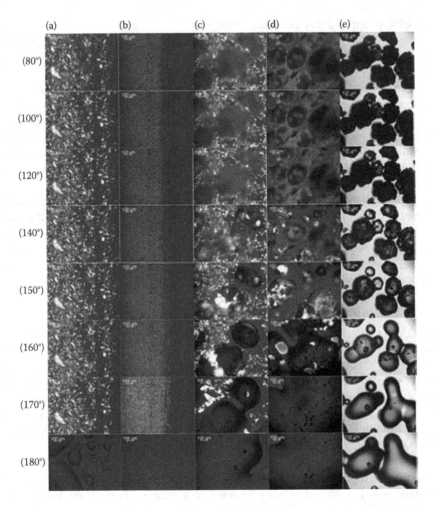

FIGURE 13.6 Hot-stage, polarized light microscopy of (a) original acetaminophen: 16 μm, (b) milled acetaminophen: 2 μm, (c) original acetaminophen + Soluplus®, (d) milled acetaminophen + Soluplus® and (e) Soluplus. (Adapted from Li, M., Gogos, C. G., and Ioannidis, N. (2015). *International Journal of Pharmaceutics*, 478(1), 103–112.)

Even though moisture content is not a critical factor to consider, the ambient moisture can become a critical issue if the polymer stabilizer is very hygroscopic. Such polymers can absorb moisture from the environment and cause phase separation of the polymer and drug substance or crystallinity of the drug.

13.4.1.1.5 Drug Loading

Drug loading can impact both kinetic and thermodynamic stability of an amorphous solid dispersion. Generally, drugs have a lower T_g compared to the T_g of polymers; therefore, in terms of kinetic stability, higher drug loading shifts the composite (drug-polymer) T_g lower, which lowers the kinetic stability of the composition. For a thermodynamically stable amorphous solid dispersion, increasing drug loading can saturate bonding sites between the drug and polymer, which results in a less stable amorphous solid dispersion due to the instability of the unbound drug. As drug loading impacts both stability mechanisms, it is critical to conduct stability studies at different drug loading to formulate a physically stable amorphous dispersion with an acceptable drug loading. There is no definite rule about drug loading to achieve stable amorphous solid dispersion. For example, Nair et al. (2001) have studied the effect of drug loading on the behavior of amorphous solid dispersion for acetaminophen, naproxen, carbamazepine, salicylamide, propranolol hydrochloride, and griseofulvin in poly(vinylpyrrolidone) (PVP K-90). As shown in Figure 13.7, acetaminophen could remain amorphous in PVP K-90 even up to drug loading of 50%. On the other hand, griseofulvin showed a crystalline peak at drug loading as low as 30%.

13.4.1.1.6 Ionization Behavior of API

Sarode et al. (2014a) have studied the poorly soluble drugs felodipine (FLD), a neutral drug, and itraconazole (ITZ), a weak base drug, in various polymers including Eudragit EPO, Eudragit L-100-55, hydroxypropylmethylcellulose acetate succinate (HPMCAS)-LF, Pharmacoat 603, and Kollidon VA64 from an HME process. The DSC and powder x-ray diffraction (PXRD) results show conversion from original crystalline API to amorphous solid dispersion with all polymer stabilizers as shown in Figure 13.8.

Even though the ionization behavior of the drug may not be critical in formulation selection, based on experience, it was observed that the acidity of the drug can reduce the life of the process equipment. It may also generate impurities that cause problems in the process due to oxidation of the metal surface by the drug pH. These problems can shorten the life of equipment or even cause impurities.

13.4.2 EXCIPIENTS IN HOT MELT EXTRUSION

13.4.2.1 Polymers (Carriers) in Hot Melt Extrusion

Polymers used in the HME process are thermoplastic in nature and form a polymeric binder. The properties of the polymer influence the processing conditions and the characteristics of the extruded dosage form, which can include dispersibility of the active ingredient, its stability, and release rate.

Vaka et al. (2014) have presented details of excipients for amorphous solid dispersion in recent publications. Although many of the selection criteria could be applied universally to all amorphous dispersion processing technologies, the authors have focused the discussion on the selection of excipients for amorphous solid dispersions processed using melt extrusion technology.

13.4.2.1.1 Practical Consideration in Polymer Selection

13.4.2.1.1.1 Drug-Polymer Miscibility As a rule of thumb, the glass transition temperature of the system should be at least 50°C above the storage temperature to assure acceptable physical stability of the melt extrudates. The glass transition temperature of a drug-polymer system can be estimated using the Gordon-Taylor equation and can be experimentally measured using DSC. Therefore, it is desirable to have a polymer with a higher glass transition temperature. However,

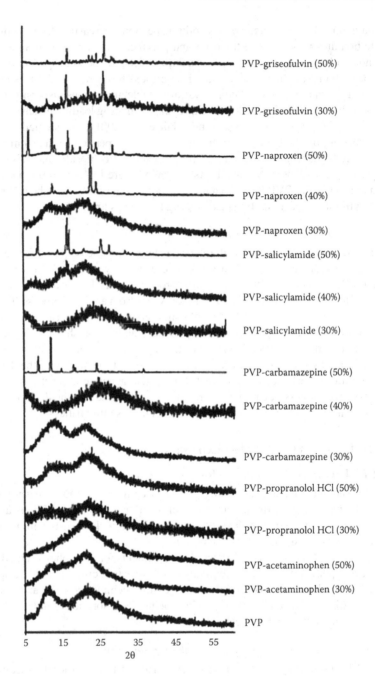

FIGURE 13.7 Powdered x-ray diffraction (PXRD) patterns for the various drug-PVP films at different drug loadings. (Adapted from Nair, R. et al. (2001). *International Journal of Pharmaceutics*, 225(1), 83–96.)

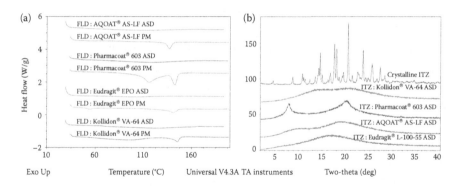

FIGURE 13.8 (a) DSC plots of FLD PMs (physical mixtures) and its AsDs and (b) PXRD plots of ITS and its AsDs. (Adapted from Sarode, A. L. et al. (2014a). *European Journal of Pharmaceutics and Biopharmaceutics*, 86(3), 351–360.)

extrusion temperatures higher than 180–200°C may cause the degradation of the polymer. For a higher melting point drug, it is essential that it is readily miscible with the polymer to enable processing below 200°C. If melt extrusion does not produce transparent extrudates, increasing the energy input of the screw by changing the screw design or using solubilizers as a plasticizer may help miscibility. Alternatively, a polymer with lower melting point (like polyethylene glycol or poloxamers) or polymers with lower glass transition temperature (such as Soluplus®) can be used. On the other hand, if the drug has a low melting point, a polymer with a higher glass transition temperature like copovidone, HPMC, HPMCAS, or polymethacrylates should be considered.

13.4.2.1.1.2 Drug-Polymer Chemical Stability and Compatibility For successfully formulating a dosage form based on HME technology, it is essential for both the drug and polymer to be chemically stable alone and compatible with each other at extrusion temperatures. During the screening stage, drug-polymer stability and compatibility at higher temperatures should be performed to assess the suitability for the melt extrusion process.

13.4.2.1.2 Commonly Used Polymers

13.4.2.1.2.1 Kollidon® VA 64 Kollidon® VA 64 is a widely used polymer for hot-melt extrusion. It is a vinylpyrrolidone [If a break is needed, break as follows: vinyl-pyrrolidone.]-vinyl acetate copolymer with a ratio of 6:4 (Table 13.2).

Vinylpyrrolidone is a hydrophilic, water-soluble monomer whereas vinyl acetate is lipophilic and water insoluble. The ratio (6:4) is balanced in such a way that the polymer is still freely water soluble. It has a molecular weight of approximately 45,000–70,000 g/mole and K-value of 25–31. It has a glass transition temperature (T_g) of 106°C. It is a matrix-forming polymer, which can also be used in combination with a surfactant. It was used in combination with sorbitan monolaurate to formulate Kaletra® (fixed-dose combination of poorly soluble drugs lopanavir and ritonavir),

Pharmaceutical Extrusion Technology

TABLE 13.2
Commonly Used Polymers as Carriers for Hot-Melt Extrusion

Chemical Name	Available Trade Name(s)	T_g (°C)	T_m (°C)
Ammonio methacrylate copolymer	Eudragit® RS/RL	64	–
Poly(dimethylaminoethylmethacrylate-co-methacrylic esters)	Eudragit® E	50	–
Poly(methyl acrylate-co-methyl methacrylate-co-methacrylic acid) 7:3:1	Eudragit® 4135F	48	–
Poly(methacrylic acid-co-methyl methacrylate) 1:2	Eudragit® S	160	–
Hydroxypropyl cellulose	Klucel®	130	–
Ethyl cellulose	Ethocel®	133	–
Cellulose acetate butyrate	CAB 381-0.5	125	157
Cellulose acetate phthalate	–	165	192
Poly(ethylene oxide)	Polyox® WSR	–67	65–80
Poly(ethylene glycol)	Carbowax®	–20	37–63
Poly(vinyl pyrrolidone)	Kollidon®	168	–
Poly(vinyl acetate)	Sentry® plus	35–40	–
Hydroxypropyl methylcellulose phthalate	–	130	–
Polyvinylpyrrolidone-co-vinyl acetate	Kollidon® VA64	107	–
Hydroxypropyl methylcellulose	Methocel® Benecel®	175	–
Hydroxypropyl methylcellulose acetate succinate	Aqoat-AS® (AS-LG)	120	–
	Aqoat-AS® (AS-MG)	130	–
	Aqoat-AS® (AS-HG)	135	–
Poly(lactide-co-glycolide)	PLGA	–	–
Polyvinyl alcohol	Elvanol®	–	–
Chitosan lactate	Sea-Cure®	–	–
Pectin	Obipektin®	–	–
Carbomer	Carbopol® 974P	–	–
Polycarbophil	Noveon® AA-1	–	–
Poly(ethylene-co-vinyl acetate)	Elvax® 40W	–36	45
Polyethylene	–	–125	140
Poly(vinyl acetate-co-methacrylic acid)	CIBA-I	–	84–145
Epoxy resin containing secondary amine	CIBA HI	80–100	–
Carnuba wax			81–86
Glyceryl palmitostearate	Precirol ATO 5®		52–55
Glyceryl trimyristate	Dynasan 114®		55–58
Triglyceride tripalmitin	Dynasan 116		61–65

Source: Adapted from Crowley, M. M. et al. (2007). *Drug Development and Industrial Pharmacy*, 33(9), 909–926; Janssens, S. and Van den Mooter, G. (2009). *Journal of Pharmacy and Pharmacology*, 61(12), 1571–1586.

and with Vitamin E TPGS for Noxafil®. The melt extrusion–based formulation approach has improved the oral bioavailability compared to the previous formulation of lopanavir/ritonavir. Kollidon® VA 64 has higher plasticity in comparison with other polymers like povidone or macrogol. Apart from the solubility enhancement, it can also be used to prepare a controlled-release formulation by embedding API in the matrix of melt extrudate (Bühler, 2008).

13.4.2.1.2.2 Hypromellose Acetate Succinate   Shin-Etsu Chemical Co., Ltd (Japan) introduced hypromellose acetate succinate (HPMCAS) in 1986 for enteric coating. It has a cellulose backbone with a substitution of hydroxypropoxy, methoxy, acetyl, and succinoyl groups. There are three major grades that are chemically distinct, varying in their acetyl and succinoyl content of the polymer, which results in differences in their pH solubility. Each grade is available in fine and granular grade. It is primarily an amorphous polymer with a glass transition temperature (T_g) of 120°C. Due to its pH-dependent solubility, it can be used to control the release of a drug in the gastrointestinal tract. Sarode et al. (2014b) evaluated different grades of HPMCAS for HME application. This study showed that HME processing did not significantly affect the glass transition temperature, semicrystalline nature, solid-state functional group properties, moisture content, or solution viscosity of these polymers. However, the increase in HME processing temperature and screw speed can cause an undesirable change in the acetate and succinate content of these polymers. At lower operating temperatures, the free acid content release was directly correlated to the speed of the extruder. In terms of stability, AS-LF was found to be the most stable, with the lowest increase in total free acid content, even at higher HME temperature and speed. From the dissolution standpoint, AS-LF and AS-MF grades were not affected by the HME processing condition, whereas it was notably increased for AS-HF, perhaps due to significant reduction of succinoyl content. It was concluded that the HME processing conditions should be determined by considering the acceptable levels of free acid in the final drug product.

13.4.2.1.2.3 Hydroxypropyl Methyl Cellulose   HPMC is less commonly used in HME due to its high glass transition temperature of 160–210°C and degradation temperature above 250°C. Because the difference between the T_g and degradation temperature is not very pronounced, the processing of HPMC in HME poses a big challenge. In order to decrease the glass transition temperature of HPMC, plasticizers have to be incorporated in large amounts to achieve satisfactory processing without significant degradation (Jani and Patel, 2015). Alderman and Wolford (1987) suggested that at least 30% w/w plasticizer should be used for successful extrusion of hypromellose.

13.4.2.1.2.4 Hydroxypropyl Cellulose   Polymers with lower glass transition temperature like HPC polymers with a glass transition temperature of 130°C can be used to manufacture solid dispersion of high melting drugs without the use of plasticizers. It is a semicrystalline polymer with amorphous and crystalline domains (Sarode et al., 2013). Since these are nonionic polymers they can be used for achieving pH-independent release from matrices. The rate of solubilization of HPC is dependent on their molecular weight. Klucel™ hydroxypropylcellulose EF and ELF are lower molecular weight grades with an approximate molecular weight of 80,000 and 60,000 Da, respectively. Due to their lower molecular weight, they can be used to aid in the release of a poorly soluble drug from the solid dispersion with these polymers. Higher molecular weight grades can be used to achieve controlled release of the drug (Mohammed et al., 2012). Low molecular weight grades of HPC like HPC-SL and HPC-SSL are also available in the market from Nisso America Inc.

13.4.2.1.3 New Polymers for Hot-Melt Extrusion

13.4.2.1.3.1 Affinisol® HPMC HME Hypromellose has been shown to be an effective recrystallization inhibitor in stabilizing amorphous drugs and can improve the bioavailability of poorly soluble drugs. The existing grades of HPMC are difficult to melt-extrude due to higher glass transition temperature, high melt viscosity, and a narrow processing temperature window due to high degradation potential above the glass transition temperature. Thus, it requires the use of plasticizer in the formulation for improving its processability. However, the inclusion of plasticizer may be detrimental for certain amorphous solid dispersion as the plasticizer may contain water and cause crystallization during storage or during the GI transit of the dosage form. In order to overcome these challenges, a modified grade of hypromellose, Affinisol™ HPMC HME (Dow), was recently introduced, which has a significantly lower glass transition temperature (117–128°C) and melt viscosity in comparison to the other available grades of hypromellose. It can be extruded at 120–180°C with the API without the need of any plasticizer. It is currently available in three grades, differing in regard to their molecular weight: HPMC HME, 15 cP; HPMC HME, 100 cP; and HPMC HME, 4M (Huang et al., 2015).

13.4.2.1.3.2 Soluplus® Soluplus® is a graft-polymer comprising polyethylene glycol, polyvinyl acetate, and polyvinylcaprolactam. It has been shown to have better solubilizing potential than other well-known solubilizers like Cremophor RH40, Tween 80, Lutrol F127, etc. Due to its excellent solubilization potential, it offers the possibility of forming a solid solution with the drug. It has a lower T_g of 70°C, allowing it to be extruded at a lower temperature, which is useful while dealing with APIs that can degrade at higher temperature. If temperatures above 200°C are required for melt extrusion, a suitable plasticizer could be added to prevent any degradation of the polymer or the API. Furthermore, the low hygroscopicity of Soluplus helps in preventing recrystallization or nucleation of API in the melt extrudate (Hardung et al., 2010).

13.4.2.1.3.3 Mesoporous Silica Mesoporous silica was recently investigated as an excipient for formulations of molecules with low water solubility. These polymeric materials have very high specific surface area and small pore size. The customized template synthesis produces highly porous silica materials which can enhance the dissolution of hydrophobic API. Surface adsorption of the molecule to the mesoporous silica not only enhances the dissolution, but also prevents the recrystallization of the amorphous drug molecules, due to the porous nature and the controlled pore size volume. Due to the relatively finite space available for the amorphous molecules, the probability to align with crystalline counterparts is low to negligible, resulting in amorphous stabilization of the drug. Van Speybroeck et al. (2010). used fenofibrate as the model drug for evaluating the SBA-15 (mesoporous silica) solid dispersion formulations. The DSC study showed the glassy nature of the fenofibrate at a 40% drug load, compared to 20% load in their previous formulations. The amorphous nature could be attributed to the decrease in the availability of pore space, decreased surface adsorption of the fenofibrate molecule, or the lack of molecular interaction with silanoyl groups. The formulations were found to be stable over six months at ambient conditions, showing that mesoporous silica could be a viable option for those drugs, which are less miscible with the traditional polymers. Wu et al. (2015) demonstrated the use of HME for preparation of a mesoporous silica/ethylcellulose mini-matrix for sustained release using fenofibrate as a model drug. Here, mesoporous silica was used as a dissolution-enhancing excipient while ethyl cellulose and xanthan gum were used as release-controlling excipients.

13.4.2.2 Plasticizers

Plasticizers are usually low-molecular-weight, water-soluble or insoluble additives that are incorporated into pharmaceutical polymers for various functions. For use in hot-melt extrusion, plasticizers are incorporated into the high-molecular-weight polymers to facilitate thermal processing and improve the physical and mechanical properties of the drug product (Follonier et al., 1994; Zhang and McGinity, 1999). Although many plasticizers are used in the chemical industry, only a few have been approved for pharmaceutical applications due to environmental and/or human health concerns attributed to plasticizer toxicity (Wu and McGinity, 1999). Since the 1940s, various theories have evolved explaining the plasticizing effect of plasticizers: lubricity theory, gel theory, free volume theory, and polarity theory. An in-depth analysis of the mechanism of plasticization is beyond the scope of this book chapter; readers are encouraged to refer to the work of (2004).

13.4.2.2.1 Selection of Plasticizers

Selection of plasticizers depends on plasticizer-polymer compatibility and plasticizer stability. In selecting the appropriate plasticizer for a polymeric material, the plasticization efficiency and compatibility must be determined by measuring the glass transition temperature of the polymeric material as a function of plasticizer concentration. Desai (2007) demonstrated the application of complementary analytical techniques such as solubility parameters, DSC, and rheology to select solid-state plasticizers for amorphous solid dispersion systems.

13.4.2.2.2 Classification Based on Chemical Structure

Materials commonly used as plasticizers that are approved by the Food and Drug Administration for use in pharmaceutical dosage forms are listed below in Table 13.3 according to their chemical structure.

13.4.2.2.3 Influence of Plasticizers in Hot-Melt Extrusion

When incorporated into a polymeric material, a plasticizer improves the workability and flexibility of the polymer by increasing the intermolecular separation of the

TABLE 13.3
Commonly Used Plasticizers in Hot-Melt Extrusion Process

Type	Examples
Citrate esters	triethyl citrate, tributyl citrate, acetyl triethyl citrate, acetyl tributyl citrate
Fatty acid esters	butyl stearate, glycerol monostearate, stearyl alcohol
Sebacate esters	dibutyl sebacate
Phthalate esters	diethyl phthalate, dibutyl phthalate, dioctyl phosphate
Glycol derivatives	polyethylene glycol, propylene glycol
Vitamin E TPGS	D-α-tocopheryl polyethylene glycol 1000 succinate
Surfactant	polysorbates, docusate sodium
Sugar alcohols	sorbitol, xylitol, lactitol, erythritol
Others	triacetin, mineral oil, castor oil, carbon dioxide, methylparaben

Source: Adapted from Crowley, M. M. et al. (2007). *Drug Development and Industrial Pharmacy*, 33(9), 909–926.

polymer molecules. This results in reduction of elastic modulus, tensile strength, polymer melt viscosity, and glass transition temperature (T_g). The polymer toughness and flexibility is improved and lower thermal processing temperatures can be employed. Methylparaben, polyethylene glycol 8000 (PEG 8000), and triethyl citrate (TEC) were efficient plasticizers for Eudragit S100 and enabled the extrusion of pellets at temperatures well below the onset of thermal degradation (Table 13.4).

TABLE 13.4
Use of Different Plasticizers in the Hot-Melt Extrusion of Eudragit® S100 Pellets at Varied Concentrations

Plasticizer	Plasticizer level (%)	Eudragit® S100	Theophylline (%)	Extrusion Temperature (°C)	Strand Diameter ± SD (μm)
None	0	70	30	220	598 ± 16
Triethyl citrate (TEC)	10	60	30	180	687 ± 19
Triethyl citrate (TEC)	20	50	30	140	655 ± 36
Polyethylene Glycol (PEG 8000)	10	60	30	180	640 ± 17
Polyethylene Glycol (PEG 8000)	20	50	30	140	625 ± 21
Methyl paraben (MP)	10	60	30	180	737 ± 17
Methyl paraben (MP)	20	50	30	140	773 ± 32

Source: Adapted from Crowley, M. M. et al. (2007). *Drug Development and Industrial Pharmacy*, 33(9), 909–926.

TABLE 13.5
Activation Energies (E_a) Obtained from Slopes of Arrhenius Plots of Unplasticized Eudragit® S100 Pellets and Plasticized with Triethyl Citrate (TEC), Polyethylene Glycol (PEG 8000), and Methyl Paraben (MP)

Formulation	None	10% TEC	10% PEG	10% MP	20% TEC	20% PEG	20% MP
E_a (KJ mol^{-1})	106.4	80.3	86.4	83.7	58.5	45.6	51.8
R^2 value	0.992	0.999	0.995	0.999	0.990	0.984	0.984

Source: Adapted from Crowley, M. M. et al. (2007). *Drug Development and Industrial Pharmacy*, 33(9), 909–926.

The E_a values (Table 13.5) for plasticized Eudragit S100 decreased to 80–86 kJ mole (10% plasticizer) and 45–59 kJ mole (20% plasticizer), respectively. This behavior was expected since plasticizers increase the chain mobility by reducing attractive forces between the polymer molecules, resulting in a lower barrier against the plastic flow during hot-melt extrusion and a reduced sensitivity of the viscosity to the processing temperature (Crowley et al., 2007).

Plasticizer can also impact the release profile of drug from the extruded matrix (Table 13.6). Zhang and McGinity (1999) have shown that the release rates of chlorpheneramine increased because of the faster hydration and dissolution of polyethylene glycol 3350 (plasticizer) compared to polyethylene oxide (polymer) from the

TABLE 13.6
Release Rates Observed Experimentally in Buffer after 45 Min and Calculated by ANOVA for Hot-Melt Extruded Eudragit® S100 Pellets Containing 30% Theophylline with Two Levels (10% or 20%) of Plasticizers and Without Plasticizers

Plasticizer	Plasticizer Level (%)	HME Yield (%)	Release in Acid after 2 Hours (%)	Release in Buffer after 45 Min (°C)	Calculated Release Rate [% hr^{-1} ± SD (μm)]	R^2 Value
None	0	6.4	5.91 ± 0.13	31.28 ± 1.88	33.60 ± 2.56	0.988
Triethyl citrate (TEC)	10	12.0	4.18 ± 0.18	28.22 ± 1.46	32.38 ± 2.02	0.998
Triethyl citrate (TEC)	20	18.3	7.14 ± 0.04	51.77 ± 1.71	59.83 ± 2.24*	0.997
Polyethylene glycol (PEG 8000)	10	9.0	18.23 ± 0.42	41.32 ± 3.51	31.52 ± 4.85	0.980
Polyethylene glycol (PEG 8000)	20	15.5	83.24 ± 1.98	90.69 ± 0.95	–	–
Methyl paraben (MP)	10	13.3	5.66 ± 0.17	36.66 ± 1.56	41.78 ± 2.09*	0.997
Methyl paraben (MP)	20	23.3	3.85 ± 0.08	61.61 ± 0.82	78.44 ± 0.91*	0.997

* Significantly higher values (one-way ANOVA with $\alpha = 0.05$ and $p < 0.0001$, Tukey Kramer *post hoc*).

polyethylene oxide (PEO) extruded tablet. It was also demonstrated that the decrease in viscosity of the hydrated layer, due to the presence of polyethylene glycol (PEG), facilitated the diffusion of the drug in the surrounding media. Strong plasticizer-polymer interactions could disrupt the polymeric structures and increase the local mobility of the carboxylic acid groups, making them more accessible for ionization and promoting film dissolution. It was further observed that methyl paraben plasticized Eudragit S100 showed an increased tendency for elastic recovery upon die exit, since the extruded strands exhibited a significantly larger diameter (Table 13.4). This elastic expansion of the matrix might decrease the packing density of the polymeric chains and facilitate water penetration in buffer pH 7.4, resulting in faster drug release rates.

13.4.2.3   Solubilizers and Wetting Agents

Surfactants are most commonly used as solubilizers or emulsifying agents to increase the apparent aqueous solubility and bioavailability of the drug. In the case of hot-melt extrusion, surfactants can also have a plasticizing effect, which allows processing at lower temperatures. Some of the commonly used surfactants include polysorbate 20, polysorbate 80, vitamin E polyethylene glycol succinate, polyoxyl 40 hydrogenated castor oil, etc. (Padden et al., 2011). Ghebremeskel et al. (2007) demonstrated the effect of Tween 80 and docusate sodium on the physical stability of API-PVP solid dispersions. They concluded that the two surfactants evaluated on API-PVP dispersions were very similar in their plasticization, water uptake, and consequently their physical stability. It was suggested that the surfactant's ability to lower the viscosity of the melt and increase the API solubility and homogeneity in the carrier polymer might be the reason for such observations. Since, the plasticizers lower the T_g as well as absorb water, it is possible that physical stability of the system can decrease; however, this study showed that this effect was minimal (Ghebremeskel et al., 2007).

Albano et al. (2012) demonstrated that the incorporation of docusate sodium in melt extruded solid dispersion helped improve dissolution rate and reduce motor load and process temperatures (Albano et al., 2012). On the other hand, Janssens et al. (2008) have shown that the addition of even 10% of TPGS 1000 to the polyvinyl pyrrolidone co-vinyl acetate (PVPVA) 64 carrier matrix causes destabilization of the molecular dispersion of itraconazole and leads to the formation of crystalline itraconazole clusters. Therefore, the choice and concentration of surfactant should be judiciously selected by considering their effect on processing conditions, solid-state physical stability, and the physical stability of amorphous solid dispersions during exposure to *in vitro* dissolution media or gastrointestinal fluid.

13.4.2.4   Antioxidants

The excessive temperatures needed to process unplasticized or under plasticized polymers may lead to polymer degradation. The stability of polymers that are susceptible to degradation can be improved with the addition of antioxidants, acid receptors, and/or light absorbers during HME (Table 13.7). One manufacturer of these materials recommends the incorporation of an antioxidant into formulations containing low-molecular-weight hydroxypropylcellulose (Klucel™). Similarly, polyethylene oxide can be protected from free radical and oxidative degradation by the incorporation of an antioxidant (Crowley et al., 2002).

TABLE 13.7
Common Processing Aid

Chemical Name	Trade Name
Saccharose monopalmitate	Sucroester
Glycerolester and PEG esters	Gelucire 44/14
Glyceryl monostearate	Imwitor
d-α-tocopherol (Vitamin E)	–
Vitamin E Succinate	–
Vitamin E TPGS	–
Butylated hydroxy anisole	–
Methyl paraben	–
Mixture of hydrogenated castor oil and soyabean oil	Sterotek® K
Glyceryl palmitostearate	Precirol® ATO 5

Source: Adapted from Crowley, M. M. et al. (2007). *Drug Development and Industrial Pharmacy*, 33(9), 909–926.

Antioxidants are most effective in stabilizing oxygen-sensitive drug formulations. They have the ability to inhibit or slow down chain reaction oxidative processes at relatively low concentrations. This property of antioxidant substances is of considerable importance, with respect to formulations, because of the large number of chemically diverse medicinal agents known to undergo oxidative decomposition. Antioxidants are classified as preventive antioxidants or chain-breaking antioxidants based on their mechanism. Preventive antioxidants include materials that act to prevent initiation of free radical chain reactions. Reducing agents, such as ascorbic acid, are able to interfere with autoxidation in a preventive manner since they preferentially undergo oxidation. The preferential oxidation of reducing agents protects drugs, polymers, and other excipients from attack by oxygen molecules. Chelating agents such as edetate disodium (EDTA) and citric acid are another type of preventive antioxidant that decreases the rate of free radical formation by forming a stable complex with metal ions that catalyze these reduction reactions.

Hindered phenols and aromatic amines are the two major groups of chain-breaking antioxidants that inhibit free radical chain reactions. Commonly used antioxidants such as butylated hydroxyanisole (BHA), butylated hydroxytoluene (BHT), and vitamin E are hindered phenols. Because the O-H bonds of phenols and the N-H bonds of aromatic amines are very weak, the rate of oxidation is generally higher with the antioxidant than with the polymer (Crowley et al., 2007).

13.4.2.5 Lubricants

Waxy materials like glyceryl monostearate have been reported to function as a thermal lubricant during hot-melt processing. Vitamin E TPGS has been reported to plasticize polymers and enhance drug absorption (Table 13.3) (Crowley et al., 2002).

13.4.2.6 Other Excipients

Some of the approaches to modify the release of the drug embedded in the solid dispersion are the addition of superdisintegrants like Explotab®, the use of pH-dependent polymers in conjunction with matrix polymers, and the use of viscosity-increasing agents that limit and reduce the initial burst often observed with these systems (Crowley et al., 2007; Meng et al., 2015).

Flowability of the premix in the hot-melt extruder is also essential for ensuring uniformity of the drug content in the melt extrudates and processability. Glidants like colloidal silicon dioxide can be added to promote the flowability of the drug and polymer mixture.

13.5 PROCESS CONSIDERATIONS

For the preparation of amorphous solid dispersion, a typical HME process (Figure 13.9) includes

- Feeding,
- Conveying of the solid feed,
- Melting the drug-polymer mixture,
- Mixing the molten liquid in order to create an intimate mixture (one-phase system),
- Devolatilization, and
- Rapid cooling at a rate that will convert and restrict the drug to an amorphous form.

For the preparation of an amorphous solid dispersion, as mentioned in the previous sections, the API needs to be miscible with the polymer. During the melting of the polymer, the API progressively dissolves in the now molten polymer and

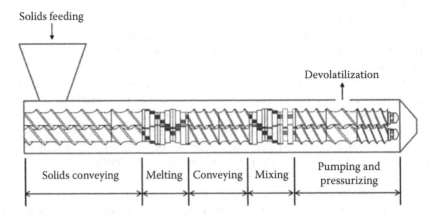

FIGURE 13.9 Schematic diagram of the hot-melt extrusion process for the manufacturing of molecular dispersion. (Adapted from Brown, C. et al. (2014). *Amorphous solid dispersions* (pp. 197–230) Springer.)

fully dissolves in the mixing step. After this step, devolatilization may be needed to remove entrapped air, moisture, and/or residual solvent. Finally, pressure is built up due to the small opening of the die, and the molten blend is forced through it. After the material exits the die, it is cooled down (solidified) rapidly to arrest the drug in an amorphous form during solidification. Further downstream processes include milling or pelletization before capsule filling or tablet compression. Alternatively, the extrudate may be shaped directly into a dosage form.

In order to ensure a homogeneous blend of components, pharmaceutical scientists usually prefer a fine powder grade of materials over larger pelletized materials for melt extrusion processes. The finer materials are either preblended prior to loading into a powder feeder or fed separately from individual feeders. The liquid components (typically plasticizer and solubilizer) could also be metered/pumped directly into the extruder using a liquid addition port. A side stuffer and an additional feeder have been explored and employed to feed low-density materials. The modular design of melt extruders has allowed the feeding of thermolabile materials in the later sections of the extruder, closer to the exit die, reducing residence time and exposure to elevated temperatures.

Of many available feeding technologies, gravimetric feeding has been well adopted in the pharmaceutical industry for melt extruder feeding. The finer powder blend of the API, polymer, and other excipients tends to have poor flow properties, leading to challenges in precise feeding of the powder blend. Gravimetric feeding can compensate for variations in density, poor flow, and feeder load, providing a controlled discharge rate of the powdered blend.

13.5.1 ROLE OF HME EQUIPMENT VARIABLES

13.5.1.1 Equipment Type Selection

Both single-screw and twin-screw extruders are widely used in pharmaceutical research. Compared to single-screw extruders, twin-screw extruders can produce higher shear during mixing, maintain tight residence time distributions (RTD), and minimize material stagnation (McCrum et al., 1997; Tadmor and Gogos, 2006). In addition, the short residence time, self-wiping screw profile, and versatility of twin-screw extruders have propelled the use of twin-screw extruders for manufacturing of amorphous solid dispersions.

The twin-screw extruder has two agitator assemblies mounted on parallel shafts. These shafts are driven through a gearbox to rotate together in the same direction (corotating) or in the opposite direction (counterrotating).

Corotating twin-screw extruders have been widely employed in the pharmaceutical industry to produce molecular dispersions due to their superior efficiency of mixing and self-wiping action, ensuring first-in-first-out material flow (Bigert and Smith-Goettler, 2011; Sandhu et al., 2014).

Compared to corotating twin-screw extruders, counterrotating twin screw extruders impart extensional flow along the entire length of the screw because of the diverging geometry at the intermesh and can be designed to provide a greater degree of positive displacement. Keen et al. (2014) showed that a counterrotating extruder formed amorphous solid dispersions at a slightly lower temperature and with a narrower residence time distribution, which also exhibited a more desirable shape, compared to corotating. It was concluded that the amorphous content in solid dispersions depended on the combination of screw speed, temperature, and operating mode. In the case of high-melting-point compounds, where decomposition occurs as a function of time and temperature, the impurity formation is minimized due to the narrow distribution and more uniform time exposures that are seen in the counter-rotating system. Therefore, counterrotating extruders may prove advantageous for the production of solid dispersions.

13.5.1.2 Screw Design Role, Importance, and General Guidance on Design

Most melt extruders consist of modular screws and can be assembled in many different configurations. The manner in which the screw profile is designed generally causes changes to parameters like mechanical shear and residence time. A typical screw design will consist of conveying elements, kneading elements, and special mixing elements.

There are different types of conveying elements based on the depth and length of the pitch. Similarly, screws have various types of mixing elements, which impart two types of mixing—distributive mixing and dispersive mixing. Distributive mixing ideally maximizes the division and recombining of the material while minimizing energy. Dispersive mixing ideally breaks droplet or solid domains to fine morphologies using energy at or slightly above the threshold level needed. This mixing aids in efficient compounding of two or more materials in the twin-screw extruder. Since the amorphous solid dispersion formulation requires breaking of the crystal lattice of API to render it amorphous and homogeneously mix it with a stabilizing polymer matrix in molten form, dispersive mixing elements are preferred. Intensive mixing may also lead to an excessive increase in microenvironmental temperature, which may lead to API or polymer degradation.

As part of the HME process development of amorphous solid dispersion formulations, scientists should start with the least aggressive mixing screw design and gradually increase the number of mixing elements to increase the dispersion mixing capacity of screws.

Specialized screw elements such as shovel elements (to increase the feed rate), fractional-lob elements, and dynamic stir elements (to increase mixing efficiency while reducing peak shear and peak pressures) can be used to aid challenges associated with manufacturing of amorphous solid dispersions using melt extrusion (Steerworld).

Generally, an extruder consists of one or two rotating screws inside a stationary cylindrical barrel(s). There are mainly four types of barrels used for pharmaceutical applications: (a) feeding blend from top, (b) feeding solids from the side of extruders, (c) liquid injection, and (d) venting (Figure 13.10). Further details can be found in other chapters of this book.

13.5.1.3 Die Design Shaping from Downstream Processing and Back Pressure

The extrusion die (Figure 13.11) is a processing tool that gives the required structure and dimensions of the extrudate. Based on the necessary downstream processing,

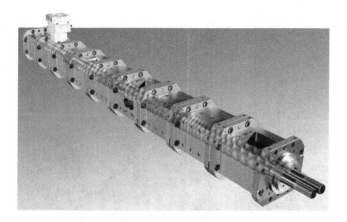

FIGURE 13.10 Material flow in a hot-melt extruder.

the die can be designed to yield extrudates in long spaghetti forms or as continuous ribbons. Die heads could be designed with multiple outputs of different shapes based on the capacity of the extruder. Melt pressure and extruder load should be taken into account while selecting a die design. The diameter of the strands will determine the output and die pressure.

13.5.2 Downstream Processing

In order to transform melt extruded amorphous solid dispersions into desirable dosage forms, downstream processing of melt extrudates is necessary, unless profile extrusion techniques or direct shaping such as calendaring is employed as a postextrusion step. The typical downstream process includes cooling, cutting, and collecting of extrudates. Process analytical technology such as near infrared (NIR), Raman, ultrasound, and DSC systems are also integrated to continuously monitor the critical quality attributes of the melt extruded products.

13.5.2.1 Pelletizer

For amorphous solid dispersion systems, rapid cooling of melt extrudates is necessary to reduce the mobility of amorphous API and arrest the amorphous form in the viscous polymeric matrix. Extrudates shaped from the die head can be directed on a moving conveyor belt with air-drying capacity or a chiller to aid the rapid cooling process. Conveyor belts can be equipped with a roller, which helps to increase the surface area and air-drying efficiency of the extrudates. At the other end of the conveyor belt, the dried brittle extrudates are guided into a pelletizer for further downstream operations, like milling. The density of extruded material has a significant impact on the design and performance of the finished dosage form. Higher density of extrudates could help to reduce the overall size of a final dosage form. By the same token, the density of extruded material could also impact the release of the API from the solid dispersion system. In order to optimize the bulk properties of extruded systems, foam extrusion technology has been evaluated to aid the manufacturing of amorphous solid dispersion systems.

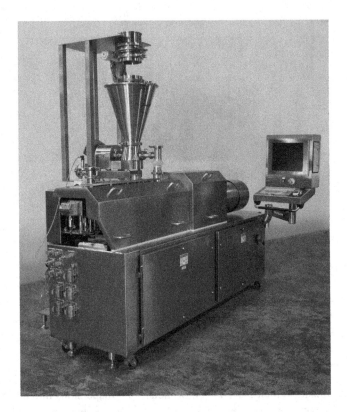

FIGURE 13.11   Twin-screw extruder with a melt strand die.

13.5.3 FOAM EXTRUSION

Foaming has been used in many polymer applications. The advantage of using foaming material in polymer processing is the reduction of raw material cost. Besides the economic issue, the porous structure offers many superior properties, including high thermal insulation, low dielectric coefficient, and excellent damping properties.

One of most common foaming agents is carbon dioxide due to its lower toxicity and environmental aspects.

Carbon dioxide can act as a plasticizer by reducing the glass transition temperature for a number of amorphous and semicrystalline polymers. Carbon dioxide is absorbed between the polymer chains and increases volume while decreasing chain entanglement. Carbon dioxide can also act as a molecular lubricant that reduces melt viscosity.

Foaming can be used in pharmaceutical applications to improve surface area to increase bioavailability or even improve the milling ability (Terife et al., 2012). The foaming process can improve the process conditions by reducing the viscosity of the melt material and the temperature of the process. Polymeric foams are produced by a phase separation process, as a result of a sudden change in temperature or pressure in the homogeneous polymer (with or without the drug) or blowing agent system (Verreck et al., 2006). Usually the formation of a gas cell takes place via three steps: nucleation, growth, and coalescence.

13.5.4 Practical Considerations for Processing for Molecular Dispersion

13.5.4.1 Melting Stage

13.5.4.1.1 Processing Section/Barrel Temperature

As a rule of thumb, the set barrel temperature during the melting stage should be 30–50°C higher than the glass transition temperature of the polymer, or above its melting point. An increase in temperature decreases the melt viscosity; however, it increases the possibility of degradation of the drug, polymer, or other incorporated processing aids. An addition of plasticizer can decrease the melt viscosity. It should be noted that much of the energy utilized in melting is obtained from the rotation of the screws, especially at large scales. During the conveying of the solids, heat is generated through frictional energy dissipation, which is followed by a combination of plastic and viscous energy dissipation in fully filled kneading blocks (Tadmor and Gogos, 2006; Todd, 1998b).

13.5.4.1.2 Feed Rate and Screw Speed

Feed rate and screw speed should be adjusted such that the input material has sufficient time to melt, mix, and solidify (cool down). It should ideally partially fill the free volume. A higher feed rate with a lower barrel speed can jam the extruder. On the other hand, a lower feed rate and higher barrel speed can expose the physical mixture to the higher surface area of the barrel at a higher temperature, which may result in degradation of the drug, polymer, or other incorporated processing aids. It should be noted that when the barrel is partially filled, the residence time of the melt is dependent on the rate, screw speed, and screw design; however, when the barrel is completely filled, the residence time is dependent on the screw speed (Todd, 1998b).

13.5.4.2 Mixing Stage

Sufficient kneading elements should be incorporated into the section after the melting compartment. Kneading elements allow intimate mixing of the drug and polymer, forming weak or strong physical interactions. These interactions form the basis for the enhanced physical stability of the amorphous solid dispersion. An increase in the kneading elements may expose the system to higher localized shear, which may lead to chemical degradation. In some cases, the combination of kneading and conveying elements are incorporated to minimize localized energy input. In other cases, reverse conveying elements are also incorporated for efficient mixing; however, it increases the localized temperature due to higher shear and may cause degradation.

13.5.4.3 Devolatilization Stage

If any solvents are used during melt extrusion, the vapors of the solvents can be released through a vent on one of the barrels after mixing.

13.5.4.4 Cooling (Solidification)

After exiting the die, the molten mass needs to be cooled at a fast rate to prevent the drug from recrystallizing. The molten mass usually cools at ambient temperature if the drug does not recrystallize; i.e., the extrudates appear transparent. If the extrudates appear translucent or opaque, the residence time and/or mixing speed should be increased to allow for complete mixing of the drug and polymer or the cooling rate should be increased with the help of chiller to prevent the crystallization of the amorphous form of the API. In the latter case, it will be essential to store the extrudates at lower temperature for further processing.

If the glass transition temperature of the molecular dispersion is less than 50°C, the extrudates will soften due to the heat produced during milling. In such cases cryomilling or air-jet milling are quite useful. Compared to other techniques, like spray drying, melt extrusion produces material with a high density and low compressibility. Therefore, a high quantity of compressible excipients is required to produce acceptable tablets. Alternatively, foam extrusion using liquefied carbon dioxide is a viable option in producing porous extrudates.

For working with a small quantity of API, small scale extrusion can be carried out using a Haake Mini-Lab MicroCompounder. It can provide an estimate of the processing parameters and predict the quality of an HME product that can be manufactured using bigger versions such as a Leistritz extruder. However, scale-up to larger versions requires optimization of processing parameters, characterization and performance evaluation of the product, and assessment of its stability for successful application of HME in pharmaceutical formulations.

13.5.5 OTHER THERMAL PROCESSING TECHNOLOGIES FOR AMORPHOUS SOLID DISPERSION PROCESSING

13.5.5.1 Kinetisol®

Generally, plasticizers are required to improve the flow property of the molten material during the HME process. Kinetisol® dispersing (KSD) is a rapid, high energy thermal manufacturing process. It has been developed to produce amorphous solid dispersions without plasticizer. In this process, the equipment is a closed, fixed-volume chamber containing blades that can rotate at high radial velocities. The materials (drug and polymer) are mixed at a very high speed with short durations of exposure to elevated temperature. Since the system is unplasticized, it has a higher T_g and eventually leads to a greater solid-state stability compared to the plasticized system that is manufactured using the traditional hot-melt extrusion process (DiNunzio et al., 2010).

13.5.5.2 Injection Molding

Injection molding (IM) is a common polymer processing technique in the plastic industry. Many products from injection molding, including bottles, toys, and plastic equipment, are available in the market. It has slowly been adapted for pharmaceuticals. Parts made by injection molding that are widely used in the pharmaceutical industry include caps, seals, closures, valves, syringes, and inhalers. Biomedical industries have started using injection molding to manufacture biodegradables for medical devices like scaffolds and microneedles. Injection molding is now gaining popularity for manufacturing more complex device parts and is even the platform of choice for preparing certain proprietary drug products.

The versatility of the IM technique can be exploited for the production of drug delivery systems with defined shape and/or dimension characteristics. The process does not require the use of solvents, which is advantageous with respect to manufacturing times, costs, and stability.

Numerous product patents have been filed with IM, which demonstrates the potential of this technology. However, the number of products that are at an advanced development stage or already on the market is still limited (e.g., Capill®, Chronocap TM, Egalet®, Septacin™), but room for improvement and in-depth investigation exists.

13.6   SCALE-UP CONSIDERATIONS

Due to the fact that HME is a continuous pharmaceutical process, only a small amount of API is required at early developmental stages to perform various formulation screening. In addition, extrusion of small scale batches significantly decreases the time and cost of formulation and process development. Therefore, HME processing on a laboratory scale is a powerful tool for rapid drug product development in comparison to other pharmaceutical solid dispersion technologies like spray drying, bead layering, and solvent precipitation (Patil et al., 2016). Once a successful proof of concept (POC) formulation is obtained, the scale-up of the successful pivotal HME formulation is essential for the commercialization of the product to meet the increasing needs of the market. Scale-up issues during commercial manufacturing can cause delay in the launch of a product, costing the pharmaceutical industry millions of dollars. Therefore, product development using a quality by design (QbD) approach, recommended by regulatory agencies, is essential to provide insight into potential problems that may be encountered during scale-up and subsequent commercial production. Using the knowledge gained during the QbD approach for product development, scaling-up of the successful pivotal formulation becomes more predictable by establishing a correlation and identifying the design operating space of the processing parameters like screw speed, feed rate, barrel temperature, pressure, melt viscosity, and drive amperage. State-of-the-art extruders utilize programmable logic controllers (PLCs) for logic functionality that implements graphical touchscreens, data acquisition, and recipe management as standard features (Martin, 2013).

The U.S. Food and Drug Administration (FDA) defines the highest quality drug product as one that consistently and reliably delivers the clinical performance and is free of contaminants. The FDA's critical path initiative, launched in March 2004 (http://www.Fda.gov/Science Research), encourages utilizing scientific tools to understand and control each unit operation involved in the manufacturing of drug products. It emphasizes modernizing scientific advancement of the product development process. QbD is an essential element of it. As defined by the FDA, QbD is a systematic approach to pharmaceutical product development that begins with predefined objectives and emphasizes product and process understanding and process

control, based on science and quality risk management. It is very important to identify and control critical process parameters (CPP), which affect the critical quality
attributes (CQAs) of intermediate and finished product quality (Gupta and Khan,
2012; Martin, 2013). In summary, applying QbD principles to product development
can facilitate product development by

- Understanding Knowledge Space from Laboratory-Scale Batches
- Defining Process Design Space Using DOE Experiments and Software
  Tools
- Determining the Control Space and Application of Control Strategy to the
  Established Process

The key to scale up the melt extrusion process for ASD formulations is to
optimize the process early in development, fix key parameters, maintain geometric similarity between the scales, and maintain a constant specific energy (SE).
Control of key process parameters of melt extrusion for manufacturing of molecular dispersion has been discussed earlier, but to reiterate, these parameters are
feeding material properties, feed configuration (volumetric/gravimetric feeder),
process length, screw/barrel design, temperature profile, die design, and feed rate
to screw speed ratio. Identifying target specifications and acceptable operating
spaces for each of these parameters will significantly increase the likelihood for
successful process transfer between scales. Table 13.8 lists some of the important
intermediate CQA and finished product CQA that can have an impact on the safety
and efficacy of a drug product.

In general, during scale-up, the HME variables that are used to confirm the reproducibility of the process parameters are listed below (Patil et al., 2016):

- Melt temperature,
- Melt viscosity,
- Mechanical strength of the die,
- Distribution of melt within the zones of the extruder, and
- Geometry of the dies.

TABLE 13.8
Critical Quality Attributes of HME Process

Critical Process Parameters (CPPs)	Critical Quality Attributes (CQAs)
Screw speed	Amorphous/crystalline nature of the API
Feed rate	Dissolution rate and extent *in vitro* and *in vivo*
Barrel temperature	Physical nature of the API
Residence time	Chemical degradation of API and polymer
Melt pressure	
Torque	

13.7 SUMMARY

In the last few decades, HME has rapidly transformed itself from the traditionally adapted technology in the plastic, rubber, and food industries to a pharmaceutical manufacturing platform due to its advantage of being a continuous, solvent-free process. It facilitated development of several successful drug delivery systems and enabled online process characterization in conjunction with advanced analytical techniques (e.g., Raman and NIR spectroscopy). The introduction of specialized stabilizing polymers for amorphous solid dispersion by melt extrusion is a testament to the fact that HME has been instrumental in solving the complex manufacturing needs of amorphous solid dispersions. Thorough understanding of excipients and processes can help achieve stabilization of the amorphous drug throughout its shelf-life and maintain supersaturation of the drug solution. Appropriate selection of downstream processes is required to achieve finished dosage forms with desirable physicochemical properties. The modular design and continuous manufacturing are natural enablers for successful scale-up. With growing interest, HME technology is expected to evolve in the areas of newer materials with wider thermal stability and to solve the challenges of the pharmaceutical industry for newly discovered molecules (e.g., solubility and bioavailability enhancement, taste masking, shape delivery, etc.) that are yet unresolved by conventional pharmaceutical technology.

ACKNOWLEDGMENTS

The authors would like to thank Dr. Hemlata Patil for the review and comments that greatly improved the chapter.

REFERENCES

Albano, A., Desai, D., DiNunzio, J., Go, Z., Iyer, R. M., Sandhu, H. K. et al., (2012). *Pharmaceutical Composition.*

Alderman, D. A., and Wolford, T. D. (1987). *Sustained release dosage form based on highly plasticized cellulose ether gels*, U.S. Patent No. 4,678,516, U.S. Patent and Trademark Office, Washington, DC.

Alhalaweh, A., Alzghoul, A., and Kaialy, W. (2014). Data mining of solubility parameters for computational prediction of drug-excipient miscibility. *Drug Development and Industrial Pharmacy*, 40(7), 904–909.

Baird, J. A., and Taylor, L. S. (2012). Evaluation of amorphous solid dispersion properties using thermal analysis techniques. *Advanced Drug Delivery Reviews*, 64(5), 396–421.

Bellantone, R. A., Patel, P., Sandhu, H., Choi, D. S., Singhal, D., Chokshi, H. et al., (2012). A method to predict the equilibrium solubility of drugs in solid polymers near room temperature using thermal analysis. *Journal of Pharmaceutical Sciences*, 101(12), 4549–4558.

Bigert, M., and Smith-Goettler, B. (2011). PAT to support the hot melt extrusion platform. *6th Annual Leistritz Pharmaceutical Extrusion Seminar*. Leistritz, Clinton, NJ. p. 41.

Brown, C., DiNunzio, J., Eglesia, M., Forster, S., Lamm, M., Lowinger, M. et al., (2014). Hot-melt extrusion for solid dispersions: Composition and design considerations. *Amorphous solid dispersions* (pp. 197–230) Springer.

Bühler, V. (2008). Kollidon® polyvinylpyrrolidone excipients for the pharmaceutical industry; 2008. *BASF SE, Ludwigshafen, Germany,*

Cabral, A., Cardoso, A., and Zanotto, E. (2003). Glass-forming ability versus stability of silicate glasses. I. Experimental test. *Journal of Non-Crystalline Solids*, 320(1), 1–8.

Chiou, W. L., and Riegelman, S. (1971). Pharmaceutical applications of solid dispersion systems. *Journal of Pharmaceutical Sciences*, 60(9), 1281–1302.

Craig, D. Q. (2002). The mechanisms of drug release from solid dispersions in water-soluble polymers. *International Journal of Pharmaceutics*, 231(2), 131–144.

Crowley, M. M., Zhang, F., Koleng, J. J., and McGinity, J. W. (2002). Stability of polyethylene oxide in matrix tablets prepared by hot-melt extrusion. *Biomaterials*, 23(21), 4241–4248.

Crowley, M. M., Zhang, F., Repka, M. A., Thumma, S., Upadhye, S. B., Kumar Battu, S. et al., (2007). Pharmaceutical applications of hot-melt extrusion: Part I. *Drug Development and Industrial Pharmacy*, 33(9), 909–926.

Desai, D. (2007). Solid-state plasticizers for melt extrusion.

DiNunzio, J. C., Brough, C., Miller, D. A., Williams III, R. O., and McGinity, J. W. (2010). Applications of KinetiSol® dispersing for the production of plasticizer free amorphous solid dispersions. *European Journal of Pharmaceutical Sciences*, 40(3), 179–187.

DiNunzio, J. C. and Miller, D. A. (2013). Formulation development of amorphous solid dispersions prepared by melt extrusion. in: M. A. Repka, N. Langley, J. DiNuzio. *Melt Extrusion: Materials Technology and Drug Product Design*, (pp. 161–203) Springer, New York.

Djuris, J., Nikolakakis, I., Ibric, S., Djuric, Z., and Kachrimanis, K. (2013). Preparation of carbamazepine–Soluplus® solid dispersions by hot-melt extrusion, and prediction of drug–polymer miscibility by thermodynamic model fitting. *European Journal of Pharmaceutics and Biopharmaceutics*, 84(1), 228–237.

Docoslis, A., Huszarik, K. L., Papageorgiou, G. Z., Bikiaris, D., Stergiou, A., and Georgarakis, E. (2007). Characterization of the distribution, polymorphism, and stability of nimodipine in its solid dispersions in polyethylene glycol by micro-raman spectroscopy and powder X-ray diffraction. *The AAPS Journal*, 9(3), E361–E370.

Follonier, N., Doelker, E., and Cole, E. T. (1994). Evaluation of hot-melt extrusion as a new technique for the production of polymer-based pellets for sustained release capsules containing high loadings of freely soluble drugs. *Drug Development and Industrial Pharmacy*, 20(8), 1323–1339.

Forster, A., Hempenstall, J., Tucker, I., and Rades, T. (2001). Selection of excipients for melt extrusion with two poorly water-soluble drugs by solubility parameter calculation and thermal analysis. *International Journal of Pharmaceutics*, 226(1–2), 147–161.

Friesen, D. T., Shanker, R., Crew, M., Smithey, D. T., Curatolo, W., and Nightingale, J. (2008). Hydroxypropyl methylcellulose acetate succinate-based spray-dried dispersions: An overview. *Molecular Pharmaceutics*, 5(6), 1003–1019.

Ghebremeskel, A. N., Vemavarapu, C., and Lodaya, M. (2007). Use of surfactants as plasticizers in preparing solid dispersions of poorly soluble API: Selection of polymer–surfactant combinations using solubility parameters and testing the processability. *International Journal of Pharmaceutics*, 328(2), 119–129.

Greenhalgh, D. J., Williams, A. C., Timmins, P., and York, P. (1999). Solubility parameters as predictors of miscibility in solid dispersions. *Journal of Pharmaceutical Sciences*, 88(11), 1182–1190.

Gupta, A., and Khan, M. A. (2012). Hot-melt extrusion: An FDA perspective on product and process understanding. *Hot-Melt Extrusion: Pharmaceutical Applications*, 323–331.

Hancock, B. C., and Parks, M. (2000). What is the true solubility advantage for amorphous pharmaceuticals? *Pharmaceutical Research*, 17(4), 397–404.

Hancock, B. C., Shamblin, S. L., and Zografi, G. (1995). Molecular mobility of amorphous pharmaceutical solids below their glass transition temperatures. *Pharmaceutical Research*, 12(6), 799–806.

Hardung, H., Djuric, D., and Ali, S. (2010). Combining HME and solubilization: Soluplus®— the solid solution. *Drug Deliv Technol*, 10(3), 20–27.

Huang, S., O'Donnell, K. P., Keen, J. M., Rickard, M. A., McGinity, J. W., and Williams III, R. O. (2015). A new extrudable form of hypromellose: AFFINISOL™ HPMC HME. *AAPS Pharmscitech*, 1–14.

Jani, R., and Patel, D. (2015). Hot melt extrusion: An industrially feasible approach for casting orodispersible film. *Asian Journal of Pharmaceutical Sciences*, 10(4), 292–305.

Janssens, S., and Van den Mooter, G. (2009). Review: Physical chemistry of solid dispersions. *Journal of Pharmacy and Pharmacology*, 61(12), 1571–1586.

Janssens, S., Nagels, S., De Armas, H. N., D'autry, W., Van Schepdael, A., and Van den Mooter, G. (2008). Formulation and characterization of ternary solid dispersions made up of itraconazole and two excipients, TPGS 1000 and PVPVA 64, that were selected based on a supersaturation screening study. *European Journal of Pharmaceutics and Biopharmaceutics*, 69(1), 158–166.

Karmwar, P., Bøtker, J. P., Graeser, K., Strachan, C., Rantanen, J., and Rades, T. (2011). Investigations on the effect of different cooling rates on the stability of amorphous indomethacin. *European Journal of Pharmaceutical Sciences*, 44(3), 341–350.

Kauzmann, W. (1948). The nature of the glassy state and the behavior of liquids at low temperatures. *Chemical Reviews*, 43(2), 219–256.

Keen, I., Rintoul, L., and Fredericks, P. M. (2002). Raman microspectroscopic mapping: A tool for the characterisation of polymer surfaces. *Macromolecular Symposia* 184(1), 287–298.

Keen, J. M., Martin, C., Machado, A., Sandhu, H., McGinity, J. W., and DiNunzio, J. C. (2014). Investigation of process temperature and screw speed on properties of a pharmaceutical solid dispersion using corotating and counter-rotating twin-screw extruders. *Journal of Pharmacy and Pharmacology*, 66(2), 204–217.

Khatri, P. (2011). *Improving dissolution rate of pyrimethamine via solid dispersion technique*. St. John's University.

Klucel™ hydroxypropylcellulose physical and chemical properties http://www.ashland.com/file_source/Ashland/Product/Documents/Pharmaceutical/PC_11229_Klucel_HPC.pdf

Laitinen, R., Priemel, P. A., Surwase, S., Graeser, K., Strachan, C. J., Grohganz, H. et al., (2014). Theoretical considerations in developing amorphous solid dispersions. *Amorphous solid dispersions* (pp. 35–90) Springer.

Law, D., Wang, W., Schmitt, E. A., and Long, M. A. (2002). Prediction of poly (ethylene) glycol-drug eutectic compositions using an index based on the van't hoff equation. *Pharmaceutical Research*, 19(3), 315–321.

Leuner, C., and Dressman, J. (2000). Improving drug solubility for oral delivery using solid dispersions. *European Journal of Pharmaceutics and Biopharmaceutics*, 50(1), 47–60.

Li, M., Gogos, C. G., and Ioannidis, N. (2015). Improving the API dissolution rate during pharmaceutical hot-melt extrusion I: Effect of the API particle size, and the co-rotating, twin-screw extruder screw configuration on the API dissolution rate. *International Journal of Pharmaceutics*, 478(1), 103–112.

Lipinski, C. A. (2000). Drug-like properties and the causes of poor solubility and poor permeability. *Journal of Pharmacological and Toxicological Methods*, 44(1), 235–249.

Maddineni, S., Battu, S. K., Morott, J., Soumyajit, M., and Repka, M. A. (2014). Formulation optimization of hot-melt extruded abuse deterrent pellet dosage form utilizing design of experiments. *Journal of Pharmacy and Pharmacology*, 66(2), 309–322.

Marsac, P. J., Shamblin, S. L., and Taylor, L. S. (2006). Theoretical and practical approaches for prediction of drug-polymer miscibility and solubility. *Pharmaceutical Research*, 23(10), 2417–2426.

Martin, C. (2013). Twin screw extrusion for pharmaceutical processes. in M. A. Repka, N. Langley, and J. DiNunzio. *Melt Extrusion: Materials Technology and Drug Product Design*, (pp. 47–79) Springer, New York.

McCrum, N. G., Buckley, C., and Bucknall, C. B. (1997). *Principles of Polymer Engineering*. Oxford University Press, Oxford, USA.

Meng, F., Dave, V., and Chauhan, H. (2015). Qualitative and quantitative methods to determine miscibility in amorphous drug–polymer systems. *European Journal of Pharmaceutical Sciences*, 77, 106–111.

Mohammed, N. N., Majumdar, S., Singh, A., Deng, W., Murthy, N. S., Pinto, E. et al., (2012). Klucel™ EF and ELF polymers for immediate-release oral dosage forms prepared by melt extrusion technology. *AAPS Pharmscitech*, 13(4), 1158–1169.

Nair, R., Gonen, S., and Hoag, S. W. (2002). Influence of polyethylene glycol and povidone on the polymorphic transformation and solubility of carbamazepine. *International Journal of Pharmaceutics*, 240(1), 11–22.

Nair, R., Nyamweya, N., Gönen, S., Martınez-Miranda, L., and Hoag, S. (2001). Influence of various drugs on the glass transition temperature of poly (vinylpyrrolidone): A thermodynamic and spectroscopic investigation. *International Journal of Pharmaceutics*, 225(1), 83–96.

Padden, B. E., Miller, J. M., Robbins, T., Prasad, L., Spence, J. K., and LaFountaine, J. (2011). Formulation development-amorphous solid dispersions as enabling formulations for discovery and early development. *American Pharmaceutical Review*, 14(1), 66.

Papageorgiou, G., Papadimitriou, S., Karavas, E., Georgarakis, E., Docoslis, A., and Bikiaris, D. (2009). Improvement in chemical and physical stability of fluvastatin drug through hydrogen bonding interactions with different polymer matrices. *Current Drug Delivery*, 6(1), 101–112.

Parikh, T., Gupta, S. S., Meena, A. K., Vitez, I., Mahajan, N., and Serajuddin, A. (2015). Application of film-casting technique to investigate drug-polymer miscibility in solid dispersion and hot-melt extrudate. *Journal of Pharmaceutical Sciences*, 104(7), 2142–2152.

Patil, H., Tiwari, R. V., and Repka, M. A. (2016). Hot-melt extrusion: From theory to application in pharmaceutical formulation. *AAPS Pharmscitech*, 17(1), 20–42.

Patterson, J. E., James, M. B., Forster, A. H., Lancaster, R. W., Butler, J. M., and Rades, T. (2007). Preparation of glass solutions of three poorly water soluble drugs by spray drying, melt extrusion and ball milling. *International Journal of Pharmaceutics*, 336(1), 22–34.

Paudel, A., Geppi, M., and Mooter, G. V. d. (2014). Structural and dynamic properties of amorphous solid dispersions: The role of solid-state nuclear magnetic resonance spectroscopy and relaxometry. *Journal of Pharmaceutical Sciences*, 103(9), 2635–2662.

Rumondor, A. C., Ivanisevic, I., Bates, S., Alonzo, D. E., and Taylor, L. S. (2009). Evaluation of drug-polymer miscibility in amorphous solid dispersion systems. *Pharmaceutical Research*, 26(11), 2523–2534.

Sandhu, H., Shah, N., Chokshi, H., and Malick, A. W. (2014). Overview of amorphous solid dispersion technologies. *Amorphous solid dispersions* (pp. 91–122) Springer.

Sarode, A., Wang, P., Cote, C., and Worthen, D. R. (2013). Low-viscosity hydroxypropylcellulose (HPC) grades SL and SSL: Versatile pharmaceutical polymers for dissolution enhancement, controlled release, and pharmaceutical processing. *AAPS Pharmscitech*, 14(1), 151–159.

Sarode, A. L., Obara, S., Tanno, F. K., Sandhu, H., Iyer, R., and Shah, N. (2014b). Stability assessment of hypromellose acetate succinate (HPMCAS) NF for application in hot melt extrusion (HME). *Carbohydrate Polymers*, 101, 146–153.

Sarode, A. L., Wang, P., Obara, S., and Worthen, D. R. (2014a). Supersaturation, nucleation, and crystal growth during single- and biphasic dissolution of amorphous solid dispersions: Polymer effects and implications for oral bioavailability enhancement of poorly water soluble drugs. *European Journal of Pharmaceutics and Biopharmaceutics*, 86(3), 351–360.

Savjani, K. T., Gajjar, A. K., and Savjani, J. K. (2012). Drug solubility: Importance and enhancement techniques. *ISRN Pharmaceutics, 2012*.

Sekiguchi, K., and Obi, N. (1961). Studies on absorption of eutectic mixture. I. A comparison of the behavior of eutectic mixture of sulfathiazole and that of ordinary sulfathiazole in man. *Chemical and Pharmaceutical Bulletin*, 9(11), 866–872.

Serajuddin, A. (1999). Solid dispersion of poorly water-soluble drugs: Early promises, subsequent problems, and recent breakthroughs. *Journal of Pharmaceutical Sciences*, 88(10), 1058–1066.

Shah, M. K., Madan, P., and Lin, S. (2014). Preparation, in vitro evaluation and statistical optimization of carvedilol-loaded solid lipid nanoparticles for lymphatic absorption via oral administration. *Pharmaceutical Development and Technology*, 19(4), 475–485.

Shah, N., Iyer, R. M., Mair, H., Choi, D. S., Tian, H., Diodone, R. et al., (2013). Improved human bioavailability of vemurafenib, a practically insoluble drug, using an amorphous polymer-stabilized solid dispersion prepared by a solvent-controlled coprecipitation process. *Journal of Pharmaceutical Sciences*, 102(3), 967–981.

Singh, S., Gamlath, S., and Wakeling, L. (2007). Nutritional aspects of food extrusion: A review. *International Journal of Food Science and Technology*, 42(8), 916–929.

Steerworld. *Steer's patented 'fractional-lobe' EPZ technology*. http://steerworld.com/epz-technology.html

Tadmor, Z., and Gogos, C. (2006). *Principles of polymer processing*. A John Wiley and Sons, Inc., Publication.

Tadmor, Z., and Gogos, C. G. (2013). *Principles of polymer processing*. John Wiley and Sons.

Terife, G., Wang, P., Faridi, N., and Gogos, C. G. (2012). Hot melt mixing and foaming of Soluplus® and indomethacin. *Polymer Engineering and Science*, 52(8), 1629–1639.

Tiwari, R. V., Patil, H., and Repka, M. A. (2016). Contribution of hot-melt extrusion technology to advance drug delivery in the 21st century. *Expert Opinion on Drug Delivery*, 13(3), 451–464.

Todd, D. (1998a). *Introduction to compounding* Polymer Processing Institute Books from Hanser Publishers, DB Todd.Hanser/Gardner Publications, Inc., Cincinnati, 1–12.

Todd, D. B. (1998b). Practical aspects of processing in intermeshing twin screw extruders. *Journal of Reinforced Plastics and Composites*, 17(18), 1607–1616.

Vaka, S. R. K., Bommana, M. M., Desai, D., Djordjevic, J., Phuapradit, W., and Shah, N. (2014). Excipients for amorphous solid dispersions. *Amorphous solid dispersions* (pp. 123–161) Springer.

Van Speybroeck, M., Mellaerts, R., Mols, R., Thi, T. D., Martens, J. A., Van Humbeeck, J. et al., (2010). Enhanced absorption of the poorly soluble drug fenofibrate by tuning its release rate from ordered mesoporous silica. *European Journal of Pharmaceutical Sciences*, 41(5), 623–630.

Vasconcelos, T., Sarmento, B., and Costa, P. (2007). Solid dispersions as strategy to improve oral bioavailability of poor water soluble drugs. *Drug Discovery Today*, 12(23–24), 1068–1075.

Verreck, G., Decorte, A., Li, H., Tomasko, D., Arien, A., Peeters, J. et al., (2006). The effect of pressurized carbon dioxide as a plasticizer and foaming agent on the hot melt extrusion process and extrudate properties of pharmaceutical polymers. *The Journal of Supercritical Fluids*, 38(3), 383–391.

Wu, C., and McGinity, J. W. (1999). Non-traditional plasticization of polymeric films. *International Journal of Pharmaceutics*, 177(1), 15–27.

Wu, Q. L., Quan, G. L., Hong, Y., Wu, L. N., Zeng, Y. M., Li, G. et al., (2015). Preparation and release behaviour of mesoporous silica/ethylcellulose sustained-release mini-matrix. *Yao Xue Xue Bao = Acta Pharmaceutica Sinica*, 50(4), 492–499.

Wypych, G. (2004). *Handbook of plasticizers*. ChemTec Publishing.

Yuan, X., Sperger, D., and Munson, E. J. (2013). Investigating miscibility and molecular mobility of nifedipine-PVP amorphous solid dispersions using solid-state NMR spectroscopy. *Molecular Pharmaceutics*, 11(1), 329–337.

Zhang, F., and McGinity, J. W. (1999). Properties of sustained-release tablets prepared by hot-melt extrusion. *Pharmaceutical Development and Technology*, 4(2), 241–250.

14 Process Modeling and Simulation of Extrusion Operations

David Johnson, Rick Peng, and James DiNunzio

CONTENTS

14.1 INTRODUCTION

Following Moore's Law, computational power has increased exponentially and opened up new opportunities for moving experimental testing from the lab to the computer. Process modeling and simulation packages to assess extrusion operations are now commercially available through a number of vendors. These packages rely on fundamental material and energy balances to simulate process conditions for a given set of material attributes. The nature of the calculations can vary from simpler one-dimensional balances to computationally intensive multidimensional simulations.

Within the pharmaceutical industry, computational simulation has been increasingly relied upon to enhance development. Applications of these types of software platforms to unit operations include roller compaction (Muliadi et al. 2012), tablet compression (Sinha et al. 2010), film coating (Ketterhagen 2011), and spray drying (Dobry et al. 2009). For pharmaceutical melt extrusion, simulation software has been utilized to assess material flow, residence time distribution and the level of mixing within processing systems. The selection of the type of model is driven by the nature of the output. Owing to the simplified nature of the calculations, one-dimensional models have been predominantly used for the complete process modeling to support the calculation of pressure, temperature, and fill ratio along the extruder. These

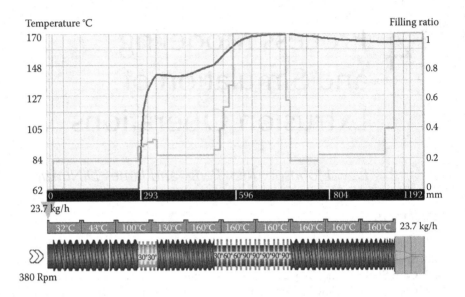

FIGURE 14.1 Temperature and fill profile across the process section of a simulated extruder.

packages can also be deployed to execute *in silico* experimental designs ahead of real-world manufacturing, helping to enhance the study design and identify high risk regions of the process space. An example output from a commercially available software package is shown in Figure 14.1, which describes the temperature and fill ratio across the length of the process section.

Beyond axial performance understanding, more complex higher resolution simulations are utilized based on computational fluid dynamics (CFD) or discrete element modeling (DEM). These simulations are capable of providing detailed performance information and have been used successfully to describe mixing within fully filled kneading sections; however, at this time it is not possible to simulate an entire extruder with this approach. A representative output from a CFD simulation in a 90° kneading section, shown in Figure 14.2, illustrates the velocity profile as a function of spatial orientation. Relative to the one-dimensional counterparts, these simulations provide a greater level of local understanding about processing dynamics and can be used to answer specific microscale questions about process performance. Clearly, successful simulation requires an understanding of material properties as well as an appreciation of the questions one is trying to ask.

The objective of this chapter is to provide the fundamental principles for simulation technology and illustrate the practical application of simulation software for addressing process challenges in the manufacture of amorphous solid dispersions.

14.2 SPATIAL EQUATIONS FOR MODELING AN EXTRUSION SYSTEM

The mass, momentum, and heat flows within an extrusion system are all in balance during steady state operation of extrusion processes. Accounting for these

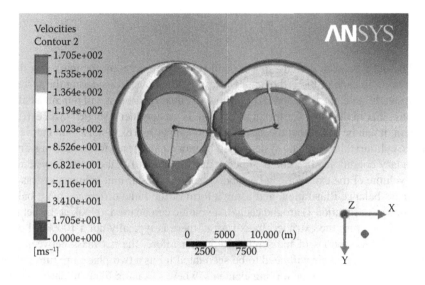

FIGURE 14.2   Velocity profile within fully filled 90° kneading section.

relationships by including the corresponding information of rheological and thermal properties enables the development of representative models that are able to describe operating conditions and material properties. Noting that these models are derived from first principles balances, the modeling process can be approached initially using a finite unit volume to balance the mass flow through the system as shown in Figure 14.3 (Deen 1998).

Summing the mass flow in and out of the x, y, and z directions, it is possible to generate a finite difference relationship, Equation 1, which can be further refined to its differential and more commonly associated form, which is shown in Equation 2.

$$\rho v_x\big|_x \Delta y \Delta z \Delta t - \rho v_x\big|_{x+\Delta x} \Delta y \Delta z \Delta t + \rho v_y\big|_y \Delta x \Delta z \Delta t - \rho v_y\big|_{y+\Delta y} \Delta x \Delta z \Delta t +$$
$$\rho v_z\big|_z \Delta x \Delta y \Delta t - \rho v_z\big|_{z+\Delta z} \Delta x \Delta y \Delta t = \rho\big|_{t+\Delta t} \Delta x \Delta y \Delta z - \rho\big|_t \Delta x \Delta y \Delta z \tag{14.1}$$

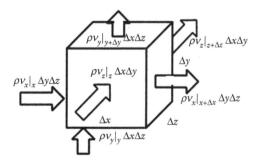

FIGURE 14.3   Finite element mass balance illustration.

$$\frac{\partial}{\partial x}(\rho v_x) + \frac{\partial}{\partial y}(\rho v_y) + \frac{\partial}{\partial z}(\rho v_z) = -\frac{\partial \rho}{\partial t} \tag{14.2}$$

The mass balance uses the density and velocity to represent the mass flux that is happening in each of the orthogonal Cartesian directions. Considering the system to be at steady state, the time derivative term will equal zero, but it will remain a balance of mass flux in the three Cartesian directions. If we consider a single barrel extrusion system, it can be noted that the system would appear more cylindrical in nature, and hence cylindrical coordinate systems will be more appropriate for developing simpler boundary conditions. In a three-dimensional simulation of an extrusion system, the free volume of the extruder can be subdivided into similar unit volumes as was used for mass balance illustration, and using a form of the finite difference mass balance (as shown in Equation 1) around each unit volume can be used to look at the net mass flux effect across the extruder. In extrusion, there is typically not a 100% fill of the melt in some sections of the screw profile. Therefore, the net mass between polymer and interstitial air will need to be accounted for as a two-phase mixture moving through the system. In the mixing elements, where it is more likely to have complete fill with polymer melt, a single-phase representation can be sufficient.

The balance of momentum is typically represented by the Cauchy-momentum balance, where the viscoelastic nature of a fluid's properties can be applied to the shear terms in the equation.

$$\rho\left(\frac{\partial v_x}{\partial t} + v_x \frac{\partial v_x}{\partial x} + v_y \frac{\partial v_x}{\partial y} + v_z \frac{\partial v_x}{\partial z}\right) = -\frac{\partial p}{\partial x} - \left(\frac{\partial \tau_{xx}}{\partial x} + \frac{\partial \tau_{yx}}{\partial y} + \frac{\partial \tau_{zx}}{\partial z}\right) + \rho g_x \tag{14.3}$$

$$\rho\left(\frac{\partial v_y}{\partial t} + v_x \frac{\partial v_y}{\partial x} + v_y \frac{\partial v_y}{\partial y} + v_z \frac{\partial v_y}{\partial z}\right) = -\frac{\partial p}{\partial y} - \left(\frac{\partial \tau_{xy}}{\partial x} + \frac{\partial \tau_{yy}}{\partial y} + \frac{\partial \tau_{zy}}{\partial z}\right) + \rho g_y \tag{14.4}$$

$$\rho\left(\frac{\partial v_z}{\partial t} + v_x \frac{\partial v_z}{\partial x} + v_y \frac{\partial v_z}{\partial y} + v_z \frac{\partial v_z}{\partial z}\right) = -\frac{\partial p}{\partial z} - \left(\frac{\partial \tau_{xz}}{\partial x} + \frac{\partial \tau_{yz}}{\partial y} + \frac{\partial \tau_{zz}}{\partial z}\right) + \rho g_z \tag{14.5}$$

To illustrate a couple of case studies of analytical solutions to simple representations of an extruder system, we will simplify these to their Newtonian equivalent—the Navier-Stokes equations—and use cylindrical coordinates to better represent a single barrel extrusion system. These equations can be seen below, in which the x and y coordinates have been replaced with r and θ (which represent radial and theta components). These equations can be found in standard transport theory or in textbooks (Geankoplis 2003).

$$\rho\left(\frac{\partial v_r}{\partial t} + v_r \frac{\partial v_r}{\partial r} + \frac{v_\theta}{r} \frac{\partial v_r}{\partial \theta} - \frac{v_\theta^2}{r} + v_z \frac{\partial v_r}{\partial z}\right) = -\frac{\partial p}{\partial r}$$

$$+ \mu\left[\frac{\partial}{\partial r}\left(\frac{1}{r} \frac{\partial(r v_r)}{\partial r}\right) + \frac{1}{r^2} \frac{\partial^2 v_r}{\partial \theta^2} - \frac{2}{r^2} \frac{\partial v_\theta}{\partial \theta} + \frac{\partial^2 v_r}{\partial z^2}\right] + \rho g_r \tag{14.6}$$

$$\rho\left(\frac{\partial v_\theta}{\partial t} + v_r \frac{\partial v_\theta}{\partial r} + \frac{v_\theta}{r}\frac{\partial v_\theta}{\partial \theta} - \frac{v_r v_\theta}{r} + v_z \frac{\partial v_\theta}{\partial z}\right) = -\frac{1}{r}\frac{\partial p}{\partial \theta}$$
$$+\mu\left[\frac{\partial}{\partial r}\left(\frac{1}{r}\frac{\partial(r v_\theta)}{\partial r}\right) + \frac{1}{r^2}\frac{\partial^2 v_\theta}{\partial \theta^2} + \frac{2}{r^2}\frac{\partial v_r}{\partial \theta} + \frac{\partial^2 v_\theta}{\partial z^2}\right] + \rho g_\theta$$

(14.7)

$$\rho\left(\frac{\partial v_z}{\partial t} + v_r \frac{\partial v_z}{\partial r} + \frac{v_\theta}{r}\frac{\partial v_z}{\partial \theta} + v_z \frac{\partial v_z}{\partial z}\right) = -\frac{\partial p}{\partial z}$$
$$+\mu\left[\frac{1}{r}\frac{\partial}{\partial r}\left(r\frac{\partial v_z}{\partial r}\right) + \frac{1}{r^2}\frac{\partial^2 v_z}{\partial \theta^2} + \frac{\partial^2 v_z}{\partial z^2}\right] + \rho g_z$$

(14.8)

To begin looking at an extrusion-like system, one can develop several limited case studies of analytical solutions to begin to describe this system.

14.3 CASE STUDY 1: THE SIMPLE POISEUILLE SYSTEM

Let's consider first the simple system of pressure-driven flow in a single cylinder (Figure 14.4). Assuming the system is Newtonian with laminar flow, the z-direction Navier-Stokes equation (Equation 8) simplifies to the following equation (note that the inertial terms in the left-hand side of the equation tend to disappear in laminar flow systems):

$$0 = -\frac{\partial p}{\partial z} + \mu\left[\frac{1}{r}\frac{\partial}{\partial r}\left(r\frac{\partial v_z}{\partial r}\right)\right]$$

(14.9)

At steady state, there should only be flow in the z direction, but due to frictional losses it is expected that this variable will be in the r direction only. With boundary conditions of the velocity derivative being zero at $r = 0$ and the velocity being zero at the wall ($r = R$) due to no slip, the expression can be integrated into the following (assuming constant pressure drop):

$$v_z = \frac{1}{4\mu}\frac{\partial p}{\partial z}\left(r^2 - R^2\right) = -\frac{R^2}{4\mu}\frac{\partial p}{\partial z}\left[1 - \left(\frac{r}{R}\right)^2\right]$$

(14.10)

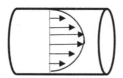

FIGURE 14.4 Simple flow illustration.

By integrating the velocity over the cross-sectional area to get the average velocity and integrating the pressure drop across the length of the tube, the Hagen-Poiseuille relationship is derived:

$$v_{z,av} = -\frac{R^2}{8\mu}\frac{\partial p}{\partial z} = \frac{1}{A}\iint_A v_z dA = \frac{1}{\pi R^2}\int_0^{2\pi}\int_0^R v_z r\,dr\,d\theta \qquad (14.11)$$

$$\frac{\Delta P}{L} = \frac{8\mu v_{z,av}}{R^2} \qquad (14.12)$$

14.4 CASE STUDY 2: FLOW BETWEEN CONCENTRIC CYLINDERS

In the case of pressure-driven flow between the central shaft of a single extruder barrel (Figure 14.5) and its wall (assuming no rotation of the shaft), a similar solution scheme can be developed (Geankoplis 2003). Utilizing the same analysis as for the simple Poiseuille case study, but now needing to consider that the velocity derivative will not be going to zero at $r = 0$ but at $r = R_{ZM}$, it is possible to derive a solution. Returning to the cylindrical Navier-Stokes equations, assuming a laminar and Newtonian system for simplicity in this case, it can be shown that the same differential relationship in Equation 9 represents this system as well. Integration using the R_{ZM} boundary conditions yields the following expression:

$$\frac{\partial v_z}{\partial r} = \frac{1}{\mu}\frac{\partial p}{\partial z}\left(\frac{r}{2} - \frac{1}{r}\frac{R_{ZM}^2}{2}\right) \qquad (14.13)$$

Integration from either the inner wall (R_0) where velocity equals zero or the outer wall (R) where velocity also equals zero (due to a no-slip assumption), the following two velocity relationships can be shown:

$$v_z = \frac{1}{2\mu}\frac{\partial p}{\partial z}\left(\frac{r^2}{2} - \frac{R_0^2}{2} - R_{ZM}^2 LN\left(\frac{r}{R_0}\right)\right) \qquad (14.14)$$

$$v_z = \frac{1}{2\mu}\frac{\partial p}{\partial z}\left(\frac{r^2}{2} - \frac{R^2}{2} - R_{ZM}^2 LN\left(\frac{r}{R}\right)\right) \qquad (14.15)$$

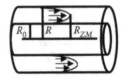

FIGURE 14.5   Concentric cylinders illustration.

From these two equations, it is possible to solve for R_{ZM} and substitute back into one of the equations above.

$$R_{ZM} = \sqrt{\frac{R^2 - R_0^2}{2LN(R/R_0)}} \tag{14.16}$$

$$v_z = \frac{1}{2\mu}\frac{\partial p}{\partial z}\left[\frac{r^2}{2} - \frac{R^2}{2} - \frac{R^2 - R_0^2}{2LN(R/R_0)}LN\left(\frac{r}{R}\right)\right] \tag{14.17}$$

In the limited case where $R_0 \to 0$, the last term ends up dropping to zero, which yields the same solution as the simple Poiseuille case.

14.5 CASE STUDY 3: FLOW BETWEEN CONCENTRIC CYLINDERS WITH ROTATION

Consider an extruder barrel where the inner shaft is spinning and the barrel wall is stationary (Figure 14.6). In the absence of pressure-driven flow in the axial direction, the theta component for velocity can be examined to assess the rotational effect. Simplifying the theta equation from the Navier-Stokes formula (assuming Newtonian and laminar flow), we get the following relationship:

$$0 = \frac{\partial}{\partial r}\left[\frac{1}{r}\frac{\partial(rv_\theta)}{\partial r}\right] \tag{14.18}$$

Since the derivative of the theta velocity is not known, the Dirichlet boundary conditions of having no slip at the moving ($r = R_0$) and stationary wall ($r = R$) must be applied. This results in having $v_\theta(r = R_0) = \omega R_0$ and $v_\theta(r = R) = 0$. By integrating the above equation (Equation 18) and applying integration constants, the following solution can be shown:

$$v_\theta = Ar + \frac{B}{r} \tag{14.19}$$

Applying the boundary conditions to solve for A and B,

$$A = \frac{\omega R_0^2}{R_0^2 - R^2} \tag{14.20}$$

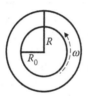

FIGURE 14.6 Rotating concentric cylinder illustration.

$$B = -\frac{\omega R_0^2 R^2}{R_0^2 - R^2} \tag{14.21}$$

$$v_\theta = \frac{\omega R_0^2 R}{R_0^2 - R^2}\left(\frac{r}{R} - \frac{R}{r}\right) \tag{14.22}$$

This solution is similar to an example by Geankoplis 2003, where the outer cylinder is rotating instead of the inner. Through this example Geankoplis mentions that torque on the cylinder can be calculated by using the shear component in the radial-theta direction and applying it to the area of contact on the cylinder.

$$\tau_{r\theta} = -\mu\left[r\frac{\partial(v_\theta/r)}{\partial r} + \frac{1}{r}\frac{\partial v_r}{\partial \theta}\right] = -\frac{2\mu\omega R_0^2}{R^2 - R_0^2}\left(\frac{1}{r^2}\right) \tag{14.23}$$

$$Torque = (2\pi R_0 L)(-\tau_{r\theta})\big|_{r=R_0}(R_0) = \frac{4\pi\mu\omega L R_0^2 R^2}{R^2 - R_0^2} \tag{14.24}$$

In a real extrusion system, it should be kept in mind that each of these phenomena described in the case studies may be happening in parallel, and the system is likely not undergoing laminar flow nor is the fluid a simple Newtonian fluid. While, with each of the case studies the intent is to show how, with adding additional features to the motion of the system, a direct solution of the equations becomes less likely, and a numerical method is preferred for approaching the appropriate solution. The more complex geometries that are used for the extrusion screws, and using a double barrel screw design, do make it much more challenging to design an analytical solution for the system. Using 3D simulation software, the differential balances can be applied to the many different finite volumes or elements to enable convergence to a solution that fits the mass and momentum equations (note that heat balancing is also applied where heat transfer and friction effects are being accounted for in the system of equations).

14.6 APPLICATION OF 1D SIMULATION SOFTWARE FOR EXTRUSION OPERATIONS

One-dimensional extrusion process modeling is one of the computational simulation tools available to scientists and engineers studying and developing pharmaceutical extrusion processes. The single dimension of one-dimensional modeling is the position along the axis of material flow within an extruder that is effectively bound on one end by a material inlet (i.e., feed point) and on the other end by a product outlet (i.e., extruder die). Simulation results provide continuous, quantitative profiles of process and product parameters along this dimension. While lacking the fundamental granularity of more complex, multidimensional modeling methods, one-dimensional modeling provides a readily accessible view of intraprocess macroscopic phenomena that are directly relevant to understanding observable process performance.

Ludovic® is computational software developed by Sciences Computers Consultants, Inc. (Saint-Étienne, France) for one-dimensional, thermomechanical modeling and simulation of corotating twin-screw extrusion processes. Other simulation packages, including WinTXS™ by PolyTech (Bradford, Connecticut, USA), are also available and provide similar features; however, this section will focus on examples utilizing Ludovic® with the intention of providing a comprehensive overview on the application of 1D simulation in the development of pharmaceutical extrusion processes. The utilization of Ludovic® as the software package for illustration does not constitute an endorsement of that platform versus other commercially available software packages.

14.6.1 USING SOFTWARE

Ludovic® generates results based on a user-specified model of an extrusion system. The three categories of user inputs for basic model specification are extruder geometries (screws, barrels, and die); product material properties (thermal, physical, and rheological); and controlled process parameters (screw speed, temperature setpoints, material throughput).

Extruder geometry is specified using known or measured dimensions of an extruder's various elements. Barrel geometry is specified using internal diameter, centerline, and clearance as well as heating zone segment length. Screw profiles are constructed using prebuilt screw elements that include options for type (e.g., conveying, kneading, combing); flights; forwarding or reversing; and stagger angle (where applicable). Dies are constructed using basic geometric elements such as 8-0 pipes, circular pipes, and rectangular slits.

Material properties may either be obtained through a prepopulated library of commonly extruded materials or, as would be the case for most pharmaceutical applications, through experimental characterization. The required product material thermal properties include solid phase bulk density, melting point, temperature-independent liquid phase density, liquid phase heat capacity, and thermal conductivity. In terms of rheological properties, software packages require viscosity data in the form of a viscosity law (e.g., power law, Carreau-Yasuda law) or a set of points (viscosity vs. shear rate for a range of temperatures that spans the range of simulated process temperatures). Typical methods for obtaining these data include differential scanning calorimetry for thermal properties and strain-controlled and/or capillary rheometry for melt viscosity and density.

Simulation packages such as Ludovic® typically use an iterative computation method to generate quantitative results. First, the software geometrically discretizes the extruder's internal free volume into individual elements based on the specified geometries for various screw, barrel, and die elements. The boundaries of the computed volume are defined as the outlet of the die and the first restrictive element (i.e., the first reverse conveying, kneading, or combing element), where the melt may be assumed to be fully melted at the melting temperature. With initial outlet conditions of zero pressure and outlet temperature equal to user-estimated outlet temperature, the software computes the change in pressure and temperature for the melt within each discretized volume element, starting from the extruder outlet and moving upstream, sequentially updating the pressure and temperature within each discretized element. This calculation iterates until one of two convergence criteria is reached: the computed melt temperature at the first restrictive element equals the user-specified melting point or the computed temperature in the inlet zone equals the user-specified inlet temperature. Thermomechanical parameters at each point within the extruder are computed based on the temperature and pressure in each discretized element. Subsequent interpolation between the discretized elements effectively generates a continuous end-to-end profile for each parameter.

Simulation results include residence time distribution, a summary of quantitative results for the overall process, and profiles along the extruder length dimension for thermomechanical parameters such as temperature, pressure, viscosity, shear rate, fill ratio, local residence time, change in temperature, etc. The results for one or multiple simulations may be viewed, compared, and analyzed within the software interface or exported into common spreadsheet formats for additional processing and analysis.

Additionally, some software packages may also feature a design-of-experiment (DOE) tool for generating results in a multivariate format similar in form and function to typical experimental DOEs. By specifying the variations of geometric parameters or process parameters to change and computing batch results for all combinations of the variable model elements, the software can generate a multivariate analysis of the interactions of various simulation parameters.

14.6.2 APPLICATION TO DEVELOPMENT—CASE STUDY USING LUDOVIC®

Process simulation played an important role during the process development of an extrusion-formulated product. The extrusion process for the product featured a devolatilization section that used the elevated temperature of the extruder as well as a vacuum vent to remove residual solvent from the melt within the extruder. Due to limitations in intraprocess direct measurement, limited materials, and insufficient opportunity for full-scale experimentation, process simulation was essential for guiding the experimentation process during development by refining hypotheses and thereby increasing the likelihood that experimentation and resulting process changes would yield practically favorable outcomes.

The two problems addressed using simulation software were a vent flow issue (upstream raw material feed being drawn downstream into the devolatilization vacuum vent) and the optimization of devolatilization efficiency, defined as the percentage of incoming residual solvent removed by extrusion devolatilization.

To address the vent flow issue, where molten material was observed to discharge from the vent zone, simulations were used to verify the hypothetical mechanism and subsequently develop a new screw design that effectively mitigated the issue. A schematic of the different processing designs is shown in Figure 14.7. Leveraging general understanding of common phenomena in extrusion troubleshooting, it was hypothesized that the issue was caused by vent flow that could occur due to the pressure difference and possible lack of separation between an upstream feed zone and an adjacent downstream vacuum vented devolatilization zone. Although the pressure difference was directly measurable, the lack of separation between the two zones could not be directly observed or measured. Therefore, simulation was used to model

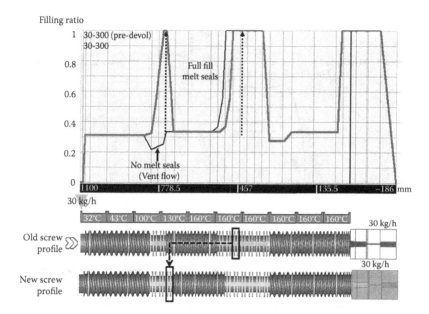

FIGURE 14.7 Simulation of different screw design configurations showing fill ratio differences across the process section length.

the process and generate *in silico* results for the level of fill for the entire length of the extruder. The results indicated that the given screw design and process parameters did not provide the sufficient amount of local residence time prior to the devolatilization zone to form an effective melt seal between the feed zone and the devolatilization zone, thus confirming the hypothesized lack of interzone separation and giving more credibility to the hypothesis. The software was subsequently used to design a screw profile modification that ensured the formation of a melt seal. After implementing this design change in the process, the vent flow problem and its symptoms were observed to be effectively mitigated.

To address the optimization of devolatilization efficiency, simulations were used to analyze existing devolatilization process data and thereby modify an existing hypothesis on the mechanisms that determine devolatilization efficiency for the given materials system. Previous understanding of devolatilization mechanisms, largely based upon literature research, asserted that the primary mechanism of devolatilization efficiency is the kinetics of mass transfer. Process modeling was used to retrospectively analyze existing devolatilization efficiency data by generating profiles for the process parameters (e.g., level of fill, residence time) that were directly relevant to the kinetics hypothesis as well as profiles for other parameters that were not directly related to the kinetics hypothesis. A summary of the temperature profile for the different processing conditions is shown in Figure 14.8. Analysis of correlation between simulation results and devolatilization efficiency data indicated that the kinetics-determining parameters correlated poorly with devolatilization efficiency in comparison to other parameters (e.g., local melt temperature, devolatilization vacuum pressure) that were more related to the thermodynamic state of the system.

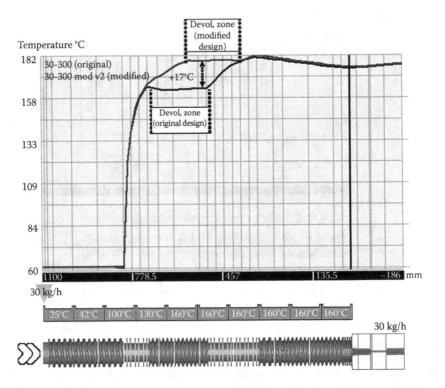

FIGURE 14.8 Simulation of different screw design configurations showing fill ratio differences across the process section length.

Therefore, the previous mechanistic hypothesis was revised to state that devolatilization efficiency for the given materials system may be better maximized by ensuring that the thermodynamics of the system are optimized.

14.7 MULTIDIMENSIONAL MODELING OF EXTRUSION OPERATIONS

The application of multidimensional modeling can also serve as a powerful tool for greater understanding of extrusion operations. Although the ability to simulate an entire extruder with this technique is not possible, the detailed high fidelity understanding for certain sections of the process can be of seminal importance. These techniques can provide useful advantages for characterizing the degree of mixing and important flow characteristics within dies during advanced forming operations. In one recent example (Gonçalves et al. 2013), researchers used CFD modeling to simulate the extrusion processing during a complex compounding and shaping application for the production of medical catheters. Through the application of the simulation package it was possible to better understand complex flows and drive for a more effective design of the process. Similar studies have been conducted by other researchers (Eitzlmayr and Khinast 2015) to investigate the mixing dynamics in fully filled and partially filled screws along with the subsequent impact on processing characteristics. Utilizing tracers it was possible to track the evolution of mixing and confirm the model accuracy. With this approach it was possible to show how the mixing rate per revolution and residence time govern performance. While these two examples are general in nature, the detailed understanding provided through the use of multidimensional simulation can provide fundamental insights into process performance that directly drive material attributes.

14.8 SUMMARY

Process modeling and simulation is a powerful tool for increasing the understanding of extrusion operations. Given the relative ease of use, the limitations of direct experimental measurements for extrusion, and the costliness of pharmaceutical extrusion experimentation, one-dimensional extrusion modeling is a powerful but also cost-effective tool for pharmaceutical process development. Although one-dimensional modeling and simulation can never be a direct replacement for experimentally generated evidence, it does serve as an effective means for screening and improving hypotheses on macroscopic intraprocess mechanisms, thereby increasing the speed and lowering the costs associated with the development of pharmaceutical extrusion processes. Further granularity of process characteristics can be achieved through the application of multidimensional models, allowing for greater understanding of microscale phenomena that may impact product performance. Overall, modeling and simulation is a powerful tool that can greatly enhance the development of extruded products.

REFERENCES

Deen, W., *Analysis of Transport Phenomena*, Oxford University Press, New York, 1998

Dobry D.E., Settell D.M., Baumann J.M., Ray R.J., Graham L.J., Beyerinck R.A., A model-based methodology for spray drying process development, *Journal of Pharmaceutical Innovation* 4 (3) 2009, Pages 133–142

Eitzlmayr A., Khinast J., Co-rotating twin-screw extruders: Detailed analysis of conveying elements based on smoothed particle hydrodynamics. Part 2: Mixing, *Chemical Engineering Science*, 134, 2015, Pages 880–886

Geankoplis C.J., *Transport Processes and Separation Process Principles (Includes Unit Operations)* 4th Edition, Prentice Hall, Upper Saddle River, NJ, 2003

Gonçalves N.D., Carneiro O.S., Nóbrega J.M., Design of complex profile extrusion dies through numerical modeling, *Journal of Non-Newtonian Fluid Mechanics*, 200, 2013, Pages 103–110

Ketterhagen W.R., Modeling the motion and orientation of various pharmaceutical tablet shapes in a film coating pan using DEM, *International Journal of Pharmaceutics*, 409 (1), 2011, Pages 137–149

Muliadi A.R., Litster J.D., Wassgren C.R., Modeling the powder roll compaction process: Comparison of 2-D finite element method and the rolling theory for granular solids (Johanson's model), *Powder Technology*, 221, 2012, Pages 90–100

Sinha T., Bharadwaj R., Curtis J.S., Hancock B.C., Wassgren C., Finite element analysis of pharmaceutical tablet compaction using a density dependent material plasticity model, *Powder Technology*, 202 (1), 2010, Pages 46–54

15 Devolatilization via Twin-Screw Extrusion

Theory, Tips, and Test Results

Charles Martin and Brian Haight

CONTENTS

In a twin-screw extruder (TSE), the mixing/blending of polymers/additives and devolatilization are mass-transfer operations dependent upon shear/energy that is being imparted into the materials being processed by rotating screws. Devolatilization (DV) refers to the removal of unreacted monomer, solvent, water, and other undesirable materials from the process melt stream. In pharmaceutical applications, DV could refer to the removal of residual solvents from an active pharmaceutical ingredient (API), removal of water from the process that could cause degradation through hydrolysis, or even simply removing air to reduce entrapped bubbles in the final product. It is a mass transfer process driven by a combination of thermodynamic and diffusional variables that superheat the volatile components and expose the melt to rapid decompression. There are many devices that perform DV, including extruders. Almost always, the TSE includes the provision for devolatilization, sometimes as a critical factor in the process, and sometimes as an afterthought. Factors that affect devolatilization efficiencies, in any device, include:

1. Residence time under the vent or vents: longer is better but...
   a. Oxygen, shear, time, and temperature may contribute to degradation and side reactions (understand kinetics of degradation)
2. Surface area of the melt: higher is better
   a. Rolling pools and film effects
   b. Function of screw geometry and operating parameters

3. Surface renewal: higher is better
   a. Renewed surfaces come from rolling pools and partially filled screw channels
4. Bubbles are key: nucleation, growth, and rupture
   a. Stripping agents can be injected to facilitate bubbles
5. Vacuum level applied to vent zone(s): it can make a big difference
   a. Low-viscosity material may require decreased vacuum levels

Materials are metered into the twin-screw extruder and the screws' rpm is independent and set to optimize processing efficiencies. Melt pools are bounded by screw flights and barrel walls, which makes extrusion, by definition, a "small mass" continuous process that results in a high surface area of the polymer melt. Rotating screws (Figure 15.1) result in rolling pools and thin films, both of which improve DV.

Process control parameters include screw speed (rpm), feed rate, barrel/die temperatures, and vacuum level. Typical readouts include melt pressure, melt temperature, motor amperage, and in-line optical sensors. Depending on how the TSE is configured and operated, residence times can be as short as 5 seconds, as long as 10 minutes, and are typically in the 20-second to 2-minute range.

Starve feeding refers to the extruder being fed at a rate less than the forwarding efficiency of the screws. The independence of feed rate from the screws' rpm facilitates control of surface area generation, residence time, and mixing (to eliminate temperature gradients) and is what makes the TSE an effective tool for stripping volatiles from polymer melts.

Barrel segments include the provision for venting. The pressure gradient in the twin-screw extruder is controlled and, to a significant degree, determined by the selection of screws. Flighted elements are strategically placed so that the screw channels are not filled, which results in zero pressure underneath vent sections that prevents vent flooding, and also allows downstream feeding of fillers and fibers (Figure 15.2).

The intense mixing associated with the short interscrew mass transfer characteristics inherent with a TSE makes it ideal to perform intimate mixing/blending. Simultaneously, entrapped air, moisture, and volatiles are removed by devolatilization, driven by the superheating of the volatile component and exposing the melt pool to a rapid decompression under a vent.

The length/diameter ratio (L/D) represents the overall length of the process section divided by the screw diameter. The L/D ratio is matched to downstream unit operations that need to be performed, and typically ranges from 24/1 to 60/1+. Extended L/Ds allow for multistage venting; allow stripping agents (i.e., water or sCO_2) to be injected; and increase DV efficiencies, as well as the feeding, mixing, and pumping functions inherent to the TSE process.

There are an infinite number of TSE screw element types. There are, however, only three basic types of screw elements: flighted elements, mixing elements, and

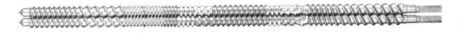

FIGURE 15.1   Corotating intermeshing twin-screw extruder screw set.

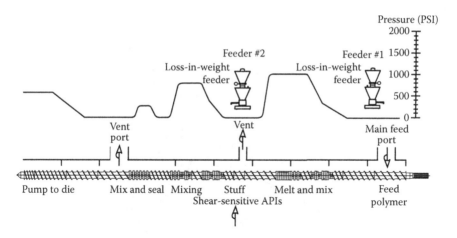

FIGURE 15.2 Pressure gradient in a starve-fed twin-screw extruder.

zoning elements. Flighted elements are strategically placed to forward materials. Zoning elements isolate two operations within the extruder, such as to facilitate a melt seal prior to a vacuum venting zone (Figure 15.3). Mixing elements can be dispersive and/or distributive in nature and often serve a dual purpose as zoning elements. Distributive elements are typically used to mix stripping agents upon injection into the TSE process section (Figure 15.4). Adequate pumping elements are required under vents and at the TSE discharge to prevent vent flooding.

Screws are segmented and assembled on splined shafts. Torque is limited by the cross section of the shaft and its design. Free volume is related to the OD/ID ratio, which is defined by dividing the outside diameter (OD) by the inside diameter (ID) of each screw. Asymmetrical splined shafts isolate the tangential force vector being transmitted by the motor into the process and result in higher torque capabilities from a smaller diameter shaft.

Therefore, a 1.5 or 1.66/1 OD/ID ratio is common (and higher is possible), and deeper flights are possible without decreased torque. Increased flight depths help prevent the melt from flying up the vent, and a higher free volume results in a higher surface area, which is preferred for DV processes. See Figure 15.5 below for a comparison of common OD/ID ratios.

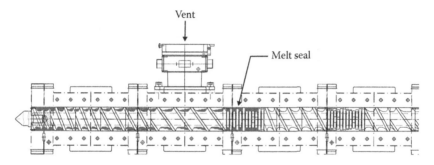

FIGURE 15.3 Vent/discharge from TSE.

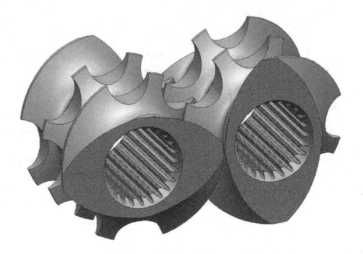

FIGURE 15.4   Example of a distributive mixing element.

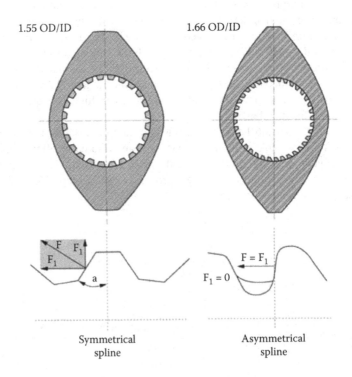

FIGURE 15.5   A comparison of TSE OD/ID ratios.

Two equations to better understand surface area generation are

$$SA = \left(V_y\right) * (n * Z * H) \tag{15.1}$$

representing the surface area generation from a rolling bank where

V_y = face velocity of rolling bank
n = number of screw channels
Z = helical length of open zone
H = channel depth, and

$$SA = \left(1 - f\right) W * nZ * N \tag{15.2}$$

representing the surface area generation from the barrel film where

W = channel width
f = fill fraction
n = number of screw channels
Z = helical length of open zone
N = screw speed

Sometimes a stripping agent, such as water or a supercritical CO_2, is injected into the TSE to augment DV efficiencies. For example, 500 ppm water as vapor (1 mm bubbles) at 250°C and 0.1 atm would provide 27 times more transfer area than the atmospheric vent alone. However, the L/D must be lengthened to accommodate this task, and the liquid should be injected over distributive mixers to prevent flashing or ponding. In the decompression zones bubbles grow and rupture, releasing volatiles.

It's evident that increasing the screws' rpm and/or decreasing the rate generally improves DV efficiencies within the constraints of the formulation. Vents can be atmospheric, or vacuum can be applied to further enhance devolatilization effects.

To help quantify how various extrusion factors impacted DV efficiencies, the following tests were performed.

15.1 TEST #1: DEVOLATILIZATION OF COPOVIDONE (KOLLIDON® VA 64)/API/SOLVENT (METHANOL) FORMULATIONS

A formulation using typical pharmaceutical ingredients was selected and a solvent was injected and then removed via DV to determine the results for different operating conditions. Specifically, copovidone and griseofulvin, the API, were metered into the TSE feed throat, and 5% of a solvent was injected into the melt, mixed, and then devolatilized in the TSE process section.

Experiments were performed at 2 and 4 kg/hr and 200 and 400 screw rpm, with and without vacuum. The temperature zones for the barrels were 60°C at the feed throat, transitioned to between 100 and 140°C for the barrels, and 180°C at the die. The motor load was 40%–50% for all runs. The melt temperature was around 180°C.

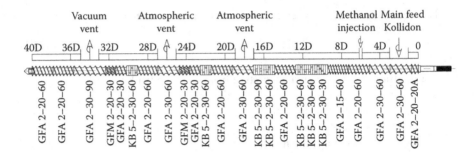

FIGURE 15.6   ZSE-27 MAXX screw/process section design.

The following is a summary of the equipment: two loss-in-weight (LIW) metering feeders for polymer and API; piston pump to inject the solvent; ZSE-27 MAXX corotating, intermeshing twin-screw extruder (28.3-mm-diameter screws, 1.66/1 OD/ID ratio) with 40 to 1 L/D; two atmospheric vents and one vacuum vent; strand die; air quench conveyor; and pelletizer. Figure 15.6 represents the TSE process section and screw design used for the experiments.

All samples were characterized using gas headspace chromatography and are shown in Figure 15.7.

From the results, the following conclusions may be stated:

1. There is a linear correlation between rpm and feed rate and reduction in volatiles concentration.
2. The application of vacuum resulted in a significant reduction in concentration of volatiles.

15.2   TEST #2: PROCESSING UNDRIED PLA IN A COROTATING TWIN-SCREW EXTRUDER

Polylactic acid (PLA) was metered into the extruder at a rate of 180 kg/hr and processed at 250 screw rpm. The temperature zones for the barrels were between 180 and

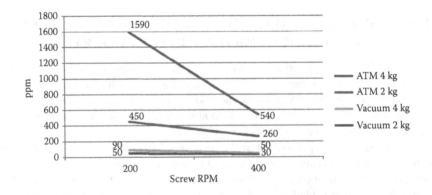

FIGURE 15.7   Residual solvent (in PPM) for various operating conditions.

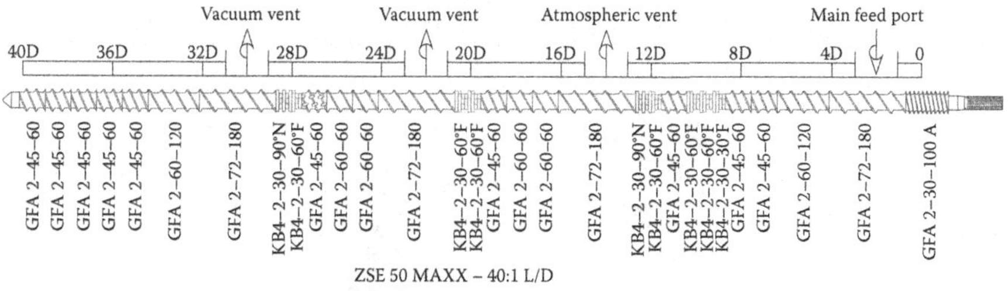

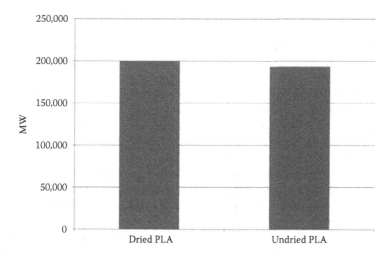

FIGURE 15.8 ZSE-50 MAXX screw/process section design.

190°C. The motor load was approximately 70%. The melt temperature was 200°C. Moisture analysis indicated the PLA pellets had 1600–4000 PPM moisture content.

The following is a summary of the equipment: loss-in-weight (LIW) metering feeder, ZSE-50 MAXX twin-screw extruder (51.2-mm-diameter screws), 1.66/1 OD/ID ratio, 40 to 1 L/D with a screw/barrel design to optimize venting efficiencies, gear pump front-end attachment, slide plate screen changer (120-mm-diameter breaker plate), 800-mm-wide flexible lip sheet die, three-roll stack with pull roll station, and torque winder. Three venting sections were integrated into the process section, shown in Figure 15.8.

The sheet sample was dimensionally stable with an acceptable appearance. Analysis of the sheet samples indicated a molecular weight loss of between 5 and 8%, as indicated in Figure 15.9, which was deemed successful for this application.

15.3 VACUUM SYSTEM DESIGNS/APPLICATIONS

Vacuum systems require preventative maintenance. Each system component must be carefully specified for the intended purpose with regard to protecting the pump

FIGURE 15.9 Comparison of molecular weights, dried vs. undried samples.

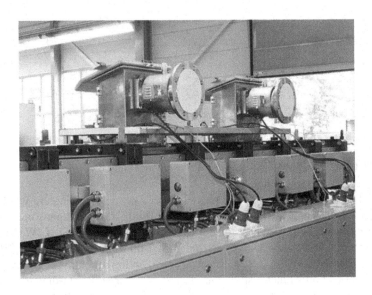

FIGURE 15.10   Heated vent stack.

and cleaning/maintenance. These are typical system components that are part of a vacuum system:

Vent stack: The vent stack is a housing that incorporates several devices, including sight glass in a hinged cover, O-ring seal, pipe connection for vacuum hose, connections for air bleed valve, vacuum transducer, etc. At the bottom of the vent stack is a barrel insert, which has one or more slots, and is angled and contoured to prevent vent flow. The vent stack is usually heated enough by conduction from the barrel; however, for some polymers it is heated to make it semi-self-cleaning (Figure 15.10).

Interconnection plumbing: Typically, this is a stainless-steel pipe or hose. Sometimes it helps to heat the plumbing to prevent the melt from freezing off and blocking the pipe. Plumbing should be pitched downward toward the knock-out pot to allow materials to fall by gravity into the pot.

Knock-out pot: The "K/O" pot is the first vessel the vent stream encounters after exiting the extruder vent and will collect the most solids/liquids, if present. The K/O pot should be situated as close to the extruder vent as possible.

Liquid condenser: A liquid condenser, typically cooled by water, is required based on the composition of the vent stream. Low-viscosity liquids will drain from the housing simply by opening a valve at the bottom, whereas "gelled" liquids require the vessel to be opened and manually cleaned. To design the system, it is important to define the residual materials being condensed.

Dry filter: A dry filter is the last line of defense to protect the pump and is simply a filter element inside a sheet-metal canister with quick-release clamps. Filter elements are often stainless steel or polyester, with many other materials of construction also available.

Vacuum pump: The vacuum pump is what pulls the vacuum that removes volatiles from the extruder vent. Larger motors/pumps only increase volumetric pumping capacities, so beyond a certain capacity there's little benefit for a larger pump since

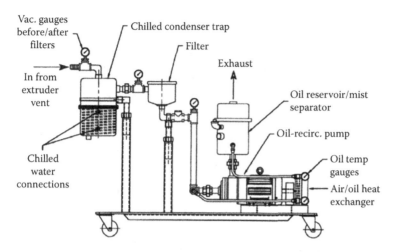

FIGURE 15.11   Example of vacuum venting system components.

it is pulling a vacuum in a finite/closed area. For most processes, a moderate vacuum (i.e., 130–60 millibar) is acceptable. That being said, some processes benefit from a higher vacuum level, in which case a two-stage pump to facilitate deeper vacuum levels may be specified.

An example of a vacuum venting system can be seen in Figure 15.11.

To approximate the level of vacuum needed to remove a certain number of residual volatiles from the process, the Flory-Huggins relationship for partial pressure above polymer solvent systems can be used:

$$\ln\left(\frac{P}{P_o}\right) = \ln\left(1 - V_p\right) + V_p + xV_p^2 \qquad (15.3)$$

where

P = absolute pressure
P_o = pressure of pure solvent at same temperature
$1 - V_p = V_s$ = solvent volume fraction
V_p = polymer volume fraction
x = Flory-Huggins interaction parameter; if solvent and polymer are mutually soluble, $x \leq 0.5$

For example, with 1000 ppm residual solvent at 260°C, with $P_o = 10.5$ atm and $x = 0.5$,

$$\ln\left(\frac{P}{P_o}\right) = \ln\left(1 - 99.999\right) + 1 + 0.5 = -6.908 + 1.5$$

$$= -5.408; \frac{P}{7980} = 0.0045; P = 36 \text{ torr}$$

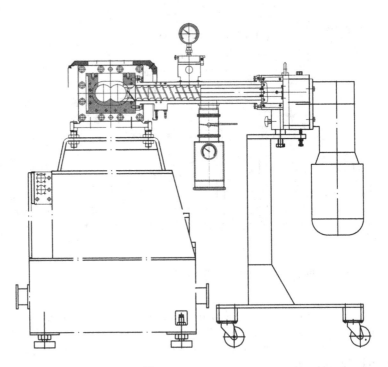

FIGURE 15.12   Vacuum vent stuffer.

An absolute pressure of approximately 48 millibar is required to remove 1000 ppm of residual solvent.

The following are some tips and techniques to assist the venting process:

Vent stuffer: A vent stuffer is a corotating intermeshing twin-screw auger that pushes materials back into the extruder process section that might "fly out" due to a high vent vapor velocity and/or low melt viscosity materials being pulled by the vacuum. It can be designed to operate with vacuum or to allow downward discharge/draining, as might be the case if 10%+ water is being devolatilized (Figure 15.12).

Vent position: The vent should be situated about 6 to 10 L/D back from the discharge, allowing for stable pumping, and is generally acceptable for the required venting efficiencies.

Multiple vents: Each vent can decrease the level of volatiles by at best an order of magnitude. For example, 10% volatiles in the system will decrease to 1% at the first vent and then will decrease to 0.1% at the second vent, etc. Early vents are typically atmospheric, while vacuum is often applied to later vents. For each vent, the overall L/D of the extruder must become longer.

Instrumentation: A vacuum transducer should be integrated into the vent piping. The transducer can be connected to a PLC system for control, data acquisition, and alarming.

Vent cleaning tips: Operators should only use plastic scrapers when cleaning the vent stack/insert. Also, only use a flashlight and a mirror attached to a pole to visually check a vent to avoid hazardous vapors and burns.

15.4 SUMMARY

Any extruder with a vent is devolatilizing something. Curiously, despite the commercial significance of devolatilization, there are only three texts on the subject. One is out of print, one is translated from German, and the third, *Devolatilization of Polymers* by Dr. Joseph Biesenberger, was published in 1983. It is also generally recognized that there is a lack of current DV modeling available. That being said, TSEs are well proven in wide-ranging industrial settings and broad know-how exists, as indicated by the extensive patent literature on the subject.

The test results reflected above are synced with generally accepted DV principles and practices. Understanding basic thermodynamic principles, functions and maintenance of the vacuum system, and some tricks goes a long way to ensure successful utilization and improvement of devolatilization via twin-screw extrusion.

Twin-screw extrusion continues to evolve and become more integrated in the pharmaceutical industry in research, development, and manufacturing. However, while extrusion applications and techniques have risen to the forefront, devolatilization is currently underutilized in pharmaceutical installations. Nevertheless, as understanding of the technology and realization of its importance becomes apparent (i.e., removing residual solvents from API, preventing hydrolysis degradation pathways, etc.), devolatilization will become more commonplace.

BIBLIOGRAPHY

1. Biesenberger J.A., *Devolatilization of Polymers: Fundamentals—Equipment—Applications*, Hanser Publishers (1983).
2. Jerman R.E., Devolatilization of polymers via TSE, *Leistritz Twin Screw Extrusion Workshop proceedings* (2006).
3. Todd D.B., Zhu L., Polymer devolatilization, *Leistritz Twin Screw Extrusion Workshop proceedings* (2011).
4. Martin C., Twin screw extrusion system developments to process bioplastics, SPE Bioplastics (2012).
5. Martin C., Devolatilization via twin screw extrusion: theory, tips and results, PPS (2014).

16 Continuous Oral Solid Dose Manufacture

Mayur Lodaya and Michael Thompson

CONTENTS

16.1 INTRODUCTION

While the primary focus of this chapter is on continuous wet granulation, salient aspects of other critical unit operations involved in the manufacture of oral solid dosage forms such as drying and tableting have been included. Some aspects of melt granulation are included to highlight differences in the process, though much of the knowledge in wet granulation translates well to the melt. In addition, a brief discussion of regulatory and quality considerations is also included in this chapter.

Drug formulations are rarely limited to their active pharmaceutical ingredient (API) solely. Excipients are provided along with the API to ensure that ingestion of administered medicine is palatable, targeted in its release within the body, and that its delivery maximizes bioavailability while minimizing toxicity. The many ingredients involved in solid oral dosage forms of drugs have differences in their particle size, shape, hydrophilicity, and water sorption characteristics, all of which impact the manufacturing process. As a result, granulation becomes a necessary step in the preparation of drugs to ensure compositional, handling, and dissolution properties meet stated specifications.

Granulation refers to "the buildup of clusters from powder or powder/binder mixtures to produce a free-flowing, cohesive material that can be further processed by compression or encapsulation" (1). Granulation is done to improve flow and handling, bulk density, appearance, solubility, resistance to aggregation, and/or reduction in the propensity for dust formation. The four general methods of preparing materials for oral solid dosage forms are direct compression, dry granulation, melt granulation, and wet granulation; the terms *wet granulation* and *wet massing* are often used interchangeably in the pharmaceutical literature. When feasible, direct compression is the first method of choice for obvious economic reasons because it involves many fewer processing steps. However, the majority of actives are not amenable to direct compression due to poor flow or lack of compressibility. Wet granulation permits the formulation of a very broad range of actives that lack the desired attributes for direct compression as well as those low-dose actives that are difficult to distribute uniformly. It is the most common granulation process and is among the most widely used unit operations in the preparation of pharmaceutical solid dosage forms. In cases where the active is moisture-sensitive, melt or dry granulation methods are considered as alternatives to wet granulation. Melt granulation involves the use of a molten polymer rather than a liquid form to bind the powder ingredients in granules. It requires equipment capable of reaching high temperatures and handling a viscous medium, but it is generally as easy to use as wet granulation. Dry granulation utilizes compaction for particle enlargement similar to direct compression, but involves a separate unit operation. Roller compaction and moisture-activated dry granulation (MADG) are examples of processes involving dry granulation.

Traditionally, pharmaceutical processing is done in batch mode. Some unit operations such as milling, tableting, encapsulation, etc. are inherently continuous in nature; i.e., as raw materials are fed continuously at a predetermined rate, the product is produced at a specified rate. Others such as wet granulation, drying, etc., as practiced today, are primarily batch operations. In these cases, a batch of raw materials is charged to the equipment; all ingredients are processed simultaneously for a predetermined time under a set of processing conditions to yield the desired product. While continuous processing has long been established in the food, chemical, and plastics industries, this is not so in pharmaceutical processing. The main reasons include tradition; know-how (or lack thereof); impact of regulations for any new process (however, over the last several years, this is changing and these aspects are further discussed later in this chapter); and lack of equipment/processes that can provide justification in terms of improvement in quality while achieving a lower overall cost structure. With the advent of high-speed tableting machines, an increase in current good manufacturing practice (cGMP) awareness, and an overall drive toward a superior quality of the finished dosage form at a lower cost of manufacture, it has become necessary to develop granulation processes having fewer steps while yielding consistent and high-quality products; transitioning to continuous processing can positively impact all of these desired improvements.

Batch processes like high-shear granulators, which are the most commonly used equipment for wet granulation, have some serious shortcomings in that they tend to lead to uncontrolled granule growth and material degradation owing to localized high temperatures. These disadvantages stress the need for a robust wet granulation equipment/process that has a broad applicability and is easy to scale up. The desired characteristics of one such piece of equipment can be listed as follows:

1. Applicability for processing powder blends with diverse characteristics;
2. Reduction of the level of excipients and granulation liquid required;
3. Provision of reproducible processing history resulting in consistent quality from granule to granule;
4. Short processing times; and
5. Ease of scale-up.

Attempts have been made to modify fluid bed machines and other equipment to achieve these characteristics. In a recent article, Bonde (2) summarized the technical aspects of continuous processing. He classified the batch and continuous processing equipment as mechanical/fluidized bed/other type, and briefly described continuous fluidized bed granulators. The paper contends that while batch processing will continue to be important, continuous processing will increase its share. Continuous processes with minimal product holdup and the ability to produce consistently predictable quality product are expected to supplant batch processes going forward, particularly for high-volume products. While the continuous fluidized bed and the Iverson mixer have some advantages over the batch processes discussed earlier, they do not meet all of the characteristics described above. The twin-screw extruder (TSE), on the other hand, possesses all of the above attributes and does have the potential to replace high-shear granulators as the preferred equipment for wet granulation. In addition to possessing the desired characteristics mentioned above, the TSE allows process optimization at a small scale using the final equipment.

16.2 DEFINITIONS

16.2.1 CONTINUOUS PROCESS

Continuous process refers to a process in which there is a continuous feeding of raw materials and a removal of product from the production line.

16.2.2   DISTRIBUTIVE MIXING

For a given powder blend being processed in a twin-screw extruder (TSE), the term *distributive mixing* refers to a spatial rearrangement of species that involves the reorientation/generation of new surfaces without any change in the domain size. Domain refers to a unit quantity of material fed to the extruder.

16.2.3   DISPERSIVE MIXING

For a given powder blend being processed in a TSE, the term *dispersive mixing* refers to rearrangement of species through a reduction in the size of domains with/without spatial reorientation. This mechanism may refer to breakage or erosion of the granule and/or domain reduction of the liquid binder.

16.2.4   EXCIPIENTS

An excipient is any component of a drug other than the active pharmaceutical ingredient. In solid oral dosage forms, this may include, but is not limited to, fillers, diluents, glidants, lubricants, disintegrants, binders, and taste-masking and coating agents.

16.2.5   MELT GRANULATION

Melt granulation is a comparable process to wet granulation with the purpose of producing a free-flowing cohesive material that can be further processed by compression or encapsulation but does not require a drying step to follow. The method uses a binding polymer that can be either melted and poured into the process or fed in as a solid with all other ingredients and heated till it melts/softens. Unlike wet granulation, melt granulation does not involve water or alcohols and hence may be used for moisture-sensitive ingredients.

16.2.6   RESIDENCE TIME DISTRIBUTION

Residence time distribution (RTD) is the probability distribution that describes the amount of time until a mass or fluid element exits a process. It can be used to predict the propagation of material or disturbances through the system.

16.2.7   TRACEABILITY RESOURCE UNIT

A traceability resource unit (TRU) is an optional unit used to define material processed in a continuous process. It can be specified as a segment of material that flows through the process as a unit and can then serve as a unique identifier from a process history perspective to achieve traceability throughout the integrated process in question.

16.2.8   TWIN-SCREW GRANULATOR

A twin-screw granulator (TSG) is a twin-screw extruder, most commonly the corotating intermeshing variant, which is used for the continuous granulation of pharmaceutical formulations. The machine is modular in construction, allowing multiple configurations of use specific to the needs of the granulation process. It has no die to extrude (pressurize) the mass at the exit.

16.2.9 WET MASSING

Wet massing is an agglomeration technique where powders are mixed with aqueous, alcoholic, or hydroalcoholic solution and agitated/mixed to produce a pasty product. The final product has a very broad size range starting from less than a millimeter to strands that may be a few millimeters in diameter. It tends to use a higher amount of liquid relative to solids compared to wet granulation.

16.2.10 WET GRANULATION

Wet granulation is the buildup of clusters from powder or powder/binder mixtures to produce, following drying, a free-flowing cohesive material that can be further processed by compression or encapsulation. The particles generally have a low aspect ratio and range from a few hundred microns to less than 1–2 mm in diameter.

16.3 CONTINUOUS WET GRANULATION

While traditional batch high-shear granulation still accounts for the large majority of products that use wet granulation, they have major shortcomings as discussed in the previous section. TSGs have the following important characteristics that make them a very attractive alternative:

1. Closely confined flow spaces and relatively small amounts of material being processed at a given time ensure consistent processing history and resulting granule quality.
2. Modular construction allows flexibility in the configuration with respect to process section and screw design (discussed at length later in this section). This in turn makes it applicable for processing powder blends with diverse characteristics.
3. Highly efficient mixing results in reduction of the level of excipients and granulation liquid required.
4. Short residence time (several seconds to less than a minute) further enhances its ability to ensure consistent processing history and minimizes exposure of ingredients to high temperatures in the case of melt granulation.
5. Ability to use operating time as another parameter allows the use of the same equipment for a much broader throughput range and, ultimately, ease of scale-up.

Details of the process are discussed below starting with background and equipment design considerations, followed by the mechanism of granule growth, discussion of key process parameters, and examples.

16.3.1 BACKGROUND

Broadening the use of screw extrusion machinery from extrusion spheronization to direct granulation started at least a decade before the introduction of the FDA guidance document on continuous manufacturing, 21CFR Part 211 *Current Good Manufacturing Practice for Finished Pharmaceuticals.* The transition began in the late 1980s when it was first disclosed that a twin-screw extruder had been considered for continuous granulation in place of a single-screw extruder for improved product consistency (3–7). By the late 1990s, the twin-screw extruder was being considered for direct tableting by internally compacting the wetted mass produced by wet granulation, though results showed that internal pressures were inadequate for this purpose (8). It was in later studies within a series of publications by Keleb et al. (9–11) when the first equivalence to the modern twin-screw granulator was demonstrated by removing any restrictive components from the end of the machine and directly granulating. Nowadays, numerous equipment vendors offer twin-screw extruder configurations suitable as TSGs.

The first known patent for the twin-screw granulation of powders was in the field of energetics, US 5,114,630A assigned to the U.S. Navy, whereas pharmaceutical granulation was originally described in US 6,499,984B1 for the Warner-Lambert company. The Warner-Lambert patent described a twin-screw extruder with no die, auxiliary feeders, controller(s), and downstream operations of drying and milling, all used together for continuously granulating pharmaceuticals. Further patents describing the equipment for pharmaceutical granulation are US 7,910,030B2, US 8,231,375B2, and CN 101,400,341B.

The barrel sections of a TSE consist of blocks made of hardened metal, integrating cooling and heating as well as containing port openings for solids and liquid addition. The screws constitute the heart of the machine, made up of numerous screw elements described in the following section that are assembled together on two splined shafts. The two screws are housed within the assembled barrel and engage with a gearbox at the rear of the machine. Figure 16.1 shows a common machine configuration complete with stainless steel paneling for easy wash-down.

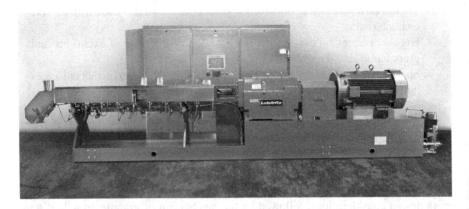

FIGURE 16.1   Photo of a twin-screw granulation process (courtesy of Leistritz).

TABLE 16.1
Extruder Models of TSG Noted in Publications

Manufacturer and Model	Machine Size (diameter, mm)	Journal Principal Author and Year
Thermo Fisher Pharma 16	16	El Hasgrasy, 2013
Prism Eurolab 16	16	Dhenge, 2011
APV Baker MP 19 TC 25	19	Keleb, 2004
GEA ConsiGma-25	25	Vercruysse, 2012
Leistritz ZSE 27	27	Sun, 2010
Leistritz	34 and 50	Shah, 2005

A distinctive feature of any TSG is that no die is used at the end of the machine, unlike other extrusion processes, but rather a special restraining plate is recommended that holds the screws in place axially without restricting powder exit. Any restriction or cause for granules to dwell in the barrel past where the flights of the screws end will invariably lead to uncontrolled agglomeration and must be minimized. Table 16.1 lists referenced TSEs in the literature that have been used to develop granulated pharmaceutical formulations. The list contains extruders of differing sizes from lab scale (12–16 mm) to pilot scale (18–19 mm) and to production scale (25–30 mm) from many major twin-screw extruder manufacturers, and notably includes the GEA ConsiGma™, which like the Bohle Conti Granulator BCG® is an integrated twin-screw granulator and drying system, dedicated to pharmaceutical granulation. Figure 16.2 shows segmented isometric views of a ConsiGma pilot-scale integrated system built by GEA.

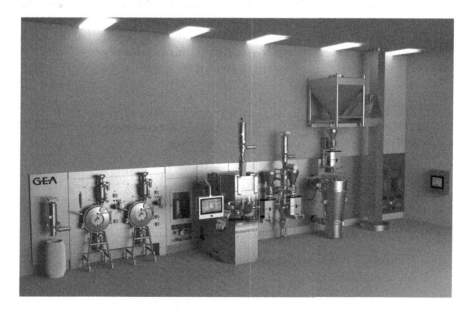

FIGURE 16.2 ConsiGma tableting line (courtesy of GEA Processing Engineering).

Powders and liquids are introduced into the extruder at multiple entry points by feeders and pumps surrounding a TSG. Single- or twin-screw gravimetric feeders are commonly used for highly accurate continuous metering of individual ingredients or blends of ingredients into the TSG. Manufacturers such as K-Tron, Brabender Technologies, and Schenck AccuRate are among the leaders in North America, supplying gravimetric feeders designed for different dosing rates and for handling powders of differing bulk density and flow properties. A good review of powder handling features for gravimetric feeders was provided in the study by Cartwright et al. (12). Difficult-to-flow powders may require special options included with the feeder such as a flexible wall hopper, bridge breaker or vibrating pan. Liquid handling into a granulation process requires a high-pressure (500–1000 psig recommended) metering pump that allows operation that is compliant with cGMP. Positive displacement type pumps are preferred for accurate delivery in the presence of varying pressures at the injection site along the barrel of the TSG.

16.3.2 EQUIPMENT DESIGN CONSIDERATIONS

While TSEs have multiple designs, to this point, corotating intermeshing TSEs are the only type that have been successfully used as TSGs and the remaining discussion will focus on this design.

Modular construction refers to both barrel and screws for the TSE, which may be readily configured to the needs of the process. This *design-as-needed* philosophy makes the TSG a flexible manufacturing platform for both drug development and production. Figure 16.3 shows a common machine configuration featuring feeders and pumps around a TSG to add powders and liquids into the process. The barrel is comprised of several barrel sections connected in an end-to-end fashion. The process length is generally measured as the ratio of length of the screw shaft to its diameter (L:D). For wet granulation, this is generally in the range of 20:1–30:1, with some examples of very short (L:D = 10:1) or long (L:D = 40:1)

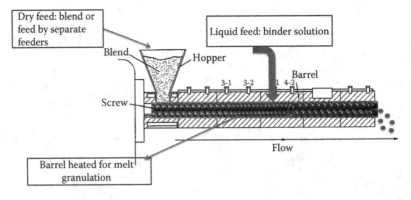

FIGURE 16.3 Common machine configuration featuring feeders and pumps around a TSG to add powders and liquids into the process.

process sections. Adjusting the placement of those auxiliary units means that pow-ders and liquids can be added at multiple positions along the process. In addition, there may be a low-shear dry blending unit upstream of TSG when a very large number of solids are to be metered into the process. Ingredients that constitute a small fraction of formulation are preblended upstream of the TSG to further improve the homogeneity of the blend as it is metered into the granulation process. Any restriction or cause for granules to dwell in the barrel past the flighted screw length of the process will invariably lead to uncontrolled agglomeration and must be minimized.

16.3.3 SCREW ELEMENTS AND SCREW DESIGN

As mentioned before, the term modular refers to both the barrels and the screws. The screw elements used for granulation can be largely broken into two types, namely, conveying (transfer) and mixing type elements.

Conveying elements are further differentiated based on the pitch, with several ele-ments of differing design shown in Figure 16.4. While the larger pitch elements are generally used in the feeding section to provide a high contact area (to ensure smooth intake of materials being fed, maximize wetting of powder in the liquid intake sec-tion, etc.), smaller pitch elements provide a higher level of distributive mixing to improve spreading of the binder liquid and allow granule growth while maintaining high porosity. Conveying elements are also instrumental after a mixing element to control granule size, with smaller pitches creating smaller particles (13).

There are multiple types of mixing elements and the type/length of the mixing section determines the level of dispersive/distributive mixing as well as compaction of the granulation mixture. The main two types used within TSGs are kneaders and

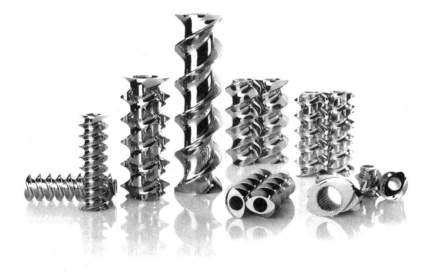

FIGURE 16.4 Different conveying elements showing differing flight pitch (courtesy of Leistritz).

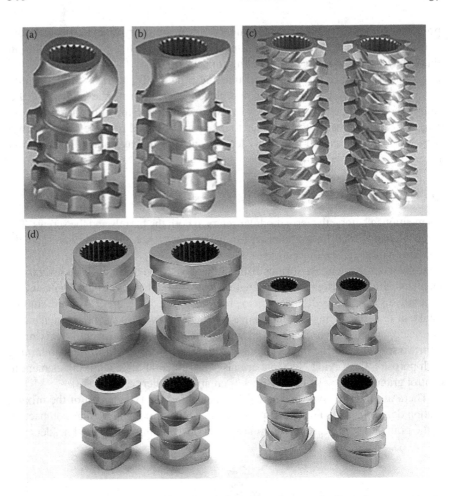

FIGURE 16.5   (a)–(d) Photos of kneaders and combing elements for the twin-screw extruder (courtesy of Leistritz).

combing (also referred to as gear) elements. While the use of kneaders has been discussed extensively in the literature (14–16), combing elements have received less attention but have been used successfully (10,17). Figures 16.5(a)–(d) show photos of these elements. The combination of distributive and dispersive mixing imparted to the granule as it is processed through the mixing section results in its compaction and fragmentation. This is ultimately critical to the liquid distribution, granule size, and granule strength. This is discussed further in the section "Mechanism of Granule Growth."

In the case of a kneader section, the size of an individual kneader disc and overall length of the mixing section determine the level of distributive vs. dispersive mixing imparted. For example, a relatively short mixing section, comprised of kneaders with thin discs (each ≤1/16D) stacked together at a small off-set angle (≤30°) in the forward direction, will favor distributive mixing. On the other hand, a relatively long mixing section, comprising kneaders with thick discs stacked at a higher off-set angle, will favor dispersive mixing. Adding more kneading elements to increase the section length produces better distribution of the granulation liquid and denser granule formation; however, excessive shear stress can lead to granule attrition and reduced granule size (18,19) or the production of very dense granules with poor compression properties (20). Additionally, increasing the number of kneading elements and/or increasing the L/S ratio results in higher mean residence times (21). The configuration of the kneading discs in a kneader section can be customized to form 30, 60, or 90° angles. The increase in disc angle was shown to increase the fill level in these kneading blocks (22) and can result in an increased fraction of coarse particles and lower granule friability (16), but the effect of the angle is only evident at high degrees of fill (15). Van Melkebeke et al. evaluated the location of the kneading elements along the screw and saw that discharging granules immediately after kneading elements resulted in larger agglomerates, indicating that the conveying elements helped break down the large consolidated granules that exit the kneading elements (16). Liu Y et al. found that this relationship between the kneader and downstream conveying element was specific to the angle of the conveying flight, with small pitches producing smaller granules (13).

Within the combing element design, the type of gear mixer in Figure 16.5(c) does not have any conveying capability and results in high levels of compaction and fragmentation, whereas the gear mixer in Figures 16.5(a) and (b) provide some forward conveying capability (much less compaction, relatively speaking), along with fragmentation (sizing of the granule). For this reason, the latter elements are preferred at discharge. Combing elements are less commonly used than kneading elements, but they were shown to have improved liquid distribution and produce more monomodal particle size distributions (PSD) (21,23).

16.3.4 METHODS OF WETTING

The closely confined space inside a TSE provides improved product consistency as a result of all particles experiencing a similar shear history compared to a high-shear batch mixer (7). However, that limited free space complicates how liquids are introduced into a TSG for the wetting of powders. In high-shear batch mixers and fluidized beds, a low-viscosity binding liquid is sprayed as fine droplets of comparable size over dry contacting powder blends in order to minimize oversaturation. The physical state sought is known as *pendular saturation*, where the amount of local liquid relative to nearby solids is just sufficient to form bridges between particles without excess. In practice, however, the wetted powders will initially be oversaturated for a short period since sprays have a limited coverage area and the liquid needs to be added as quickly as possible to control the final particle size. In an extruder, one cannot spray a liquid like in a batch mixer since powders would be pushed out of their path, creating substantial flow surging. However, the alternative of directly injecting liquids over top of the solids will invariably cause highly localized oversaturation (10).

As a result of processing issues related to liquid addition into a TSG, two wetting methods have arisen in the literature, known as *direct injection* and *foam delivery*; both methods are specifically meant for use with low-viscosity liquids. Direct injection is familiar to TSE users, in which liquids are metered by pump into the

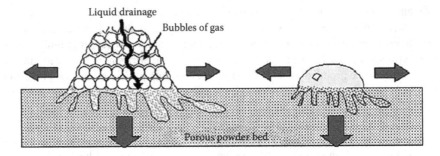

FIGURE 16.6   Conceptual diagram of powder wetting by direct liquid injection versus foam delivery. (From Tan MXL et al. *Chem Eng Sci.* 2009; 64: 2826–2836 (60).)

process. Powders have an inherent tendency to block these injection sites unless pressurized, which means the added liquid is normally provided to the extruder with sufficient force that a broad dispersal pattern is possible, such as a fan shape; no gases are used in the dispersal of the liquid. To minimize oversaturation, Shah (10) proposed multiple injection sites along the screw length but this can present issues with the growth characteristics of granules and is not likely to be a commonly selected approach. Foam delivery for TSG (11) originates from the method of foam granulation devised for high-shear batch mixers (24). A semirigid foam with the consistency of shaving cream, comprised of the binding liquid and a foaming agent (ex. hypromellose serves both purposes), will drain liquid slowly upon contact with dry powder ingredients. The wetted surface area of powders is greater by this method because it has a higher spread-to-soak ratio compared to direct injection, and the released liquid has a droplet size close to the dry powder excipients (~100 μm). A mechanical foam generator is required in addition to a pump and the rigidity of the resulting foam requires that it be fed as a solid into a TSG, namely, using a side-stuffer. Differences in wetting by these two techniques are highlighted in Figure 16.6.

Both methods of wetting can produce granules of similar properties provided the compressive forces inside the TSG are compensated depending upon the uniformity of the saturated powders (11). However, it is when powders are poorly wetted that a unique process consideration for TSG is highlighted, not observed with other granulation methods. The closely confined space that serves to complicate liquid addition yet improve product consistency also increases the likelihood of high frictional forces between the solids and barrel unless the powder is well lubricated. It is typical of normal processing conditions that flowing powders will increase in temperature by 5–15°C above the barrel setpoint but when poorly wetted solids enter a kneader or combing mixer, it has been observed that temperatures can rise as much as 70°C (11,20). Therefore, good dispersion of the binding liquid should precede compaction in TSG processes.

16.3.5   MECHANISM OF GRANULE GROWTH

Within a closed, batch system such as a high-shear granulator and fluidized bed granulator, the mechanisms of powder wetting and nucleation, consolidation and

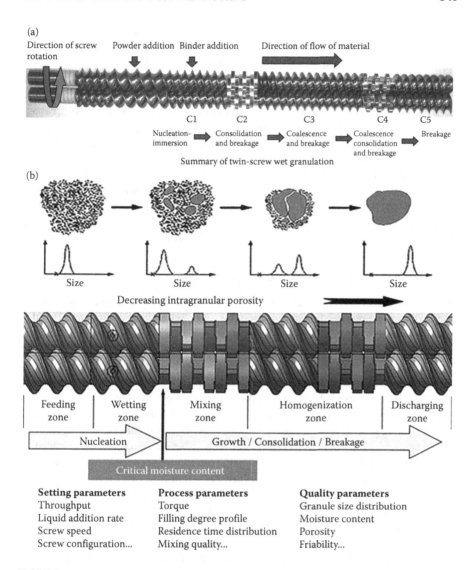

FIGURE 16.7 (a)–(b) Theoretical mechanism of twin-screw granulation. (From (a) Dhenge RM et al. *Int J Pharm*. 2012;438:20–32. (b) Kumar A et al. *Eur J Pharma Biopharma*. 2013; 85, 814–832.)

coalescence, and attrition can occur simultaneously. Dimensionless parameters and regime maps have been developed to explain the different phenomena during wet granulation to better understand and control the mechanism of granule growth (25); however, with a TSG being an open, continuous, and zoned system, the mechanisms of granule growth and attrition have been reevaluated.

Dhenge et al. tracked the progression of granulation along conveying and kneading elements (60°), as shown in Figures 16.7(a) and (b). The granulation liquid addition led to powder wetting by immersion, whereby the powder is suspended within larger liquid droplets to form loose, large agglomerates that are rich in liquid content. When these large agglomerates entered a kneader section (C2), compression or squeezing of these droplets led to denser granules and the liquid moved to their surfaces. The liquid now on the surface of the granule allowed for more coalescence during conveying (C3). When these particles again entered a kneader section (C4), they actually continued to grow, most probably due to the continued consolidation and with less breakage due to the smaller agglomerate size compared to those entering C2 (26). Kumar et al. found that the second kneading section was more influential in reshaping the granules, rather than sizing (27). The use of a larger particle size molten binder within the blend, such as high molecular weight polyethylene glycol, also resulted in immersion powder wetting (28). The use of a molten granulating agent was highlighted in the patent US 20110092515, filed by Novartis, describing the formation of a preferred anhydrous polymorph of quinolone via TSE for granulation (29), highlighting areas for potential intellectual property (IP) opportunities using TSE for granulation.

16.3.6 IMPACT OF PROCESS PARAMETERS

The processing parameters associated with TSE include length to diameter ratio (L/D), screw design, screw speed, material throughput rate, barrel temperature, and liquid to solids ratio (L/S) (30). These processing parameters affect other important processing attributes, including mean residence time (MRT), torque, and degree of fill (31).

As a general rule of thumb, an active that is easier to wet and compressible would require a shorter process length (low L:D ratio) and fewer mixing sections (1 or 2) to accomplish the required objective of making a granule with the desired characteristics. On the other hand, a hydrophobic active with very low bulk density would require a relatively long process length (high L:D ratio) with a higher number of mixing sections (three or more) within it (32). Screw design (i.e., number and configuration of kneading elements) and material throughput rate, along with screw speed (to a lesser extent) and interactions of these parameters, most significantly influence MRT (28,33).

Once the overall process section length and the number of mixing sections, as well as the locations of powder and liquid addition, are in place, the remaining operational variables are material throughput rate, screw speed, screw design (fine-tuning aspects), barrel temperature, and L/S ratio. For most granulations involving the use of water as a granulation fluid, barrel temperature is preferably maintained around room temperature and subsequently it has not been studied extensively. This is however not true when considering melt granulation (discussed separately) or when binders like HPMC are used, where water sorption properties are temperature dependent.

The amount of liquid addition required for TSG is much lower than that required for high-shear or fluid bed granulation (8), but generally higher L/S ratios result in better binder distribution, reduced fines, more monomodal PSD, lower porosity, and stronger granules (23,34). High overall throughput rate, as well as increased L/S ratio, leads to a higher degree of fill, causing substantial buildup upstream of mixing sections with higher torque and denser granules (19,35,36).

Screw speed has been found to have minimal effect on granulation, providing only minor control over the particle size distribution (9,15,19,20,26,36). Commonly used speeds are between 200 and 400 rpm, though the literature has reported values

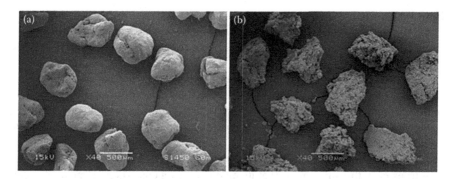

FIGURE 16.8   Images of granules from HSG (a) and TSE (b). (From Lee KT, Ingram A, Rowson NA. Comparison of granule properties produced using twin screw extruder and high shear mixer: A step towards understanding the mechanism of twin screw wet granulation. *Powder Technol.* 2013;**238**:91–8.)

as low as 30 rpm and as high as 950 rpm. It may be considered a parameter for fine-tuning granule properties for many formulations.

The viscosity of a binder has received little examination (8,9,37), possibly because of its small influence on granulation in the extruder. Mechanical forces in the extruder have been shown in numerous studies to dominate over the mechanism of liquid dispersion.

The granules produced from TSG have been found to be more elongated when compared to the spherical granules produced from conventional wet granulation methods, as shown in Figure 16.8, and tend to be more porous. However, the less dense, weaker granules prepared by TSG may be advantageous during tableting, as they have better compression properties to produce stronger tablets, due to the ease of fragmentation during compression (38). The bimodal particle size distribution obtained from TSG granulation is not necessarily a function of poor liquid-binder distribution, but may be due to the mechanism of granulation and attrition of the TSG process itself (21,39,40).

16.4   MELT GRANULATION

Melt granulation [or hot melt granulation (HMG)] refers to agglomeration processes using a polymer as a meltable binder. It is a desirable method when one or more of the ingredients in a formulation are moisture sensitive. The approach takes advantage of one of the strengths of the machine—that is, its well-controlled thermal environment. The polymeric binder is most often added as a powder along with the drug formulation to undergo sintering within the extruder, but as with high-shear batch mixers it could be pumped into the process as a melt instead. The "pumped" approach has not been demonstrated in the open literature at this point and seems unlikely to receive much attention considering the machine comes fully equipped with heaters and would otherwise require extra equipment to melt the polymer out-side of the process. The process has striking similarities to another emerging area in pharmaceutical manufacturing, which is referred to as "hot melt extrusion" (HME).

However, whereas HME primarily focuses on dissolving highly water-insoluble drugs (often BCS Class II) into hydrophilic polymers to increase bioavailability, many processes of HMG never intend to change the active ingredient from its solid state (though one could).

The TSG offers a different environment for heat transfer compared to the classical high-shear batch mixer for HMG. The shallow layer of powder in the screws of the extruder, coupled with the high power density of heaters used with extruders, reduces the temperature gradient throughout the ingredients, allowing everything to rapidly come to setpoint conditions. The rapidness of heating is necessary for this machine as its residence times are generally short (28). The other unique attribute of heat transfer in this machine is that its modular barrel construction, mentioned earlier in this chapter, allows the ingredients to experience varying temperatures along the process, customized to the needs of the formulator.

While all the points stated above indicate advantages for using an extruder in HMG, there will also be limitations. Most notably is that the powders must be well lubricated prior to a compression zone, which may require more binder than would be used in a batch mixer or fluidized bed.

16.4.1 Applications of Twin-Screw Melt Granulation

At this time, only a handful of studies have been cited in the literature on HMG with a TSG. Mu and Thompson (28) looked at a range of variables for the extruder affecting melt granulation, including screw design, polymer molecular weight, polymer concentration, and operating temperature. Examining the binder distribution in the exiting granules as well as the process dependency on binder particle size, as done by Schaefer and Mathiesen (41) for the high-shear batch mixer, the authors found no single dominant mechanism in the extruder but rather a sequential occurrence of both immersion and distribution nucleation mechanisms. Van Melkebeke et al. (42) explored conditions related to the melt granulation of a 10%–20% loaded drug (BCS Class II) using a blend of PEG 400/4000 as binder and maltodextrin as filler. XRD analysis showed the drug was crystalline in the final granules with 1% loss, which they attributed to forming a solid solution, though only 13% drug could dissolve in the PEG while molten. They concluded the drug had been finely dispersed as particles within the granules as it displayed enhanced dissolution compared to the pure drug into water. The work was done at barrel temperatures of 30–65°C, which were the lowest in the published studies for HMG. Keen et al. (43) looked at the use of Compritol® 888 ATO glyceryl behenate as a binder to develop a controlled release tablet of microcrystalline cellulose and tramadol HCl (35% load, BCS Class I, Tm 180°C). The authors found that granulation with the lipid exhibited a combination of immersion and distribution nucleation mechanisms similar to those of Mu et al. (28). Tan et al. (44) similarly looked at melt granulation with a lipid binder in their development of a direct-molded tablet with controlled release behavior, in their case for verapamil HCl (60% load, BCS Class I, Tm 160°C). The authors compared the tableting and release rate properties from granulating with different combinations of hydrophilic binders (Hypromellose K4M, PEO 1M) and hydrophobic binders (Compritol®ATO 888 glyceryl behenate and Precirol®ATO 5 glyceryl palmitostearate), with a total polymer concentration of 40% in the formulation. Lipids offer an interesting alternative to more traditional hydrophilic polymeric binders like PEG as a means of minimizing dose dumping in hydroalcoholic media. Most lipids melt well below 100°C, making them suitable in hot melt granulation without harm to the active.

Two published case studies from a group at Novartis looked at preparing products with high drug loading, using polymer binders requiring much higher melting temperatures (45,46). Vasanthavada and coworkers (45) considered HMG as a means for creating a controlled release product without the need for a high concentration of excipients to obtain the functional response. Their purpose was to produce granules consisting of 89%–94% imatinib mesylate (T_m 212°C, BSC Class II) with binders of hydroxypropylmethyl cellulose, hydroxypropyl cellulose, and ethyl cellulose. In their case, barrel temperatures of 185°C were used. Raman microscopy confirmed the drug remained as unmelted crystalline particles in the final granules and the polymer was finely dispersed. In vitro dissolution studies and in vivo human trials demonstrated that modified drug release occurred with as little as 5% polymer binder. For the second study, Lakshman et al. (46) looked at a 90% drug loading of Metformin HCl (T_m 224°C, BCS Class III) with hydroxypropylcellulose polymer (T_g 130°C). In this case, they compared their results to granules made by wet and solvent granulation. The extruder barrel temperatures were examined as a variable of study from 140 to 180°C. Once again, the approach successfully granulated the high loading of the drug while avoiding known complications with metformin related to its high solubility with water. The authors concluded that HMG with a twin-screw extruder was a suitable approach to producing small-sized tablets by neglecting the need for large amounts of excipients.

Temperature is an obvious concern for this technique of granulation as the environment increases the probability of damage to formulation ingredients. Weatherley et al. (47) explored the thermal stability of two active ingredients (15% loading), caffeine (BCS class I, T_m 147°C) and ibuprofen (BCS class II, T_m 79°C) in melt granulated products with lactose monohydrate as the filler and differing amounts of PEG 3350 or PEG 8000 (6.5%–20%) as the meltable binder. The work was done with barrel temperatures of 100°C. The ibuprofen dissolved into the molten PEG during processing (yet recrystallized upon solidification) whereas the caffeine remained as a solid suspension. Testing of the prepared granules by high-pressure liquid chromatography and XRD found no evidence of drug damage from processing at the high temperature, which was attributed in part to the short residence time of the machine.

16.5 DRYING

When it comes to drying unit operations, two techniques have been reported in the literature. These are fluidized bed and dielectric [microwave/radio frequency (MW/RF)] drying.

16.5.1 FLUIDIZED BED DRYING

Continuous fluid bed granulation with integrated drying was discussed at length in the previous edition of the book (48) and since there are no major advancements in the available equipment design, these will not be discussed.

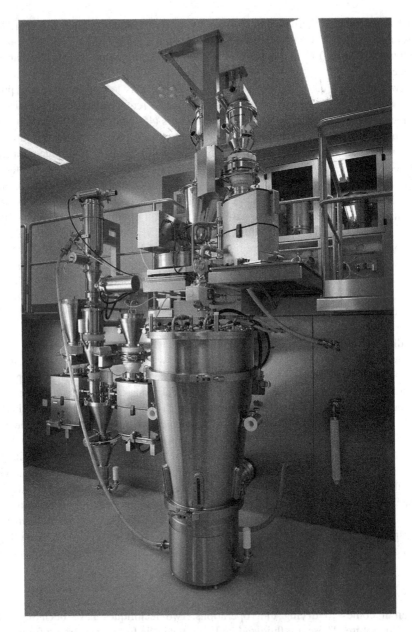

FIGURE 16.9   Photo of a ConsiGma® granulator, dryer, and evaluation unit (courtesy of GEA Processing Engineering).

One key advancement in equipment design for fluid bed drying (where the equipment is designed to dry only) is the dryer used within the ConsiGma™ continuous tableting system developed by GEA (Figure 16.9). The dryer is a segmented design (six segments) in which the continuous flow of granules is split into packages of approximately 1–3 kg (depending on the line throughput and product) by a rotating inlet valve, drying each of them in a separate segment of the dryer, thereby guaranteeing plug flow. When each of the six segments is dry, it is emptied via a rotating discharge valve and transferred to the evaluation module and refilled with a new package of wet granules. The drying curve of each package is monitored, as a fingerprint of the process, and controlled to maintain a constant end humidity over the whole batch. The end point of drying is usually determined based on time, but can also be based on product temperature or an actual online moisture measurement.

16.5.2 DIELECTRIC DRYING

As far as the use of electromagnetic energy is concerned, MW and RF have been successfully used to dry pharmaceutical granulates. While MW has also been used in some batch installations, RF has only been used in a continuous mode. Both of these techniques have been used extensively in the food industry; however, their use in the pharmaceutical industry has been minimal. L.B. Bohle (49) developed a continuous granulation system in which a planetary roller (used for granulation) was connected to a MW dryer. Use of RF dryer was disclosed by Warner Lambert/Pfizer colleagues in the continuous pharmaceutical granulation patent (17).

While dielectric drying does have a distinct advantage of no granule attrition (in comparison to FB drying), there are a few important limitations as well:

- It is not a closed system by design (i.e., generally involving a tunnel with a belt that carries the granulation as a quiescent bed and a cross flow of hot air carries away the evaporated water).
- It is challenging to make the equipment cGMP compliant, especially from a clean-in-place (CIP) standpoint.

16.6 TABLETING

Immediate and extended release formulations intended as solid oral dosages are most popular in tablet form for patient drug delivery, being palatable, portable, and easy to administer and demonstrating relatively good stability at ambient storage conditions. Tablet preparation involves a die being filled precisely with drug ingredients and then closed under great force (10–100 kN) by two opposing punches. The strength of a resulting tablet relies upon mechanical interlocking of particles; solids bridging within granulates; and intermolecular interactions including van der Waal forces, hydrogen bonding, and electrostatic forces (50). Tableting can be done manually for single pressing or automated using a rotary-style tableting machine for higher quantities. The unit is designed to compact powder ingredients into a tablet of appropriate size, weight, and hardness. Press speeds in these tableting machines have increased dramatically over the years from a few hundred tablets per hour to presently upwards of a few thousand tablets per minute (51). Weight variation is the most common defect in tableting, which occurs when powders display poor flowability to the die, uneven filling in the die, or difficulties being ejected from the die (52). As a result, solids inflow and tablet ejection play critical roles in the optimal operation of modern machines.

The predominant purpose for granulation is improved solids flowability in tablet-ing operations without ingredient segregation prior to the die press. The particle size distribution (PSD) and strength of prepared granules will influence the composition, weight, hardness, and appearance of tablets, affecting both flowability and compression. Too many fines in a supplied granulate, or occurring as a result of breakage during flow within the tableting machinery, will negatively impact tablet reproducibility and drug consistency and may introduce dust contaminates into the work environment (51). Granule porosity must be appropriate, where large pore sizes are desirable to allow for more particle rearrangement during compression in the die press (53).

Tablets prepared by TSG in comparison to a high-shear batch mixer show higher tensile strength, longer disintegration time, and less friability (7). Shah (10) showed that an acceptable 625-mg strength tablet prepared by TSG could not be comparably made by a high-shear batch mixer without the formation of a tacky mass. Lakshman et al. (46) found that melt granulation by TSG of a high-dose metformin HCl formulation minimized moisture-related issues on tablet hardness and friability compared to wet granulation. Vercruysse et al. (54) found through a series of five-hr production runs involving twin-screw granulation and tableting that granule and tablet quality were highly repeatable. The compressive forces within a TSG are far below a tableting press (i.e., <1 kN versus ~20 kN), yet some examples exist in the literature of single-step granulation/tableting processes. Keleb et al. (6) first discussed the idea of an extruder directly producing acceptable tablets, in their case with wet granulated α-lactose monohydrate. The tablets produced were highly porous and exhibited fast disintegration in comparison to those prepared by direct compression. The porosity would likely be even higher with most drug formulations by this approach as the water content would be much higher, which meant the approach was unlikely to be attractive in pharmaceutical manufacturing. However, Tan et al. (44) evaluated this idea of directly molding tablets in a TSG further but now by HMG. The authors compared offline milling and die compression versus direct molding of produced granules within their extruder, preparing a controlled release tablet with verapamil hydrochloride as the model drug. The tablets that had been molded after milling exhibited a faster release rate than the direct molded tablets.

16.7 REGULATORY AND QUALITY CONSIDERATIONS

Over the last two decades, considerable advances have been made, especially in equipment engineering, to provide a robust platform for the use of continuous processing to manufacture pharmaceuticals. In a recent review article (55), FDA colleagues concluded that continuous processing has a great deal of potential to address issues of agility, flexibility, and cost, while also providing robustness in the development and manufacture of pharmaceuticals. They argued that it is strongly aligned with the quality-by-design (QbD) paradigm and in that sense, it is a scientific and risk-based approach to pharmaceutical development. In a separate review article (56) jointly authored by colleagues from several pharmaceutical manufacturers, regulatory agencies, and others active in the field, the current regulatory environment, relevant regulations/guidelines, and their impact on continuous manufacturing were assessed. In yet another review article (57), elements of control systems engineering as applied to continuous manufacturing were discussed. This section will summarize the following key aspects as they relate to the manufacture of pharmaceuticals using continuous processes: regulatory definition, guidelines within current regulations, and control strategies.

16.7.1 REGULATORY DEFINITION

One question that is most often asked by users when discussing a batch vs. continuous approach is—how do you define a batch? The definition of a "batch" according to current good manufacturing practices (cGMP) is "a specific quantity of drug or other material that is intended to have uniform character and quality within specified limits and is produced according to a single manufacturing order during the same cycle of manufacture." Thus, the regulatory definition of a "batch" is related to the amount of material and not the mode by which it is made.

16.7.2 GUIDELINES WITHIN CURRENT REGULATIONS

The current regulatory environment supports advancing innovation including a more flexible, efficient, and cleaner continuous process. The expectation for the assurance of reliable and predictive processing resulting in consistent product quality is the same for batch and continuous processing. The emergence of ICH Q8–Q11 guidelines and accompanying points to consider, as well as Q&A documents, reinforce the adoption of risk-based, systematic, scientific approaches and a robust pharmaceutical quality system, to establish an increased level of process understanding and product knowledge. The FDA's guidance for the industry on process analytical technology (PAT) specifically identifies continuous processing as one of the outcomes from adoption of a scientific risk-based approach to process design. European Union (EU) guidelines particularly relevant to continuous manufacturing include the guidance for process validation, in which the concept of continuous process verification (CPV) is introduced. The following aspects, listed as bullet points below, are of special importance, and while they are applicable to both batch and continuous processes, they should be specifically evaluated when implementing a continuous process. One tried and true approach for this is to conduct a thorough "technical risk assessment" (TRA), where potential failure modes are clearly defined and a weighted risk priority score is calculated. This then provides a scientific and risk-based approach to define control measures for failure modes that score higher while accepting risks that score lower.

- A "batch" should be clearly defined in terms of the quantity manufactured or duration of the process.
- In-process controls (IPC) and sampling (sample size, frequency, and location) should be evaluated.
- Acceptable procedures for handling deviations should be in place.
- Raw material specifications and impact of lot-to-lot variability on the final product should be evaluated.

- All potential sources of variability should be considered during development. Specific control measures should be put in place as appropriate and their effectiveness should be confirmed during validation and continuous verification.

16.7.3 CONTROL STRATEGIES

As the regulatory environment has evolved over the past decade and concepts of product life cycle have been introduced, one key element that has been emphasized is that of defining and implementing a control strategy that provides data-based evidence of a process operating under control (55,58,59). This is what enables the manufacturer to move away from the old paradigm of testing the quality (after the fact) as the only way to accept/reject a batch to one of designing quality into the product. While this is not to say that final product testing is completely eliminated, what it does mean is that it provides a robust proof of quality at all stages of manufacture and allows room for continuous improvement while monitoring the effectiveness of any changes made.

When designing a process control strategy for a continuous manufacturing process, in addition to the points mentioned in the previous section, the following should be considered:

- The desired objective should be to ensure all critical quality attributes (CQAs) are within specification rather than process variables operating at a steady state.
- Startup and shutdown procedures should be clearly defined.
- Material traceability is an important consideration and RTD can be used in part to define this.
- Control systems employed should ensure quality in the presence of disturbances and known process constraints.

Direct measurement, first principles, use of multivariate model-based predictions, and design space approaches should be used for ensuring that CQAs remain within specified ranges.

REFERENCES

1. Lindberg NO, Tufvesson C, Olbjer L. Extrusion of an effervescent granulation with a twin screw extruder, Baker Perkins Mpf 50-D. *Drug Dev Ind Pharm.* 1987;13(9–11):1891–913.
2. Bonde M. Continuous granulation. In: Parikh DM, ed. Handbook of Pharmaceutical Granulation Technology. New York, NY, Marcel Dekker, 1998:369–386.
3. Lindberg NO, Tufvesson C, Holm P, Olbjer L. Extrusion of an effervescent granulation with a twin screw extruder, Baker Perkins Mpf 50-D—Influence on intragranular porosity and liquid saturation. *Drug Dev Ind Pharm.* 1988;14:1791–8.
4. Kleinebudde P, Lindner H. Experiments with an instrumented twin-screw extruder using a single-step granulation extrusion process. *Int J Pharm.* 1993;94:49–58.
5. Kleinebudde P, Solvberg AJ, Lindner H. The power-consumption-controlled extruder—A tool for pellet production. *J Pharm Pharmacol.* 1994;46:542–6.

6. Keleb EI, Vermeire A, Vervaet C, Remon JP. Cold extrusion as a continuous single-step granulation and tabletting process. *Eur J Pharm Biopharm.* 2001;52:359–68.
7. Keleb EI, Vermeire A, Vervaet C, Remon JP. Extrusion granulation and high shear granulation of different grades of lactose and highly dosed drugs: A comparative study. *Drug Dev Ind Pharm.* 2004;30(6):679–91.
8. Keleb EI, Vermeire A, Vervaet C, Remon JP. Twin screw granulation as a simple and efficient tool for continuous wet granulation. *Int J Pharm.* 2004;273:183–94.
9. Keleb EI, Vermeire A, Vervaet C, Remon JP. Continuous twin screw extrusion for the wet granulation of lactose. *Int J Pharm.* 2002;239:69–80.
10. Shah U. Use of a modified twin-screw extruder to develop a high-strength tablet dosage form. *Pharm Technol.* 2005;29:52–66.
11. Thompson MR, Weatherley S, Pukadyil RN, Sheskey PJ. Foam granulation: New developments in pharmaceutical solid oral dosage forms using twin screw extrusion machinery. *Drug Dev Ind Pharm.* 2012;38:771–84.
12. Cartwright JJ, Robertson J, D'Haene D et al. Twin screw wet granulation: Loss in weight feeding of a poorly flowing active pharmaceutical ingredient. *Powder Technol.* 2013;238:116–21.
13. Liu Y, Thompson MR, O'Donnell KP. Function of upstream and downstream conveying elements in wet granulation processes within a twin screw extruder. *Powder Technol.* 2015;284:551–9.
14. Djuric D, Kleinebudde P. Impact of screw elements on continuous granulation with a twin-screw extruder. *J Pharm Sci.* 2008;97:4934–42.
15. Thompson MR, Sun J. Wet granulation in a twin-screw extruder: Implications of screw design. *J Pharm Sci.* 2010;99:2090–103.
16. Van Melkebeke B, Vervaet C, Remon JP. Validation of a continuous granulation process using a twin-screw extruder. *Int J Pharm.* 2008;356:224–30.
17. Ghebre-Sellassie I, Mollan MJ, Pathak N, Lodaya M, Fessehaie M. 2002. US6499984.
18. El Hagrasy AS, Litster JD. Granulation rate processes in the kneading elements of a twin screw granulator. *AIChE J.* 2013;59:4100–15.
19. Li H, Thompson MR, O'Donnell KP. Understanding wet granulation in the kneading block of twin screw extruders. *Chem Eng Sci.* 2014;113:11–21.
20. Vercruysse J, Cordoba Díaz D, Peeters E et al. Continuous twin screw granulation: Influence of process variables on granule and tablet quality. *Eur J Pharm Biopharm.* 2012;82:205–11.
21. Vercruysse J, Toiviainen M, Fonteyne M et al. Visualization and understanding of the granulation liquid mixing and distribution during continuous twin screw granulation using NIR chemical imaging. *Eur J Pharma Biopharma.* 2014;86:383–92.
22. Lee KT, Ingram A, Rowson NA. Twin screw wet granulation: The study of a continuous twin screw granulator using positron emission particle tracking (PEPT) technique. *Eur J Pharma Biopharma.* 2012;81:666–73.
23. Sayin R, El Hagrasy AS, Litster JD. Distributive mixing elements: Towards improved granule attributes from a twin screw granulation process. *Chem Eng Sci.* 2015;125:165–75.
24. Sheskey P, Keary C, Clark D, Balwinski K. Scale-up trials of foam-granulation technology—High shear. *Pharm Technol.* 2007;31(4):94–108.
25. Iveson SM, Litster JD, Hapgood K, Ennis BJ. Nucleation, growth and breakage phenomena in agitated wet granulation processes: A review. *Powder Technol.* 2001;117:3–39.
26. Dhenge RM, Cartwright JJ, Hounslow MJ, Salman AD. Twin screw granulation: Steps in granule growth. *Int J Pharm.* 2012;438:20–32.
27. Kumar A, Vercruysse J, Bellandi G, Gernaey KV, Vervaet C, Remon JP, Nopens I. Experimental investigation of granule size and shape dynamics in twin-screw granulation. *Intern J Pharm.* 2014;475:485–95.

28. Mu B, Thompson MR. Examining the mechanics of granulation with a hot melt binder in a twin-screw extruder. *Chem Eng Sci.* 2012;81:46–56.
29. Qiu Z, Li S, Benjamin DE. 2011. US20110092515.
30. Thompson MR. Twin screw granulation—Review of current progress. *Drug Dev Ind Pharma.* 2014; doi:10.3109/03639045.2014.983931 (in-press).
31. Kumar A, Gernaey KV, Beer TD, Nopens I. Model-based analysis of high shear wet granulation from batch to continuous processes in pharmaceutical production—A critical review. *Eur J Pharm Biopharm.* 2013;85:814–32.
32. Djuric D, Van Melkebeke B, Kleinebudde P, Remon JP, Vervaet C. Comparison of two twin-screw extruders for continuous granulation. *Eur J Pharm Biopharm.* 2009;71:155–60.
33. Kumar A, Vercruysse J, Toiviainen M et al. Mixing and transport during pharmaceutical twin-screw wet granulation: Experimental analysis via chemical imaging. *Eur J Pharm Biopharm.* 2014;87:279–89.
34. Barrasso D, El Hagrasy A, Litster JD, Ramachandran R. Multi-dimensional population balance model development and validation for a twin screw granulation process. *Powder Technol.* 2015;270:612–21.
35. Dhenge RM, Cartwright JJ, Doughty DG, Hounslow MJ, Salman AD. Twin screw wet granulation: Effect of powder feed rate. *Adv Powder Technol.* 2011;22:162–6.
36. Tu WD, Ingram A, Seville J. Regime map development for continuous twin screw granulation. *Chem Eng Sci.* 2013;87:315–26.
37. Weatherley S, Thompson MR, Sheskey PJ. A study of foam granulation and wet granulation in a twin screw extruder. *Can J Chem Eng.* 2013;91:725–30.
38. Lee KT, Ingram A, Rowson NA. Comparison of granule properties produced using twin screw extruder and high shear mixer: A step towards understanding the mechanism of twin screw wet granulation. *Powder Technol.* 2013;238:91–8.
39. Barrasso D, Walia S, Ramachandran R. Multi-component population balance modeling of continuous granulation processes: A parametric study and comparison with experimental trends. *Powder Technol.* 2013;241:85–97.
40. Fonteyne M, Fussell AL, Vercruysse J, Vervaet C, Remon JP, Strachan C, De Beer T. Distribution of binder in granules produced by means of twin screw granulation. *Int J Pharm.* 2014;462:8–10.
41. Schæfer T, Mathiesen C. Melt pelletization in a high shear mixer. IX. Effects of binder particle size. *Int J Pharm.* 1996;139:139–48.
42. Van Melkebeke B, Vermeulen B, Vervaet C, Remon JP. Melt granulation using a twin-screw extruder: A case study. *Int J Pharm.* 2006;326:89–93.
43. Keen JM, Foley CJ, Hughey JR, Bennett RC, Jannin V, Rosiaux Y, Marchaud D, McGinity JW. Continuous twin screw melt granulation of glyceryl behenate: Development of controlled release tramadol hydrochloride tablets for improved safety. *Int J Pharm.* 2015;487:72–80.
44. Tan DCT, Chin WWL, Tan EH, Hong S, Gu W, Gokhale R. Effect of binders on the release rates of direct molded verapamil tablets using twin-screw extruder in melt granulation. *Int J Pharm.* 2014;463:89–97.
45. Vasanthavada M, Wang YF, Haefele T et al. Application of melt granulation technology using twin-screw extruder in development of high-dose modified-release tablet formulation. *J Pharm Sci.* 2011;100:1923–34.
46. Lakshman JP, Kowalski J, Vasanthavada M, Tong WQ, Joshi YM, Serajuddin ATM. Application of melt granulation technology to enhance tabletting properties of poorly compactible high-dose drugs. *J Pharm Sci.* 2011;100:1553–65.
47. Weatherley S, Mu B, Thompson MR, Sheskey PJ, O'Donnell KP. Hot-melt granulation in a twin screw extruder: Effects of processing on formulations with caffeine and ibuprofen. *J Pharm Sci.* 2013;102(12):4330–6.

48. Ghebre-Sellassie I, Martin C. *Pharmaceutical extrusion technology.* New York: M. Dekker; 2003, 400 pp.
49. Schroeder R. 2004, Planetary Roller, Presented at: Novel approaches for oral solid dosage forms, ISPE May 13-14, Brussels, Belgium.
50. Nyström C, Karehill PG. The importance of intermolecular bonding forces and the concept of bonding surface area. In *Pharmaceutical powder compaction technology*; Alderborn G, Nyström C, Eds. 1996. New York: Marcel Dekker, Inc., pp 17–53.
51. Tousey MD. Optimal tablet press operation—Machine versus granulation. *Pharma Technol.* 2002; 52–60.
52. Matero S, van Den Berg F, Poutiainen S, Rantanen J, Pajander J. Towards better process understanding: Chemometrics and multivariate measurements in manufacturing of solid dosage forms. *J Pharm Sci.* 2013;102:1385–403.
53. Shiraishi T, Yaguchi Y, Kondo S, Yuasa H, Kanaya Y. Studies on the granulation process of granules for tableting with a high speed mixer. 3. Analysis of the compression process. *Chem Pharm Bull.* 1997;45(8):1312–6.
54. Vercruysse J, Delaet U, Van Assche I, Cappuyns P, Arata F, Caporicci G, De Beer T, Remon JP, Vervaet C. Stability and repeatability of a continuous twin screw granulation and drying system. *Eur J Pharm Biopharm.* 2013;85:1031–8.
55. Lee SL, O'Connor TF, Yang X, Cruz CN, Chatterjee S, Madurawe RD, Moore CMV, Yu LX, Woodcock J. Modernizing pharmaceutical manufacturing: From batch to continuous production. *J Pharm Innov.* 2015;10:191–9.
56. Allison G, Cain YT, Cooney C et al. Regulatory and quality considerations for continuous manufacturing. May 20–21, 2014 Continuous manufacturing symposium. *J Pharm Sci.* 2015;104:803–12.
57. Myerson AS, Krumme M, Nasr M, Thomas H, Braatz RD. Control systems engineering in continuous pharmaceutical manufacturing. May 20–21, 2014 Continuous manufacturing symposium. *J Pharm Sci.* 2015;104:832–9.
58. Yu LX, Amidon G, Khan MA et al. Understanding pharmaceutical quality by design. *AAPS J.* 2014;16:771–83.
59. Badman C, Trout BL. Achieving continuous manufacturing. May 20–21, 2014 Continuous manufacturing symposium. *J Pharm Sci.* 2015;104:779–80.
60. Tan MXL, Wong LS, Lum KH, Hapgood KP. Foam and drop penetration kinetics into loosely packed powder beds. *Chem Eng Sci.* 2009;64:2826–2836.

17 Installation, Commissioning, and Qualification

Adam Dreiblatt

CONTENTS

17.1 INTRODUCTION

It is not within the scope of this chapter to describe validation concepts in general, but rather, to identify those aspects of melt extrusion that differentiate it from the validation of conventional pharmaceutical equipment and processes. Because melt extrusion technology is still a relatively new pharmaceutical unit operation, the installation, commissioning, and validation of extrusion equipment have not been widely discussed in the pharmaceutical literature (1). Extruders are still rather unfamiliar to those writing validation protocols, creating problems in both documentation and expectations for the users of such equipment. It is the objective of this chapter to provide an overview for developers of validation protocols as well as for project engineers responsible for installing and commissioning melt extrusion equipment.

Extruders, which were originally designed for use in the plastics processing industry, have been modified to suit the needs of the pharmaceutical industry. While suppliers of "traditional" pharmaceutical equipment are intimately familiar with cGMP requirements in terms of machine design and documentation, extruder manufacturers needed to learn and identify the unique needs of the users who, in most cases, were unfamiliar with the equipment. It is this difference that makes the commissioning and the qualification of extrusion equipment more complicated than normal.

17.2 INSTALLATION

Some aspects of the melt extrusion process, which may not be obvious but require special attention for a successful installation, are listed below.

17.2.1 FLOOR SPACE REQUIREMENTS

One major difference between extruders used for pharmaceutical applications and those used for "conventional" plastics processing is in the solubility of the polymers used in the formulations. Most thermoplastics are hydrocarbon based and are relatively insoluble as a result. This property allows water to be used in direct contact with the extruded material as a cooling medium to solidify the melt for further processing. Plastics are extruded as molten strands and are typically drawn through a water trough to cool the material below its T_g for pelletizing. Direct contact with water provides efficient cooling, thereby minimizing the residence time required in water.

Because most of the polymers used in pharmaceutical applications are water soluble or have some degree of water solubility, direct contact with water for cooling and solidification of the extruded melt is not possible. This implies cooling in air or using indirect water-cooled surfaces (e.g., cooling belts and/or chilled rolls) and longer residence times for cooling. The consequence is increased floor space requirements for these applications. It is not uncommon for downstream cooling equipment to take up more than three to four times as much floor space as the extrusion equipment. This does not include the subsequent pelletizing equipment, which would follow the cooling step. The extruded strands must be in-line with the extruder or the die can be oriented 90° to extrude at a right angle from the extruder centerline. In either case, a substantial amount of length may be needed downstream of the extruder. Thus, the floor space for melt extrusion applications should be considered prior to installation in an existing area.

17.2.2 CEILING HEIGHT

While the extruder discharge is in a horizontal plane (the standard centerline height for twin-screw extruders is approximately 1.1 m), the extruder itself does not require very much floor space nor does it require much headroom. It is the continuous operation of the feeding equipment situated directly over the extruder that can impose some height restrictions. Because the extruder is a continuous device, the feeder will need to be refilled several times. Refilling the feeder can be done manually or automatically; it is the automatic refill systems that can require considerable headroom above the feeder (refill hopper plus associated conveying equipment and refill valves).

17.2.3 FUGITIVE DUST

The material discharged from the feeder(s) into the extruder may produce some fugitive dust at the feed opening of the extruder. The refilling of the feeder may also produce some fugitive dust (especially for manual refill systems). The degree to which this dust becomes airborne depends on the material. Standard dust extraction hoods and systems should be considered in the vicinity of the feeder inlet port as well as the extruder feed opening. The extruder feed opening must be permitted to "breathe" to remove the air introduced into the extruder via the powder feed.

17.2.4 FUME EXHAUST

Depending upon the materials being processed, there may be some fumes present at the extruder discharge as a result of the material being exposed to the room environment at an elevated temperature. Whether fume extraction hoods are required will depend on the nature of the materials being processed and the product temperature at the discharge.

17.2.5 AUXILIARY EQUIPMENT

Auxiliary support equipment for the extruder (water circulator for barrel cooling, vacuum pump, etc.) can be located outside of the process area for convenience. Utility connections can be made at wall-mounted panels to connect to the extruder via quick-connect fittings and flexible hoses.

17.3 COMMISSIONING

The act of commissioning relies on a "quality by design" approach to ensure that critical aspects are designed into systems during the specification and design process. This is achieved through a planned and structured verification approach applied throughout the system's life cycle and will ensure that manufacturing systems are fit for use (2). Sufficient resources and time must be allocated in the project schedule to coordinate commissioning efforts with the construction, installation, and validation activities. It is also important to remember that all equipment must be commissioned; however, only equipment that has a direct impact upon or is critical to product quality needs to be validated.

In nonpharmaceutical applications of extrusion equipment, the commissioning process is called "startup" and is typically a "make it work" effort with no clearly defined objectives or schedule. It is often left up to the vendor to debug the system after installation. For the commissioning of melt extrusion equipment for pharmaceutical applications, commissioning includes startup, operator training, instrument calibration, verification of "as-built" documentation, etc. The commissioning of melt extrusion equipment provides an opportunity for operators, engineers, and maintenance personnel to become familiar with the equipment. At this point, there are still minor modifications that may be made to the equipment and/or installation prior to executing IQ protocols. Commissioning is also an opportunity to revise installation qualification/operational qualification/performance qualification (IQ/OQ/PQ) protocols based upon the "as-built" installation and/or equipment.

17.4   QUALIFICATION

The equipment involved in the melt extrusion process is still required to comply with cGMP regulations covered in CFR 21, Part 211.63, "equipment used in the manufacture, processing, packing, or holding of a drug product shall be of appropriate design, adequate size, and suitably located to facilitate operations for its intended use and for its cleaning and maintenance (3,4)."

The validation process is no different for an extruder; the Validation Master Plan sets the scope and the strategy for validation activities (5):

- Introduction (objective, validation scope, etc.)
- Definition of validation concepts (identify systems that require validation, definition of IQ, OQ, PQ, etc.)
- Process description (design criteria, flow diagrams, material balance, process instrumentation and control, etc.)
- Facility description (overall layout, area classification, material/personnel flow, HVAC requirements, etc.)
- Validation activities [process systems, utility systems, calibration, standard operating procedures (SOPs)]
- Validation approach (acceptance criteria, assumptions, approval procedures, etc.)
- Validation schedule
- Validation supplies
- Validation organization

An attempt will be made to identify those "issues" relating specifically to the unique nature of melt extrusion as it pertains to qualification (IQ/OQ/PQ).

It has already been mentioned that melt extrusion is a relatively new process for the pharmaceutical industry. As such, there is a lack of *fundamental* understanding as far as both process and the equipment are concerned (note that this fundamental understanding has been developed within the plastics processing industry over several decades). Without a good understanding of the melt extrusion process, a user requirements specification (URS) is difficult to create.

Without a URS, the equipment supplier's quotation then creates the specifications against which protocols are developed. This situation must change, as the validation strategy is flawed if the equipment supplier is determining the specifications for the process. At a minimum, a specification qualification (SQ) and/or design qualification (DQ) step must be included within the Validation Master Plan, where the melt extrusion process requirements are matched to equipment specifications. The vendor's equipment proposal must meet the specifications required for the process, rather than determine the specifications for the process (6).

The Validation Master Plan must also account for factory acceptance testing (FAT), an often overlooked yet important step in the project life cycle (7). Without experienced equipment specialists on-site, it becomes more difficult to resolve any technical problems after the equipment has been delivered and installed. The FAT provides an opportunity to identify any faults, prequalify draft SOPs, and verify conformance to SQ and/or DQ. A FAT protocol with extensive testing can be used to minimize the IQ/OQ effort on-site. The FAT should include dry and/or wet testing. An increased pressure to meet project deadlines is usually responsible for compromising the scope of the FAT.

17.4.1 INSTALLATION QUALIFICATION

The IQ protocol(s) are developed to challenge the extruder design and the installation. They are typically conducted in a nonoperating mode (i.e., with no power applied). There are several minor differences between an extruder used for melt extrusion and traditional pharmaceutical processing equipment that need to be addressed in an extruder IQ. Some of the typical IQ requirements are listed below.

17.4.1.1 Equipment Identification

No differences are noted; extruder nameplate data (manufacturer, model number, serial number, year of construction, etc.) are typically installed on the gearbox.

17.4.1.2 Lubricants

"Any substance required for operation, such as lubricants or coolants, shall not come into contact with components, drug product containers, closures, in-process materials, or drug products so as to alter the safety, identity, strength, quality, or purity of the drug product beyond the official or other established requirements (3)."

The extruder gearbox requires gear oil, which is contained within the gearbox housing and is isolated from product contact. Food-grade lubricants, which meet the requirements of the gearbox manufacturer, are available. No other lubricants are required.

17.4.1.3   Product Contact Materials of Construction

"Equipment shall be constructed so that surfaces that contact components, in-process materials, or drug products shall not be reactive, additive, or absorptive so as to alter the safety, identity, strength, quality, or purity of the drug product, beyond the official or other established requirements (3)."

This is one area in which extruders differ from traditional pharmaceutical process equipment. Due to the high mechanical stresses involved whereby screws rotate at a relatively high speed (up to 1200 rpm in some cases) with close tolerances (nominal 0.2 mm), it is not possible to manufacture extruder screws and barrels out of 304-type or 316-type stainless steels. These components are typically fabricated from hardenable grades of stainless alloys, similar to those used for tablet tooling (e.g., type 440B stainless steel), and are subject to corrosion if not handled appropriately. Other product contact components that do not experience high mechanical stress (feed hoppers, vent hardware, etc.) can be fabricated from 304-type or 316-type stainless steels. Other possible product contact surfaces are screw shaft seals, typically fabricated from Teflon-type materials. Documentation supporting product contact materials of construction is available from the extruder suppliers.

17.4.1.4   Utility Requirements

Most extruder drives require three-phase power and are available for 208, 230/240, or 460/480 volt service. Most drives are provided with forced-air cooling blowers, which are exhausted into the processing room. Cooling blowers and ductwork can be installed to bring air from outside the processing room and exhaust outside of the processing room.

Compressed air is rarely needed and may be used only on very large extruders for torque-limiting couplings.

The extruder barrels are typically heated using electrical heaters and cooled using a circulating coolant. The circulating coolant does not come in contact with the product and is typically treated water from a cooling tower or from a dedicated temperature control unit. The specifications for water quality are available from the extruder supplier. As the water is in direct contact with the extruder barrel, it is possible to develop some corrosion products over time. The quality of this cooling water can adversely affect the process if sediments that can block the solenoid valves used to control the flow of water through the extruder barrels are present. The installation of a filter in the circulating water system is recommended to avoid this situation. The cooling water should have a temperature control loop; cooling water temperature can vary from 10°C to 90°C.

If a vacuum pump is used as part of the extrusion system, this will also require water to maintain a vacuum seal, as well as a drain. In some instances, effluents from the extruder vent (e.g., noncondensable gases) will also be discharged to the drain, potentially creating some environmental issues.

The support equipment (water circulator, vacuum pump) can be located outside of the processing room, providing the required utilities through a wall-mounted panel.

17.4.1.5   Calibration of Critical Instruments

The critical instruments for a melt extrusion process must be identified. Instruments directly associated with the determination of product quality, which are recorded in a manufacturing batch record, are considered critical; all other instruments are regarded as noncritical. Noncritical instruments should also be calibrated for a new installation.

Those instruments that indicate and/or directly control the extrusion process include controlled parameters and response parameters:

1. *Controlled parameters* are parameters that have a set point and/or a range of set points, including:
   Screw speed
   Extruder barrel/die temperatures
   Vacuum level
   Feed rate
2. *Response parameters* are parameters whose value depends on the controlled parameters:
   Die pressure
   Product temperature
   Extruder load (torque)

There are no unique features for instruments on an extruder that would present any difference from conventional pharmaceutical equipment in terms of calibration.

17.4.1.6 Preventive Maintenance

There is nothing unique about the preventive maintenance of an extruder. The documentation accompanying extruders includes sufficient preventive maintenance information. As extruders are typically operated in a continuous environment, the preventive maintenance intervals may appear to be rather large as compared to traditional pharmaceutical process equipment.

17.4.1.7 Standard Operating Procedures

The procedures necessary for setup, operation, and cleaning of extruders require some special attention. The cleaning of an extruder used for melt extrusion poses the following challenges, which are typically not encountered with traditional pharmaceutical processes:

1. The extruder must be disassembled for cleaning while heated to a temperature above the T_g of the polymer. This can be up to 200°C for some polymers, posing unique safety hazards for the operating staff.
2. The components must be cleaned of molten polymer (versus powders that are typically encountered in traditional cleaning processes). The polymers must be dissolved, degraded, or burned to remove the residues. For controlled-release applications utilizing polymers having low solubility, there are additional challenges to find a suitable cleaning agent if the molten material is not water soluble.
3. The disassembling of the entire extruder process section (including barrels, screws, etc.) is appropriate when changing to a different product or

strength to avoid any possible cross-contamination. This can be a very time-consuming process requiring some mechanical aptitude. Because the screws in most twin-screw extruders are withdrawn from the discharge end of the barrel, the internal barrel surface cannot be visually inspected for cleanliness. Clamshell or split-barrel extruders, which may reduce some of the complexity, are available. The assembly of the segmented screws requires an equal amount of time and mechanical aptitude. Partial cleaning (e.g., between lots) can be accomplished without a disassembly of the screws or barrels.

4. As already mentioned, the major extruder components (barrels and screws) are fabricated from hardenable stainless alloys. These components will require "special" handling for cleaning, similar to tablet tooling; they will show signs of corrosion if left exposed to moisture or humidity. These components must be dried thoroughly after cleaning and maintained in a controlled humidity environment.

Because most extruders employ electrically heated barrels, standard extrusion equipment is not normally designed for wash-down. If required, extruders can be designed where the barrel temperatures are controlled using hot water or other heat transfer fluids in order to provide a wash-down environment.

17.4.1.8 Safety

Apart from the previously mentioned issues of handling the extruder components while in a heated state, there are no additional major safety issues other than site-specific requirements. As extrusion equipment is designed for an industrial environment, machine guarding for pinch points, hot surfaces, and lockout features must meet appropriate regulatory standards (OSHA, UL, CE,* etc.). Noise levels are typically within industry standards (less than 85 dBA).

17.4.2 OPERATIONAL QUALIFICATION

The objective of OQ is to challenge the operational controls, alarms, and interlocks for a given piece of equipment. The systems that should be challenged for melt extrusion need to cover the range of operation for the intended application. Thus, if the processing temperature for a given polymer/active formulation is 100°C, then the extruder temperature controls must be challenged beyond this temperature (e.g., up to 150°C) in order to accommodate the operation within the limits of OQ.

17.4.2.1 Motor Rotation

Because most extruder drives are three-phase drives, the correct rotation must be verified. Correct motor rotation must be confirmed for all other three-phase motors,

---

* OSHA = Occupational Safety and Health Administration; UL = Underwriters Laboratories; CE = mark certifying conformity to European Directives.

including the main drive motor cooling blower, vacuum pump, control panel cooling fans, etc.

17.4.2.2   Operating Controls

The controlled parameters described for calibration must be challenged for both functionality and for the range of operation. The controlled parameters and associated controls include main power disconnect, main drive motor stop/start functionality, range of operation of screw speed (with specified tolerance), vacuum pump stop/start, and range of operation of vacuum level (with specified tolerance). As previously mentioned, the testing range for temperature control of the extruder barrels and die should be outside of the intended operating range for the melt extrusion process. Both heating and cooling functions are to be challenged, with some acceptance criteria for accuracy.

Because twin-screw extruders are modular in design, with an independent control of each barrel module, the temperature limits for each temperature control zone can differ. This represents an additional degree of freedom for challenging the temperature control of the extruder. If the set points for all temperature control zones are tested at a constant value, the functionality (i.e., ability to control and to maintain set point within some degree of accuracy) of the heating and cooling systems can be verified. When the heating controls are to be tested, the extruder feed barrel can be exempted, as this barrel module is typically controlled with manual cooling only and does not have heating capability. When the cooling controls are to be tested, the dies (and associated die adapters) are typically heated only and can be exempted, as these do not have cooling capability.

The best method to test the heating and cooling systems is to verify the accuracy of each temperature control zone to maintain a set point within some acceptance criteria (e.g., ±5°C) over some specified time interval. The data can be recorded in tabular format for each temperature control zone, starting with the time when the set point is entered. The actual temperature is recorded every 10 or 15 minutes over several hours to verify not only accuracy but also temperature stability. The temperature control zones can be tested individually; however, in actual practice, the extruder barrels will all be either heated or cooled to a specific temperature profile. All temperature control zones can be set to the same set point, with several set points being tested both above and below the intended operating range for the melt extrusion process.

17.4.2.3   Alarms/Interlocks

The standard tests for emergency stop switches must be included in this section of the OQ. All extruders have specific alarm and interlock circuitry to prevent damage to the gearbox, which must be challenged:

1. Melt pressure is set up as an alarm to warn of high melt pressure at the extruder die. These are electronic signals from a pressure transducer that can be simulated to verify the alarm circuitry.

2. Melt pressure is also set up as an interlock to shut down the extruder drive when melt pressure exceeds the manufacturer's recommended maximum

limit. A signal can be generated to activate and verify the interlock circuitry.

3. Gearbox oil temperature and pressure may be set up either to signal an alarm condition or as an interlock to shut down the drive motor in the event of low or high oil pressure and high oil temperature. Signals can be generated to simulate these conditions and to verify the alarm/interlock circuitry.

4. The feeding equipment for the extruder, while not directly part of the extruder itself, must be tested for accuracy and precision. The test procedure for determining accuracy and precision involves operating the feeder with representative material(s) at a specified feed rate set point. Consecutive timed samples (e.g., one min) are obtained and weighed on a precision balance; the weights are converted to feed rates. Accuracy is then defined as a percent deviation of the mean feed rate from the feed rate setpoint. Precision is defined as relative standard deviation (RSD) and can be described at one or two standard deviations. Acceptance criteria must take into account the nature of the materials used for testing, as the accuracy and precision of feeding equipment are primarily dependent on the flowability of the material (8). If a placebo is used for OQ testing, the placebo should be representative of the materials that will actually be used in the feeding equipment.

17.4.3 PERFORMANCE QUALIFICATION

The purpose of PQ is "establishing documented evidence which provides a high degree of assurance that a specific process will consistently produce a product meeting its predetermined specifications and quality attributes" (9). This is typically accomplished through extended time studies or process runs where the system can be challenged at "worst-case" conditions. Worst case is defined as "a set of conditions encompassing upper and lower processing limits and circumstances, including those within standard operating procedures, which pose the greatest chance of process or product failure when compared to ideal conditions (such conditions do not necessarily induce product or process failure)." For a melt extrusion process, those conditions include extremes of feed rate, screw speed, barrel temperatures, and in some cases the screw design.

Performance qualification typically includes a minimum of three valid consecutive runs. The length of time required for each run can vary from hours (e.g., kilograms) to days (e.g., full batch), using either placebo or active compound. The extrusion process is a continuous process and reaches equilibrium within the first few minutes. Samples and data obtained at frequent intervals can be used to verify process stability and consistency.

Acceptance criteria should be specified for both extrusion response parameters (extruder torque, melt pressure, melt temperature) and for product performance (e.g., dissolution profile, percent crystallinity, etc.). The goal of PQ is for the product to meet the acceptance criteria at the specified extrusion operating conditions. Different lots of raw materials should also be included as part of the PQ.

17.4.4 COMPUTER VALIDATION

The relatively small volume of an extruder, coupled with an electronic batch record, provides unique capabilities that are not possible with a traditional batch process. As an example,

1. Assume a melt extrusion process with a 600-kg batch size.
2. Assume an extruder capacity of 12 kg/hr (200 g/min). The batch will take 50 hr of continuous operation for completion.
3. Assume a nominal mean residence time of approximately one min within the extruder (typical value). The volume of material contained within the extruder at any given moment is approximately 200 g (200-g/min feed rate and nominal residence time of one min).
4. A computer-based data acquisition system could record all process data approximately every 15 sec (four times per minute, or four times per 200 g).
5. The process is documented (feed rate, screw speed, temperatures, pressure, torque, etc.) for every 50 g of material throughout the 600-kg batch.

Electronic control and data acquisition systems are common in nonpharmaceutical extrusion applications where validation is not required. These systems are based on industry-standard hardware and software with application-specific software written as a "front end" for screen graphics. There are no requirements for audits, change control, documentation, etc. in the polymer processing industry.

The requirements for electronic documentation systems to comply with 21 CFR Part 11, however, can involve significant validation effort (10). The responsibility can be placed on the supplier to provide a system that is 21 CFR Part 11-compliant, thereby reducing the problems with validating noncompliant systems (11). In the end, it is the responsibility of the user to ensure compliance of electronic systems.

17.5 CONCLUSION

As more companies explore the benefits of melt extrusion technology, it is becoming more accepted as a pharmaceutical unit operation. This is evidenced by the increase in technical publications and the issuance of patents over the past five years. As a result, the extrusion equipment suppliers are responding to these new applications with improved designs and documentation.

From a regulatory perspective, there is no difference between an extruder and any other piece of process equipment. It is the users of this equipment who need to understand what is unique about an extruder as far as validation is concerned. Most of the challenges and issues are cultural rather than technical and require an industry based on batch processing to embrace a continuous technology. As with any other technology, well-written procedures (together with a documented training program) are needed for validating, operating, cleaning, calibrating, and maintaining extrusion equipment and process(es). Well-written procedures require an in-depth knowledge of materials, process, and equipment as well as the interaction between them. It will take time for the pharmaceutical industry to develop the same type of fundamental understanding for melt extrusion as currently exists for other technologies (compressing, granulating, etc.).

REFERENCES

1. Grünhagen HH, Müller O. Melt extrusion technology. *Pharm Manuf Int* 1995; 167–170.
2. Dolgin, David. Commissioning and Qualification (Verification) in the Pharmaceutical Product Process Lifecycle. 2013.
3. Food and Drug Administration. Code of federal regulations. 21 CFR Parts 210 and 211. Fed Regist 2017.
4. Cantwell J. Validation protocols. *Pharm Eng* 1999; 4:46–49.
5. Saxton B. Reasons, regulations, and rules: A guide to the Validation Master Plan (VMP). *Pharm Eng* 2001; 3:18–26.
6. Lange BH. GMP manufacturing equipment purchase and qualification: An integrated approach. *Pharm Eng* 1997; 1:18–24.
7. Roberge MG. Factory Acceptance Testing (FAT) of pharmaceutical equipment. *Pharm Eng* 2000; 6:8–16.
8. Wilson D. *Feeding Technology for Plastics Processing*. Munich: Carl Hanser Verlag, 1998.
9. Amer G. An overview of process validation (PV). *Pharm Eng* 2000; 5:62–76.
10. 21 CFR 11. Electronic records, electronic signatures final rule. *Fed Regist* 2017; 62:13430–13466.
11. Picot VS, McDowall RD. Containing the 21 CFR 11 problem: Purchase of noncompliant systems. *Am Pharm Rev* 2001; 1:91–96.

18 Extrusion Control Systems

Stuart J. Kapp and Pete A. Palmer

CONTENTS

18.1 INTRODUCTION

The extrusion control system is referred to as not only the operator-machine inter-face and monitoring center, but also all the individual motors, drives, temperature controllers, and measurement devices required to manage the extrusion process. Precise control (and monitoring) of process variables provides the ability to produce a product with repeatable accuracy, high productivity, and low waste. At the same

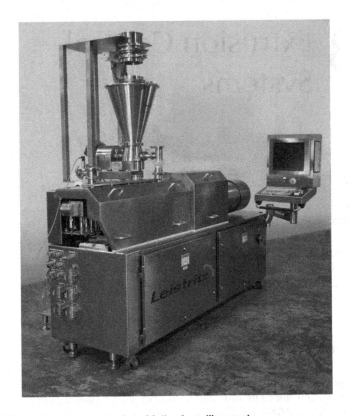

FIGURE 18.1   Twin-screw extruder with "on-board" controls.

time, accurate control and monitoring of the extrusion process is extremely important in troubleshooting, and for documentation and quality control purposes.

Typical variables that need to be *controlled* in pharmaceutical extrusions are feed rates of the individual ingredients (feedstreams), barrel/die (zone) temperatures, motor speed, and occasionally discharge pressure (Figure 18.1).

Variables and parameters that need to be *measured and monitored* during the extrusion process include screw speed, set vs. actual temperatures, motor load, "melt" pressure, "melt" temperature, and vacuum level.

Generally speaking, extruder controls can be managed by one or a combination of manual/discrete instruments, a personal computer (PC), and/or programmable logic controllers (PLCs). Specifics on each type of machine controls will be discussed in further detail in Section 18.4.

The operator would typically interface with the extruder control systems either by pressing or adjusting manual/discrete operators or by touchscreen operators on a human-machine interface (HMI) or by software control on a PC control system.

18.2   EXTRUDER TEMPERATURE CONTROL

Accurate temperature control of the extruder barrel, die, and auxiliary equipment is important for any application, but it is even more critical for pharmaceutical applications. External heating is required to bring the extruder and die up to the operating temperature, and to maintain that temperature for the duration of the process. During continuous operation, most extruders impart large amounts of energy at the screw/material/barrel interface, resulting in considerable heat rise. This mechanical energy input makes sufficient cooling of the extruder just as important as heating.

Extruders utilize one of two methods of heating: electrical or via heat-transfer fluid. Most of today's extruders are heated by means of high wattage electric heaters. A limited number of applications, particularly those that run at low temperatures (0–50°C), utilize liquid temperature control.

Cooling, when required, is accomplished through controlled quantities of either air or fluid. Heat-transfer fluids common to extrusion are oil (synthetic or hydrocarbon-based), water, glycol, or a mixture of water and glycol.

18.2.1 ELECTRIC HEATING

Electric heating is, by far, the most common method of heating modern extrusion machinery, including a vast majority of those machines processing pharmaceuticals. Electric heating offers numerous advantages over liquid, including low cost, simplistic design, wide range of temperature control, and decreased maintenance. Electric heaters, whether they are a cartridge or "band" type, are placed along the length of the extruder barrel and die. These heaters are arranged in groups called zones. Each "zone" of the extruder is independently controlled. Smaller extruders may have as few as two or three zones, while larger, longer extruders may utilize as many as 10–15 (or more) zones (Figure 18.2).

Electric resistance heaters are based on the principle of heat generation as a result of current passing through a conductor. The amount of heat generated by any

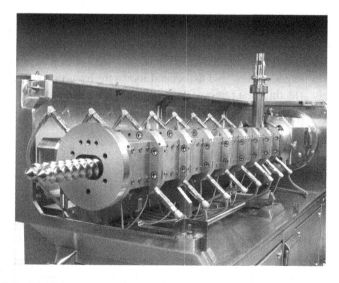

FIGURE 18.2 Multiple extruder barrel temperature zones (note supply and return piping for water cooling on each zone).

resistance-type heater is determined by the resistance of that heater and the current flow through it. Accordingly, it is the responsibility of the microprocessor-based temperature controllers to precisely control current flow.

18.2.2   LIQUID HEATING

Heating by means of liquid media offers distinct advantages in its uniformity and its absence of localized overheating or "hot spots." For these reasons, liquid heating is sometimes preferred for heat sensitive formulations. Conversely, using heat transfer fluids as a method of heating has considerable drawbacks, including high temperature limitations, possibility of leakage, costly periodic disposal of heat transfer oil, and an overall increase in maintenance.

18.2.3   AIR COOLING

Cooling of the extruder barrel can be accomplished by means of air, water, or oil. Although some dies require extremely tight temperature control and are cooled, this is the exception rather than the norm. While some very small machines may use compressed air through a regulator and solenoid valve arrangement, most air-cooled machines utilize on-board cooling fans, which are activated by their respective temperature controllers (Figure 18.3). In either case, air is forced through jackets or across fins that surround the individual barrel zones. More common, in today's modern production-scale extruders, and especially in more critical pharmaceutical applications, is the use of water as a cooling medium.

18.2.4   LIQUID COOLING

In addition to water, liquid-cooling systems may utilize oil, glycol, or synthetic heat-transfer fluids. In most cases, a mixture of water/glycol offers the best solution, as most heat transfer glycols are formulated with special additives to minimize mineral deposits and scaling commonly found in tap water. These additives prevent cooling lines, bores, passages, valves, and associated hardware from prematurely clogging and negatively affecting heat removal.

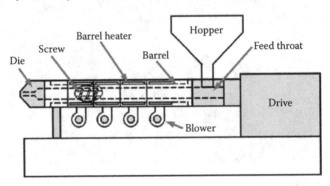

FIGURE 18.3   Extruder with barrel heaters and blowers for air cooling.

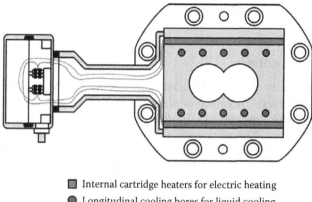

■ Internal cartridge heaters for electric heating

● Longitudinal cooling bores for liquid cooling

FIGURE 18.4 Cross section of twin-screw extruder barrel with internal cooling bores.

Liquid-cooled extruders circulate the media through passages surrounding the barrel, including the feed throat (which is often cooled-only). These passages may be internally cored in the shell of the extruder barrel or in simple systems, externally mounted bands, or jackets (Figure 18.4). A closed-loop system, consisting of a pump, filter, and heat exchanger, is commonly used to supply a constant supply of tempered water to the extruder barrels (Figure 18.5). Alternately, and typically at a higher cost, an air-cooled refrigerated chiller may be used for the same purpose, thereby

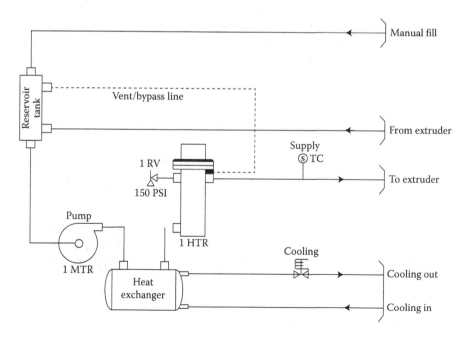

FIGURE 18.5 Closed-loop heat exchanger.

alleviating the need for a city or tower water supply to remove the process heat from the heat exchanger.

18.2.5 THERMOCOUPLES

Zone temperature is monitored by means of thermocouples or resistance temperature detectors (RTDs). Thermocouples are widely used as a result of their reliability, small size, low cost, and ease of use. Thermocouples use very low voltage to transmit their signals. Thermocouples are constructed of two dissimilar metal wires with differing thermoelectric behavior. When a variation in temperature is sensed, a small voltage is produced. The level of this millivolt signal is directly related to the temperature of the junction, and thus is a very reliable method of measuring temperature.

Thermocouples may be constructed of numerous different metals, each with their own unique thermoelectric behavior. Accepted types of thermocouples have been standardized by organizations such as the American National Standards Institute (ANSI). Each type is specified by a letter (i.e., J, K, T, E). J-type thermocouples are most commonly used in extrusion applications, while K-type thermocouples and RTDs may be utilized for higher temperature or more demanding applications (Figure 18.6).

18.2.6 TEMPERATURE CONTROLLERS

Thermocouple signals are interpreted by temperature controllers, which compare the actual measured temperature against the target setpoint. These temperature controllers then calculate the appropriate output required to achieve the desired setpoint. Most of today's temperature controllers utilize microprocessor or PLC-based proportional-integral-derivative (P-I-D) algorithms to precisely control extruder temperature (Figure 18.7).

While these PLC and microprocessor-based controllers have numerous operator selectable parameters, the three main parameters that determine the proper operation of a temperature controller are the proportional band, the integral band, and the derivative band.

The proportional band is a band or range of temperatures over which power is proportioned or reduced as the setpoint is approached. This allows for a continuous adjustment of the output power (heating or cooling) depending on the actual

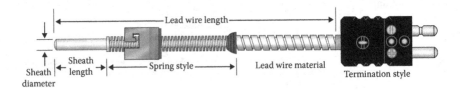

FIGURE 18.6   Type "J" control thermocouple.

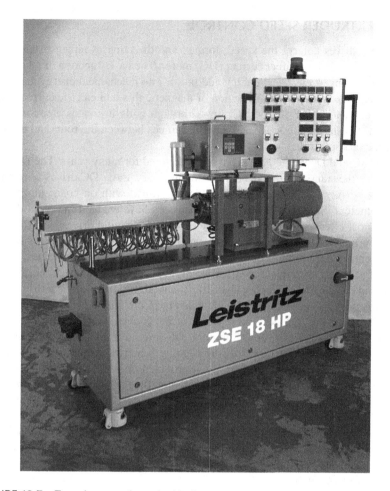

FIGURE 18.7   Extruder control panel with discrete temperature controllers.

temperature at any given time. The proportional band is adjustable to yield stable temperature control over a wide range of process conditions. The proportional band is typically specified in terms of percentage of instrument span.

The integral band is used to "automatically reset" or continuously adjust the level of the proportional band until the deviation is zero. Once this is achieved, the integrator holds the correct amount of "reset" until the process heat requirements change or the temperature is disrupted.

The derivative band helps to prevent overshooting of the temperature setpoint by compensating for the rate of change. This feature is an anticipatory function that adjusts the output, in an attempt to predict heating/cooling needs. Derivative control is critical in larger machines, where temperature changes occur slowly. Smaller extruders, on the other hand, react much more rapidly to temperature changes, and are less dependent on the derivative band.

18.3 EXTRUDER SPEED CONTROL

Electronic drives control the speed, torque, and direction of either an alternating current (AC) motor or direct current (DC) motor. The basic function of a DC or AC motor is to convert electrical energy and power into mechanical energy and power. Motors operate through the interaction of magnetic flux and electric current. When electric current, either AC or DC, flows through coils it creates electromagnetic energy; the resulting attractive and repelling forces between the rotor and the stator cause the motor to spin.

Both AC and DC technologies have been around for many years. The DC drive/ motor was the standard for extruders for many years. Early DC drives were analog electronic drives and as such were set up and tuned with on-board jumpers and potentiometers. Since the 1980s microprocessors have enabled the rapid development of cost-effective digital drives. The evolution of digital drives has brought the following advantages: improved reliability through a reduction in the number of components, elimination of drift problems associated with analog values, extreme levels of accuracy, excellent repeatability, digital communications, increased monitoring and diagnostics, complex algorithms, and ability to autotune a drive (match motor to control). The AC drive greatly benefited from digital drive technology and allowed the AC drive to perform equal to or better than the DC drive. AC motors have several advantages over DC motors. DC motors use brushes and commutators to provide electrical power to the rotating armature (rotor). This equipment requires constant maintenance and is not provided on AC motors. AC motors are also suitable for harsh, rugged environments (totally enclosed motors go up to high horsepower (HP) ranges and can be made explosion proof or wash-down rated) and have wider speed ranges (many standard inverter duty motors can go twice their base speed). The AC drive has more precise open-loop speed regulation, longer power-dip ride-through capabilities due to power storage elements on a DC bus, and a near-unity power factor regardless of speed or load. The future of extruders is AC drive/motor technology.

AC drives control speed (and torque) by converting AC to DC and then back to variable AC. AC drives convert *fixed* voltage and frequency into *variable* voltage and frequency, in order to run three-phase induction motors. Inside small AC inverter drives, power is rectified to DC using uncontrolled rectifiers. Larger AC drives rely on silicon controlled rectifiers (SCRs) to perform the same task. The DC power is then filtered and converted back to AC using solid-state transistor switches.

AC drives operate by varying the frequency and voltage to an AC motor. The frequency of the applied power to an AC motor determines the motor speed. To maintain constant torque, the drive must maintain a constant voltage-per-hertz ratio. Pulse width modulated (PWM) drive techniques (to control the inverter bridge) are by far the most popular technology for providing a simulated variable sine wave to the motor. PWM-type drives have historically required a more complex regulator than previous designs; however, the use of today's high-powered microprocessors has all but eliminated this problem. Microprocessors and other recent technological advances in digital AC variable frequency drives now allow them to support applications for which DC drive technology was traditionally the choice.

There are three basic types of AC drives: open-loop voltage/hertz drives, open-loop vector or sensorless vector drives, and flux vector or closed-loop vector drives.

1. *Open-loop voltage/Hz (V/Hz) drives:* This is the most basic type of AC drive. Open loop means there are no speed feedback devices. Motor voltage is varied linearly with frequency. Most V/Hz drives cannot separate torque-producing current from flux-producing current, so the V/Hz drive cannot regulate torque. The main drawback with voltage/Hz drives is that they cannot compensate for motor and load dynamics, resulting in poor speed regulation. V/Hz drives also lack low speed/starting torque. Advantages of V/Hz drives include easy setup, low cost, and a lack of required feedback devices.

2. *Open-loop vector or sensorless vector:* This type of drive is also open loop and does not require an encoder or tachometer to feed motor data back to the drive. Instead, open-loop vector drives utilize an advanced algorithm that creates a mathematical model of the motor's electrical characteristics to provide feedback within the drive. This configuration allows the drive to respond to sudden load changes by calling for more or less torque-producing current. Although sensorless vector drives yield higher low-speed torque, they lack the dynamic response or high-performance speed regulation of the flux vector drive.

3. *Flux vector or closed-loop vector:* This drive does require a motor-mounted feedback device to supply information to the drive on the rotor's position relative to the stator. The flux vector drive can control both the flux-producing current and torque-producing current of the motor. This allows the drive to regulate both speed and torque. This drive can provide full torque at zero speed and most can provide 150% starting torque. The flux vector drive has excellent shock load response characteristics and high-performance speed regulation. Many of today's drives can provide all three modes of operation in one drive. Changing from one mode to another mode would be a single software parameter.

Many AC drives have industrial networking capabilities. This allows the drive to digitally communicate to other drives, programmable controllers, and/or PC control systems. Digital communications to drives and devices bring numerous advantages. These include a reduction in interconnection wiring (one communications cable would replace most of the hardwired input/output to a drive or drives); the ability to display faults, settings, and feedback parameters on a central monitor for diagnostic purposes; and the increased accuracy of digital settings. Digital communications also eliminate drift associated with analog devices and inherent inaccuracies related with analog-to-digital converters. There are many different types of industrial network technologies used with digital drives. Some are proprietary and some are open networks. Open networks are accessible to anyone or any manufacturer that wants to make a product "talk" on that network. One of the more popular industrial networks is Ethernet communications using an industrial Ethernet protocol.

The AC "squirrel cage" induction motor is the fundamental workhorse of industry. The basic parts of a three-phase AC induction motor consist of a rotor, a stator, and two end shields housing the bearings that support the rotor shaft. The stator is the nonrotating component that contains the three-phase windings. The revolving section of the motor is the rotor containing steel laminations around the motor shaft. AC power is supplied directly to the stator and produces a rotating magnetic field. The motion of the magnetic field induces a magnetic field in the rotor. The induced field in the rotor rotates with the magnetic field in the stator and causes the motor to spin.

Early AC inverter drives were connected to regular AC induction motors. AC PWM inverters can yield very high switching frequencies and very rapid changes in voltage that commonly result in pinholes in the insulation, causing short circuits and premature motor failure. Many motor manufacturers introduced lines of motors they call inverter duty or vector duty motors. High dielectric strength wire insulation is typically found in these motors to resist such pinholes. Cooling performance can be increased by simply adding constant speed blowers or by using oversized frames in nonventilated motors. AC motors allow for feedback sensing and wider speed ranges.

AC motors are encased in protective enclosures. The basic protective enclosures for AC motors are totally enclosed nonventilated (TENV), totally enclosed fan cooled (TEFC), totally enclosed blower cooled (TEBC), and drip-proof force ventilated (DPFV). Much of the heat generated by an AC induction motor is in the stator. The outside frame of the motor is designed with fins to help dissipate the heat to the immediate atmosphere. Totally enclosed nonventilated motors have no ventilation. They utilize an internal fan connected directly to the motor shaft to prevent overheating. TENV motors dissipate heat through the frame of the motor, thereby requiring a larger frame as compared to the other motor enclosures of equivalent HP rating. The TENV frames are usually seen in the lower HP range. TEFC motors are totally enclosed like the TENV but have a fan on the back of the motor that blows air over the outside of the motor at the same speed as the shaft rotates. TEBC motors are also totally enclosed but provide a separate blower motor that blows air over the outside of the motor at a constant velocity. Totally enclosed motors can be provided in explosion proof construction. Totally enclosed motors are also good for environments that are excessively dusty or dirty. The DPFV motor also has a separate blower motor and provides forced cooling air through the middle of the motor. These enclosures are typically used on larger horsepower motors.

Permanent magnet motors have been around for a long time but only recently are they starting to be used in extruder applications. Permanent magnet AC motors (PMAC) have permanent magnets mounted to the rotor. Electrical power is supplied to the PMAC motor's stator windings just like the AC induction motor. However, while AC induction motors induce a field onto the stator, PMAC motors have a constant field provided by the permanent magnets. These permanent magnet stators are made from rare-earth magnets that are much more powerful that traditional ferrite magnets.

The benefits of PMAC motors are higher efficiency, more precise speed control, higher power density, and cooler operation. The higher efficiency is due to the elimination of the rotor conductor losses with the induction motor. The PMAC motor rotates at the same speed as the magnetic field produced by the stator windings or at a synchronous speed. An induction motor is considered an asynchronous motor because its rotational speed is slightly slower than the magnetic field of the stator. The synchronous speed of the PMAC results in better dynamic performance and more precise speed control. The permanent magnets provide a higher flux density than a comparable induction motor and can therefore provide more power and torque per motor frame size. Permanent magnet motors operate cooler so bearings and insulation will have a longer life and reduce the amount of heat that goes into the operating environment. Some of the disadvantages of PMAC motors include special care of the magnets and higher initial cost.

PMAC motors require an AC drive specifically designed to drive permanent magnet motors. Many of today's high-end AC drives have control algorithms capable of controlling PMAC motors and there are typically a couple of parameters that need to be set in the drive programming.

18.4 PROGRAMMABLE CONTROLLERS (PLCS AND PACS)

The programmable controller is often thought of as the brain of the control system. Programmable controllers are used on very simple control systems with relatively few inputs and outputs (I/O) to very large systems with enormous amounts of I/O and high-end communications and control features (Figure 18.8). Programmable controllers are commonly referred to as programmable logic controllers (PLC) and programmable automation controllers (PAC).

18.4.1 PLC CONTROL

The PLC has been around for the last 40 years. PLCs are still the controller of choice for most automated machinery. They have the ability to process machine logic without experiencing faults in an operating system. PLCs are ideal for critical applications (such as the manufacture of pharmaceuticals) due to their reliability.

Shortly after their introduction, PLCs began replacing relay logic, which was previously used to control machinery. Their advantage over relays was that they were programmable, whereas relays were hardwired. Relay logic required excessive space and the logic could not be changed easily. While early PLCs were also very large, expensive, and only capable of binary logic, their capabilities soon expanded to include analog I/O, thermocouple inputs, and numerous communications options. The ladder logic language used to program PLCs was the same as the ladder logic drawings used for relay wiring and was therefore well understood by electricians, further enhancing their industrial acceptance.

Advantages of PLC-based controls include reliability, low maintenance costs, ruggedness/durability, integral I/O bus design, fast boot times, and large installed base. Additionally, one specific type of visual programming language, Relay Ladder Logic, is easy to learn and understand. PLC-based controls offer a lower purchase cost for small applications (Micro-PLC), while single sourcing of hardware and software increases reliability and creates a single point of accountability.

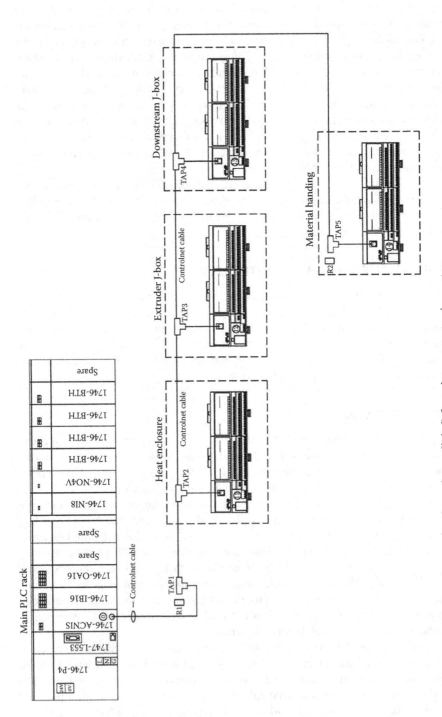

FIGURE 18.8 Flex I/O (input/output signals, analog or digital) for twin-screw extrusion system.

18.4.2 PAC Control

PAC is a relatively new term used to describe a programmable controller geared more toward complex automation systems. The PAC provides greater programming flexibility, multiple processors, larger memory, many communications options, and more PC-type features. PAC programming is very flexible, using a tag-based database for development. These tags or descriptive names can be assigned to functions before being tied to I/O, which allows it to easily scale to larger systems. PACs are also designed for tight integration with SQL and other databases.

18.5 OPERATOR INTERFACE OPTIONS

Extruder control systems must allow the operator to view, control, and adjust all functions associated with the machine. The control system must provide feedback to the operator so they know the system is performing correctly or so they can correct an undesired response. The operator interface can range from an unsophisticated manual/discrete control system to an advanced graphical user interface system or to a fully featured PC control system.

18.5.1 Manual/Discrete Control

Manual/discrete control systems use hard-wired pushbuttons, selector switches, and potentiometers, along with meters for control of all the devices associated with the extruder system. These control systems will use discrete temperature controllers to control all the heating and cooling zones associated with the extruder barrel and downstream equipment. These systems will use a PLC to manage all the logic and interlocks for the control system.

18.5.2 Human-Machine Interface

The HMI is the graphical user interface for industrial control systems. This operator interface usually consists of some type of touch screen with programmable software that allows the designer to create graphical screen pushbuttons, selector switches, potentiometers, and meters to control all the devices associated with the extruder system. The HMI can provide many of the following features for advanced control, including recipe management, trending, security, remote monitoring, and data logging. The HMI operator interface will typically communicate to an advanced programmable automation controller (PAC). The HMI with the PAC can provide digital communications to drives, feeder systems, remote access devices, company local area networks (LAN), remote I/O and downstream equipment like laser gauge systems, pelletizers, sheet lines, and other PLCs.

18.5.3 PC Control

PC-based controls utilize a personal computer acting as the brains of the system. In this scenario, the PC handles not only the HMI tasks, data handling, and communications, but also controls the entire process (Figure 18.9). The PC-based control option gives us the hardware and programming device in one unit.

PC-based controls offer the following advantages: Large memory and storage capacity, vast availability of commercial software, integral audio/video, complete HMI functionality in one platform, and the relative ease of interfacing to other systems for factory data collection. PC-based controls allow the use of off-the-shelf products from different suppliers without excessive retraining of personnel. Extensive data handling, as is typically required in pharmaceutical settings, is well suited to a PC-based control system.

The approach of combining the programmable controller (PLC/PAC) and the PC clearly provides the benefits of both systems. In this scenario, the PLC/PAC directly controls the process, while the PC handles the HMI and data logging functions. This solution is ideal for applications requiring a high level of machine control interaction by an operator and for critical process control. This is often the preferred method utilized to comply with stringent regulatory requirements, including those of the FDA.

Industrial PCs (IPCs) have several advantages over standard off-the-shelf PCs. IPCs' designs will typically include no moving parts such as solid-state hard drives versus the traditional rotating hard drive. This allows the IPC to withstand the shock and vibration sometimes found on the factory floor. The IPC's internal components are designed to have a high immunity to electrical noise and to handle higher temperatures. The industrial PC can come in many different form factors from a DIN rail mount to having integral touchscreens.

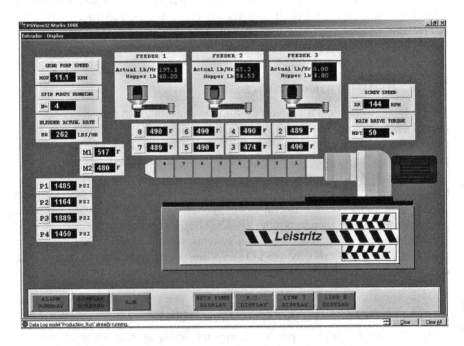

FIGURE 18.9 PC-based operator interface to PLC control system.

18.6   PROCESS MONITORING

While it is the function of the individual components (PLC's, temperature control-lers, drives, motors, and thermocouples) to precisely control their respective extruder functions, it is imperative that data are fed back to the operator, to verify that the overall process is running as expected and within acceptable limits. Basic, discrete (digital) indication of speed, temperature, pressure, and motor load is standard on almost all extruders and may be sufficient for noncritical applications and processes. Pharmaceutical processes, however, typically require constant monitoring and recording of these variables in order to satisfy stringent documentation and account-ability requirements. In this case, a personal computer is often employed to handle the tedious task of extensive data collection, organization, and manipulation. The four critical parameters that need to be monitored in any extrusion process are screw speed, motor load, pressure(s), and temperature(s).

18.6.1   SCREW SPEED

Screw speed is a critical process variable, in that it often dictates the amount of energy, the degree of mixing, the melt temperature, and sometimes the melt pres-sure of the extrusion process. In single-screw extrusion, screw speed also dictates the overall throughput, thereby affecting the dimensions of the final product. (This is not true for starve-fed twin-screw extruders, where throughput is determined by feed rate.) While DC motor/drive packages can attain control accuracy of anywhere from 0.1% to 3%, modern AC motor/drive packages can attain accuracies as good as 0.01% and thus are the preferred choice in pharmaceutical applications. Due to the drastic implications that screw speed has on the overall process, it is imperative that speed be monitored and controlled accurately.

18.6.2   MOTOR LOAD

Motor load (amperage) is a key indication of how much energy is being transmit-ted from the motor, through the screw(s), and into the material/process. A fluctuat-ing, unstable motor load often reveals problems that may otherwise be invisible. An unsteady motor load may be an indication of inconsistent feed or bridging at the feed throat, or inadequate speed control due to problems with either the motor or the drive. Conversely, a steady, stable motor load typically indicates a steady, controlled process. As with temperature and pressure, it is best to graphically plot motor load over time, as simple, instantaneous "snapshots" of the motor load will not reveal significant trends or shifts in amperage.

18.6.3   MELT PRESSURE

Pressure generation at the tips of the screws (also referred to as "head pressure") is a critical process parameter that should be monitored carefully and accurately. Some extruders will also position pressure transducers directly in the die. Variations of melt pressure can indicate process interrupts or instability, such as inconsistent

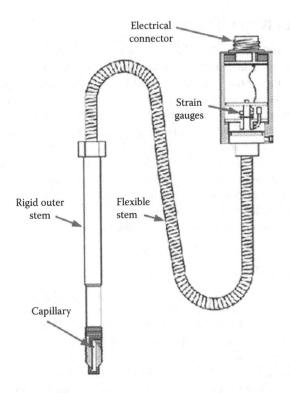

FIGURE 18.10   Strain-gauge-type pressure transducer.

feeding, melting, or throughput. Conversely, a steady, uniform pressure reading typically indicates a stable extrusion process. Accurate monitoring of an extruder's head pressure is also an important safety measure, as overpressurizing an extruder barrel can lead to serious operator injury. For this reason, most extruders are "interlocked" to the pressure indicator, so as to automatically shut down the extruder in the event that a given pressure (operator selectable) is exceeded for a given period of time.

Modern pressure transducers utilize strain gauges to detect variations in pressure on their diaphragms (Figure 18.10). Strain-gauge-type transducers offer good resolution and quick response. One limiting factor of strain gauges is their susceptibility to high temperatures. For this reason, a hydraulic membrane separates the diaphragm and the strain gauge. Mercury is the most common type of fluid used in these membranes due to its low thermal expansion and high boiling point. However, mercury-filled transducers are strictly prohibited in pharmaceutical applications, as a puncture of the diaphragm (although extremely unlikely) would be catastrophic. For this reason, sodium-filled transducers are typically utilized for food and pharmaceutical-grade applications.

18.6.4 MELT TEMPERATURE

Commonly referred to as "stock" temperature, the temperature of the product at any given point in the extruder is of vital importance, particularly as it emerges from the die. As with melt pressure, knowledge of the melt temperature will give an indication of just how stable the process is. In order to precisely measure stock temperature, a thermocouple should protrude directly into the polymer flow. Unfortunately, placing a thermocouple probe directly into the melt stream is usually impractical, as the extremely tight clearances between the screw and the barrel wall prohibit this. Even in areas of the extruder where the use of a protruding thermocouple is possible (head, adapters, die), other negative implications exist, including disrupting the flow orientation and stagnation or hang-up. The common solution to this problem is the use of a "flush-mount" thermocouple probe, where the measuring surface is flush with the barrel wall or internal die surface. It must be understood that while flush mount thermocouples are only able to detect the melt temperature of the material at the wall, they give a good indication of "apparent" melt temperature, a temperature that can be used to compare similar or identical formulations between run to run or lot to lot.

18.7 DATA ACQUISITION AND MONITORING SYSTEMS

Accurate recording of machine settings and process data is essential in pharmaceutical settings. Not only do they serve as a basis for comparison for future processes, they provide a means for accountability as required by the FDA, ISO, and other recognized industry standards.

The ability to record key process variables over time reveals important trends and shifts in process conditions that may otherwise go undetected. Prior to the evolution of the personal computer, strip charts were often used to automatically record machine and process data vs. time. These strip charts were cumbersome, prone to misinterpretation, and required manual tabulation back into numerical data for statistical process control analysis.

The personal computer revolutionized the way in which process data is recorded and manipulated. Computer-based data acquisition and monitoring systems allow the operator to instantaneously view the entire extrusion process. All measured parameters are clearly presented to the operator, either numerically or graphically. In addition, any alarms that were triggered during the run are also saved with the file. The speed and storage capabilities of today's computers allow data points to be collected several times per second, over long periods of time. This information can be stored infinitely for future recall and comparison against similar extrusion runs (Figure 18.11).

18.7.1 PROCESS ANALYTICAL TECHNOLOGY

In August 2002, the FDA released "Pharmaceutical Current Good Manufacturing Practices (CGMPs) for the 21st Century: A Risk Based Approach," widely recognized as the starting point, or initiative, for process analytical technology (PAT). The goal of the PAT initiative was to simplify the introduction of new manufacturing technologies in the pharmaceutical industry, with the ultimate objective of achieving more efficient processes. The USFDA defines PAT as "a system for designing, analyzing, and controlling manufacturing through timely measurements (i.e., during

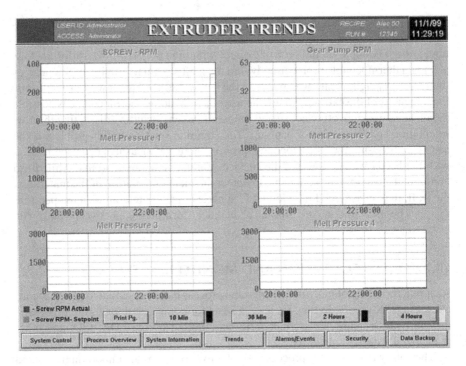

FIGURE 18.11   PC-based data acquisition, monitoring, and trending.

processing) of critical quality and performance attributes of raw and in-process materials and processes with the goal of ensuring final product quality."

Even prior to the introduction of PAT, properly equipped extrusion processes have historically monitored critical process data in a continuous manner, including screw speed, melt temperature, melt pressure, percentage of motor load, and actual vs. set temperatures. More recently, in-line and on-line analytical tools such as near-infrared, mid-infrared, and Raman spectroscopy instruments (Figure 18.12) have been utilized to evaluate the manufacturing process in real time.

Benefits of a successfully implemented PAT program include expedited development of new products, faster manufacturing cycle times, increased efficiency/productivity, and reduced waste.

18.7.2   ELECTRONIC RECORDS AND ELECTRONIC SIGNATURES

Collecting data on the conditions and events throughout a manufacturing process helps manufacturers ensure that they are making a consistent, reliable, and quality product. FDA predicate rules determine if regulated industries must document conditions and events throughout the manufacturing process to be compliant. When required, historically, these data were in the form of paper records. Title 21 Code of Federal Regulations (CFR) Part 11 was released in 1997. It allows pharmaceutical companies to store these data electronically and views these electronic records as equivalent to paper records. The FDA predicate rules also mandate that many

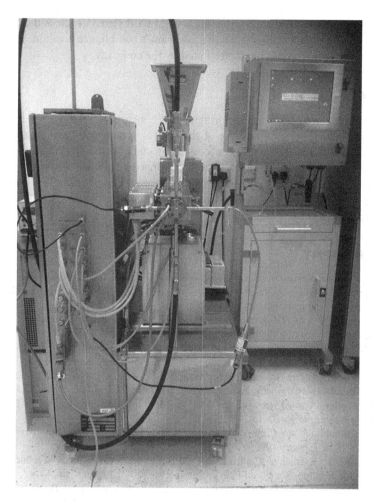

FIGURE 18.12   PAT instrument/probe.

regulated documents must be signed. 21 CFR Part 11 also allows pharmaceutical companies to provide electronic signatures in place of handwritten signatures. 21 CFR Part 11 provides guidelines on using electronic records and electronic signatures and goes into detail on providing security, audit trails, operating procedures, training, and version control. Supervisory control and data acquisition (SCADA) software, along with a computer operating system, is typically used to address many of the requirements of 21 CFR Part 11. SCADA software is an industrial automation control system that allows an operator to monitor and control machines and devices. Many SCADA software products can archive raw process and event data to data logs. SCADA software products can be linked to the computer operating system to provide many of the security requirements of 21 CFR Part 11. SCADA software cannot provide version control or maintain the data. This is typically handled from a central plant-wide software solution to keep track of changes between versions and to archive and report on the data. Other parts of 21 CFR Part 11 such as the establishment of written policies/procedures of a company's compliance position, validation, and training would have to be implemented by the company.

18.8 CONCLUSION

The extrusion control system is the primary link between the operator and the overall machine system. The main purpose of the control system is to provide an efficient means to control and monitor key process parameters, including (but not limited to) speed, temperature, and pressure. Today's pharmaceutical control systems routinely utilize cutting-edge technology, including programmable logic controllers, AC motors and drives, on-line/in-line PAT instrumentation, and sophisticated PC-based data monitoring and storage systems.

BIBLIOGRAPHY

1. P. Newtown, Drives and Servos Yearbook 1990. Control Techniques, 1989.
2. Application Guide Adjustable Frequency Drives and AC Motors. Emerson Industrial Controls, March, 1993, ADG-080B.
3. Warner SECO AC/DC Drives Application Notes. Warner Electric, October 1993, 1101.
4. N. Linder, Choosing the Right AC Drive Type. Eurotherm Drives Regional Seminar.
5. L. Cooksey, Driving Process Control with Vector Technology. Motion Control Magazine, July/August, 1999.
6. Baldor Motors and Drives Technical Handbook. Fundamentals of Inverter-Fed Motors. Baldor Electric Company, February 1996, NM780.
7. D. Morley, The History of the PLC as Told to Howard Hendricks. R. Morley Incorporated, 1996-2001.
8. L.S. Gould. When Controls Converge: CNC, PLC & PC, Automotive Design & Production, January 1999.
9. T. Fisher. Extrusion Control, The SPE Guide on Extrusion Technology and Troubleshooting. Society of Plastics Engineers, 2001, Chapter 4, pp. 1–14.
10. T. Whelan, D. Dunning. The Dynisco Extrusion Processors. 1st ed. Dynisco Inc., 1998.
11. D. Todd. Plastics Compounding Equipment and Processing. Ohio: Hanser/Gardner Publications, 1998.
12. G. Clark, FDA's PAT initiative. Pharmaceutical Technology Magazine, June, 2012.
13. A. Shirodkar, Process Analytical Technology (PAT) in pharmaceutical development and its application. Mobi moPharma Mobile Apps, HTML5, December 2015.
14. PATA—framework for innovative pharmaceutical development, manufacturing, and quality assurance. Guidance for Industry, U.S. Department of Health & Human Services/FDA, Pharmaceutical CGMP's, September, 2014.
15. Wikipedia contributors. Process analytical technology. Wikipedia, The Free Encyclopedia. August 17, 2017. Web. November 29, 2017.

Index

395

Printed in the United States
by Baker & Taylor Publisher Services